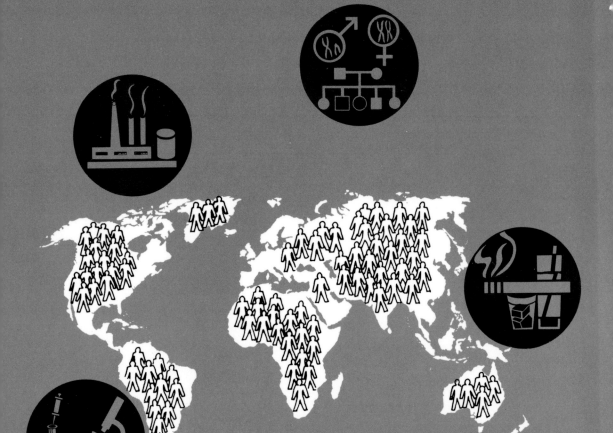

PRINCIPLES OF EPIDEMIOLOGY

A Self-Teaching Guide

L.H. ROHT ▪ B.J. SELWYN

A.H. HOLGUIN and B.L. CHRISTENSEN

ACADEMIC PRESS   A Subsidiary of Harcourt Brace Jovanovich, Publishers

PRINCIPLES OF EPIDEMIOLOGY
A Self-Teaching Guide

PRINCIPLES OF EPIDEMIOLOGY
A Self-Teaching Guide

LEWIS H. ROHT, M.D.
BEATRICE J. SELWYN, D. Sc.
ALFONSO H. HOLGUIN, JR., M.D.
BOBBE L. CHRISTENSEN, Ph.D.

University of Texas School of Public Health
Houston, Texas

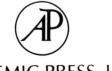

ACADEMIC PRESS, INC.

(Harcourt Brace Jovanovich, Publishers)

Orlando   San Diego   New York   London
Toronto   Montreal   Sydney   Tokyo

ACADEMIC PRESS, INC.
Orlando, Florida 32887

United Kingdom Edition published by
ACADEMIC PRESS, INC. (LONDON) LTD.
24/28 Oval Road, London NW1 7DX

Library of Congress Cataloging in Publication Data
Main entry under title:

Principles of epidemiology.

    Bibliography: p.
    1. Epidemiology. I. Roht, Lewis H. [DNLM: 1. Epi-
demiologic methods. WA 950 P956]
RA651.P24   1982   614.4   82-11639
ISBN 0-12-593180-8

PRINTED IN THE UNITED STATES OF AMERICA

85 86 87 88   9 8 7 6 5 4 3 2

In memory of Paul—who made the present possible. . .
and
for Nancy—in whose eyes the future brightly glows.

Contents

PART III. EPIDEMIOLOGIC STRATEGY

PART IV. STUDY DESIGN AND INTERPRETATION OF DATA

Acknowledgments

The authors wish to express their appreciation to the many people who helped in the preparation of this book. We are singularly indebted to Mrs. Gay Robertson whose patience, friendship, good humor, and skills with word processing equipment enabled us to attempt the preparation of this text, endure its many revisions, and finally realize its completion.

Many others have helped along the way: Mrs. Elizabeth G. Faris, who prepared several of the early drafts of the text; Betty Maxine Mathews, Dora Marks, Betty Hall, and Diane M. Loville, who helped with text revisions; Fran Garman, Bett Oaks, John Hubbard, Sandra Gerth, and Connie Harris, who assisted in the preparation of the illustrations; Sally Andrews, Robert Byington, and Barbara Divine, who assisted in the preparation of the text. And to Ms. Bett Oaks, our special appreciation for the cover design.

We are grateful to Dr. Ron Forthofer and Dr. Ron Harrist whose programmed self-instructional teaching material in Biometry provided the stimulus for developing our Epidemiology Teaching Guide. We are grateful for the interest, patience, encouragement, and suggestions of many of our students and colleagues in the evolution of the Teaching Guide to its present form. Our appreciation is also extended to the staff of Academic Press for their assistance in the preparation of the text for publication.

None of this work could have been completed without the encouragement and support of our families. To Cheryl and Claire Roht, Bob and Bea Selwyn, Hanna and Alfonso Holguin, Sr., and Art Christensen, we owe you a great deal. Thank you.

INTRODUCTION

You are about to begin the study of epidemiology, a subject that many consider the basic science of public health. The public health sciences are concerned with the management, prevention, and control of diseases and other health problems in the community. The field of epidemiology stands in the center of the public health sciences, playing an important role in identifying health problems as well as seeking measures to control or prevent the occurrence of illness in human populations. Epidemiologists also participate in teaching and research, and in the organization and administration of programs that attempt to solve actual and/or perceived health problems in the community.

The Epidemiology Self-Teaching Guide consists of a series of problem-solving exercises designed to introduce and guide you toward an understanding of the principles and methods of epidemiology, rather than the epidemiology of specific diseases or subject areas such as "infectious disease" or "chronic disease" epidemiology. The guide has been formulated to be used by itself or as a supplement to standard textbooks. It illustrates and illuminates the principles and concepts of epidemiology and provides the reader an opportunity to practice the application of these principles in a logical sequence.

The guide has two major objectives: when you have completed the exercises you should be able (1) to plan an investigation of a community health problem, and (2) to constructively evaluate research and scientific reports appearing in the literature. These skills will be useful to you whether or not you become an epidemiologist because they are applicable to a wide variety of community health activities including research, review of scientific literature, evaluation of health programs, and administration or decision making based upon the correct interpretation and application of available knowledge.

HOW TO USE THE GUIDE

The guide is divided into 14 exercises. Each exercise will help you to understand principles or methods used by epidemiologists, which are necessary to achieve the two objectives mentioned above.

1. At the beginning of each exercise one or more goals will be stated, to indicate what you should expect to learn from that exercise.

2. A list of standard textbooks keyed to the material of each exercise is provided to supplement the material presented. You are strongly urged to read one or more of these suggested references before working the exercise.

3.   Work through the exercise. Space is provided for you to answer ques-
      tions or construct tables or graphs relating to an epidemiologic problem.

4.   For each exercise suggested responses are provided. Use these to verify
      your answers. In some cases you may disagree with the suggested re-
      sponse. That does not mean your answer is incorrect or that the sug-
      gested response is the only correct answer. In fact, there may be other
      correct answers. The suggested responses are provided as a guide to
      indicate the type of response we hope would occur to you. They will also
      raise some issues that concern epidemiologists. Many of the suggested
      responses go beyond what is called for in the question. These extensive
      responses are intended to provide additional insight or to stimulate your
      thinking about the subject. A reader's ability to answer the questions
      will reflect his or her awareness of health issues and previous professional
      experience.

5.   An extensive bibliography of epidemiologic literature and some examples of
      test questions are provided in appendices following Exercise 14.

While many of the problems in the exercises will use data from actual diseases,
the reader should be aware that our goal is to illustrate a principle, concept,
or method commonly employed by epidemiologists. Do not be overly concerned
with memorizing epidemiologic facts about the diseases but try to grasp the
epidemiologic concepts. We have assumed that you have an understanding of
the pathology and other biologic features of the disease, so that emphasis will
be placed on the epidemiologic principles and concepts and not on the disease
process. For those of you who become epidemiologists or who are involved
with disease control programs or research, more complete knowledge of the
epidemiology of the specific diseases will be mandatory.

SUPPLEMENTARY REFERENCE BOOKS

There are many useful and suitable reference books concerned with epidemiology. However, no single book is likely to have universal appeal to all readers or to cover a given subject to the same degree or from the same point of
view as other textbooks. All texts in the suggested reading list are appropriate and cover the material adequately. The choice of which reference text
to use will depend upon the reader's individual preference for writing style
and the degree of sophistication required by the reader.

COURSE OBJECTIVES

For use of this guide in a formal education program (medical or public health
school, college, or graduate program) student evaluation would be based upon
an ability to demonstrate understanding of the concepts, principles, and
methods of epidemiology by achieving the two primary objectives:

1.   Planning an investigation of a community health situation and carrying out
      appropriate analyses to determine if an epidemic is present, the epidemic
      type, and the determinants.

2.   Performing a critical review to assess the quality of epidemiologic reports, investigations and studies.

Successful completion of objective 1 requires the skills developed in Exercises 1-9, and includes the abilities to:

1.   Obtain existing demographic data to describe the "population at risk."

2.   Obtain morbidity, mortality, physiologic, or behavioral data relating to the frequency of the disease or health problem in question.

3.   Prepare (or obtain if available) appropriate graphs, charts or tables relating the "disease" to the population at risk so that the pattern of disease in that population is discernible and can be described in terms of the person affected and the place and time of occurrence.

4.   Analyze and interpret data to assess whether the observed frequency of disease exceeds the normal or expected amount.

5.   Formulate and test hypotheses to explain the disease pattern and suggest measures to prevent or control present and future occurrence of that health problem.

To perform a critical review of an epidemiologic report, investigation or study (objective 2) requires the skills and knowledge developed in Exercises 10-14 and includes the abilities to:

1.   Define the health problem being investigated and describe the purpose of the study.

2.   Define the population to be studied and its method of selection.

3.   Determine if the design of the study is appropriate to the problem being investigated.

4.   Identify the potential sources of error in selection of the study population and/or data collection.

5.   Determine if the interpretations or conclusions made by the investigator are appropriate to the study design and data presented.

Use of this guide in a formal teaching program could include examinations at the conclusion of Exercises 9 and 14. Examples of an examination format are provided in Appendix 2.

By way of easing you into your studies the remainder of this introductory section will enable you to construct a definition of epidemiology and become aware of the areas of interest and concern to epidemiologists.

WHAT IS EPIDEMIOLOGY?

The ancient Greek scholar and physician Hippocrates wrote a treatise[3] "On Airs, Waters and Places" which comes close to illustrating the way epidemiologists approach health problems.

> Whoever wishes to investigate medicine properly should proceed thus: in the first place to consider the seasons of the year, and what effects each of them produces. Then the winds, the hot and the cold, especially such as are common to all countries, and then such as are peculiar to each locality. In the same manner, when one comes into a city to which he is a stranger, he should consider its situation, how it lies as to the winds and the rising of the sun; for its influence is not the same whether it lies to the north or the south, to the rising or to the setting sun. One should consider most attentively the water which the inhabitants use, whether they be marshy and soft, or hard and running from elevated and rocky situations, and then if saltish and unfit for cooking; and the ground, whether it be naked and deficient in water, or wooded and well watered, and whether it lies in a hollow, confined situation, or is elevated and cold; and the mode in which the inhabitants live, and what are their pursuits, whether they are fond of drinking and eating to excess, and given to indolence, or are fond of exercise and labor.

While Hippocrates gives us a general impression about epidemiology's content or approach, the subject requires a clearer definition. Several of those which have been proposed are listed below. You will notice that there is no single definition to which all epidemiologists subscribe. However, there are recurrent themes among them. Try to discern the notions common to these varying definitions and write them in the space provided below.

Hirsch (1883):

"A picture of the occurrence, the distribution, and the types of the diseases of mankind, in distinct epochs of time and at various points of the earth's surface; and ... render an account of the relations of those diseases to the external condition."

Frost (1927):

"The science of the mass phenomena of infectious diseases, or as the natural history of infectious diseases... an inductive science, concerned not merely with describing the distribution of disease, but--fitting it into a consistent philosophy."

Greenwood (1934):

"Epidemiology is the study of disease as a mass phenomenon."

Lilienfeld (1957):

"Epidemiology may be defined as the study of the distribution of a disease or condition in a population and of the factors that influence this distribution."

Plunkett and Gordon (1960):

"The field observation of disease under natural conditions in whole populations... medical ecology... deals with the mutual relations between man and his environment, seeing health and disease as selected instances of this total interaction."

Morris (1964):

"The study of health and disease of populations, this is the epidemiology of Farr and Snow, of Hirsch and Goldberger."

Taylor (1967):

"The study of health or ill health in a defined population."

MacMahon, Pugh, and Ipsen (1970):

"The study of the distribution and determinants of disease frequency in man ... distribution... (descriptive epidemiology) and... determinants of the noted distribution (analytic epidemiology)."

Stallones (1971):

"Epidemiology is the description and explanation of the differences in occurrence of events of medical concern in subgroups of a population, where the population has been subdivided according to some characteristic believed to influence the occurrence of the event."

Epidemiology of Non-Communicable Disease British Medical Bulletin (1971):

"Like so many words 'epidemiology' has changed its meaning over the years. It is not mentioned in Samuel Johnson's Dictionary of the English Language, although not surprising in 1775, epidemic--'that which plagues'--is mentioned. Its original usage was to describe 'that branch of medical science which treats of epidemics,' but it is now widely understood to be 'a science that deals with incidence, distribution, and control of disease in a population 'whether or not the disease in question is epidemic or communicable'... . The definition of the term may require modification again in the near future to include the critical evaluation of measures directed at treatment of disease as well as its prevention (and therefore by implication the study of prognosis)."

Epidemiology--A Guide to Teaching Methods (1973):

"Epidemiology is defined as the study of the factors determining the frequency and distribution of disease in human populations. For many years the word covered only and quite specifically, the study of the spread and decline of communicable disease in human populations and the prophylaxis and control of those diseases... the scope includes all disease acute or chronic, physical or mental; communicable or non-communicable."

Sartwell (1973):

"The study of the distribution and dynamics of diseases in human populations."

Lasagna (1975):

"The science dealing with the incidence, spread, and control of disease."

Lilienfeld (1977):

"Epidemiology is a method of reasoning about disease that deals with biologic inferences derived from observations of disease phenomena in population groups."

Frerichs and Neutra (1978):

"Epidemiology is the study of the prevalence and dynamics of stages of health in populations."

Webster's Unabridged Dictionary:

"The term epidemiology is derived from the Greek epi, on, upon; -demos-, the people; -logos, theory, source, the study of."

Stop for a moment to consider these definitions. Before you read any further, write your summary of the factors that are common to these definitions.

Your definition should include or mention that epidemiology is a basic science of preventive medicine and public health concerned with:

1.   Disease (or some health status).

2.   Frequency (enumeration of amount present or rate of development within a specific time period).

3.   Distribution (patterns produced by disease occurrence in population).

4.   Determinants (the factors affecting the distribution).

5.   Methods (processes employed to describe frequency and distribution and scientific rationale used to determine causal relationship of disease distribution in populations).

6.   Populations (a defined human population).

These definitions clearly indicate that the subjects of interest to epidemiologists (diseases and health conditions) have grown through time, and also that the range of factors that the epidemiologist considers in search for determinants of disease distribution has markedly expanded. The epidemiologist has come to recognize that patterns of diseases observed in a community reflect the interaction of multiple factors (genetic, environmental, social, physiologic, etc.).

By now you should have a feeling that epidemiology encompasses a wide range of activities, but at the same time you should also have the impression of an overall consistency among these definitions. Before laying this issue to rest, two other views bear mentioning.

Frost (1936):

"Epidemiology at any given time is something more than the total of its established facts. It includes their orderly arrangement into chains of inference which extend more or less beyond the bounds of direct observation."

Gilliam (1963):

"Epidemiology is what epidemiologists do."

APPLICATIONS OF EPIDEMIOLOGY

In your study of epidemiology you will discover that epidemiologists have played a role in many areas of public health, including the study of infectious disease, chronic disease, accidents and injury, maternal and child health, family planning, iatrogenic diseases (diseases resulting from medical treatment, as with Thalidomide), mental health, nutritional disorders, health education, medical care delivery, health services administration, and health planning. Specific activities include:

1. Collection and analysis of vital records (births and deaths).

2. Collection and analysis of morbidity data from hospitals, health agencies, clinics, physicians, and industry.

3. Surveillance of diseases or community health problems.

4. Investigation leading to control or prevention of epidemics and other community health problems.

5. Design and implementation of clinical research studies and health surveys.

6. Design and implementation of health registries for problems of interest such as birth defects, cancer incidence, or drug and medication use.

7. Screening for diseases.

8. Evaluation of the effectiveness of existing or newly proposed treatment methods.

9. Describing the clinical course as well as the natural history of specific diseases.

10. Identifying individuals or subgroups of the general population at increased risk of developing certain diseases.

11. Identifying links in the etiology of disease.

12. Identifying public health problems and measuring the extent of their distribution, frequency or effect on the public's health.

13. Evaluation of health programs.

14. Providing data necessary for health planning or decision making by health agency administrators or health policy makers.

In the guide we present some examples of the approaches and applications to the health problems that have been described. Space and the limitations on a student's time prevent a complete exposition of all of these topics. The authors' intent is to introduce the principles, concepts, and methods used by epidemiologists with the hope that you the student will be able to apply the ideas and techniques to your own areas of interest. We hope you find the exercises interesting and challenging, and that they will enable you to build a firm foundation for the development of ideas and skills that you will need in future academic and professional activities in public health.

Suggested Readings

1. Friedman, G. Primer of Epidemiology, McGraw-Hill, 1980, Chapter 1.

2. Mausner, J., and Bahn, A. Epidemiology, W.B. Saunders Co., 1974, Chapters 1,2.

3. MacMahon, B., and Pugh, T.F. Epidemiology, Principles and Methods, Little, Brown & Co., 1970, Chapter 1.

4. Paul, J.R. Clinical Epidemiology, The University of Chicago Press, 1958, Chapter 1.

5. Fisher, I. An Introduction to Epidemiology, Appleton-Century Press, 1975, Frame 1-44.

Additional References

6. Hirsch, A. Handbook of Geographical and Historical Pathology, London: New Sydenham Society, 1883.

7. Frost, W.H. Papers of Wade Hampton Frost, New York: The Commonwealth Fund, 1941.

8. Lilienfeld, A.M. Epidemiology Methods and Inferences in Studies of Non-infectious Diseases, Pub. Health Reports, 72:51, 1957.

9. Plunkett, R.J., and Gordon, J.E. Epidemiology and Mental Illness. New York, Basic Books, Inc., 1960.

10. Morris, J.N. Uses of Epidemiology. Edinburgh: E & S Livingstone, Ltd., 1964.

11. Epidemiology--A Guide to Teaching Methods, Churchill Livingstone, 1973.

12. White, K.L. Contemporary Epidemiology, Int. J. Epidem., 3:295, 1974.

13. Lilienfeld, D.E., Definitions of Epidemiology, Am. J. Epidem. 107:87, 1978.

14. Frerichs, R.R., and Neutra, R. Re: Definitions of Epidemiology. Am. J. Epidem. 108:74, 1978.

15. Frost, W.H. Introduction. In: Snow on Cholera by J. Snow. Cambridge: Harvard University Press, 1936.

16. Gilliam, A.G. Quoted in Stallones, R.A. Epidemi(olog)^{2}y. Am. J. Pub. Health 53:82, 1963.

PART I. BASIC TENETS OF EPIDEMIOLOGY

Exercises 1 and 2 will illustrate the basic tenets of epidemiology:

1. THE DISTRIBUTION OF DISEASES OCCURS IN PATTERNS IN A COMMUNITY.

2. THE PATTERN OF DISEASES IN COMMUNITIES IS PREDICTABLE.

3. CHARACTERISTICS OF THE PATTERN MAY SUGGEST OR LEAD TO MEASURES TO CONTROL OR PREVENT THE DISEASE.

An epidemiologist seeks to identify and describe the individuals or groups within a community who are ill or likely to become ill. Description includes answers to the questions WHO? WHAT? WHEN? WHERE?

Who became ill? What type of illness and under what circumstances did the illness occur? When and where did the illness occur?

The epidemiologist arranges this information to determine if patterns might exist, i.e., whether or not certain groups will be observed to have a health problem more frequently than others in that community. Based upon these observations, conclusions (the validity of which might be tested through research or experimentation) may be drawn concerning HOW? and WHY? the illness occurred in a particular group. When these questions have been answered and the relationship between the causes of a disease and factors associated with those causes becomes understood, it may be possible to develop measures that can PREVENT OR CONTROL the occurrence of that disease in human populations.

EXERCISE 1.   PATTERNS OF DISEASE

Goals

Upon completion of this exercise you ought to be able (1) to describe and discern a disease pattern and (2) to propose alternative explanations of why the pattern occurs in the observed manner.

Methods

In order to achieve these goals you will need to understand the notions of:

I.   RISK
II.   RATES
III.   POPULATION AT RISK
IV.   THE "PERSON-PLACE-TIME" MODEL
V.   THE "HOST-AGENT-ENVIRONMENT" MODEL
VI.   EPIDEMICS

Terms

Source, transmission, spread, epidemic, endemic, susceptibility, exposure, dose, etiology, pathogenicity, trend, immunity, reservoir, incubation period, infectivity, and virulence.

Suggested Reading

Lilienfeld and Lilienfeld Foundations of Epidemiology, Chapters 3, 5, 7.
Mausner and Bahn, Epidemiology, Chapters 2, 3, 4.
Friedman, Primer of Epidemiology, Chapter 5.
APHA Handbook, Control of Communicable Diseases in Man, 13th ed., 1981.
MacMahon and Pugh, Epidemiology: Principles and Methods, Chapters 7-10.
Fox, Hall and Elveback, Epidemiology, Man and Disease, Chapters 4-6, 9-11.
Elandt-Johnson, R.C., Definition of rates: some remarks on their use and
    misuse. Am. J. Epidemiol. 102:267, 1975.

Before beginning to study disease patterns you will need to understand some terms that are basic to epidemiology:

I.   RISK - A statement of the likelihood of developing a disease or some
         health problem. Risk can be stated in absolute and objective terms
         by measures called rates.

II.   RATES - A rate measures the risk of occurrence of a particular event in
         a population during a given time period. It indicates the change in
         some event that takes place in a population over a period of time,
         e.g., the development of disease or the occurrence of deaths.

A rate is expressed in the form:

$$(x/y) \cdot k \text{ per unit of time.}$$

where the numerator x is the number of events occurring in the specified time period; the denominator y, the number of persons at risk of the event during the same interval; and a unit of reference k, a convenient number or base to express the relation of x and y. It is usual to use 100; 1000; 10,000; 100,000; or 1,000,000.

An example of a typical rate is the mortality rate*:

$$\frac{\text{deaths in 1981}}{\text{midyear population in 1981}} \times 100,000$$

The rationale for using rates and other quantitative measures in epidemiology is implied in the following quotation:

> Epidemiology stands... in somewhat the same relationship to the practice of preventive medicine as do some of the more familiar basic medical sciences to curative medicine. Pathology, pathologic physiology and pharmacology are basic and introductory to the clinical care of patients; in like manner the concept of epidemiology--a science concerned with the circumstances under which a person or persons get sick or remain sick--is basic to any attempt to alter these circumstances so as to protect individuals from future illness (John R. Paul, 1958).

A physician in attempting to diagnose and treat his patient will use instruments such as a stethoscope or an x-ray machine to obtain the necessary information. The epidemiologist, whose "patient" is the community, must utilize surveys or existing health data to generate rates that reflect events occurring among a GROUP OF INDIVIDUALS.

III. POPULATION AT RISK

This is the denominator or y term found in rates. Theoretically it implies that all persons at risk are susceptible to developing the disease or problem being studied. In most instances it is impossible to determine whether every person in the group is actually susceptible to a disease; in order to overcome this difficulty, the entire population (city, state or country) may be used to denote being "at risk" of disease. Because the population size varies daily due to births, deaths, and migration, an estimate of the midyear population is usually selected as the denominator term.

---

*By convention, when calculating a mortality rate, epidemiologists use the midyear population, which is an estimate of the average number of persons who were alive in that year.

HOW DISEASES OCCUR

A useful way of thinking about how a disease might occur is in terms of:

1. a susceptible population, which is
2. exposed to the causative factors of a disease and
3. receives a dose of the causal agent sufficient to produce a disease.

The elements of <u>susceptibility</u>, <u>exposure</u>, and <u>dose</u> are useful to explain a variety of diseases, for example, infectious or communicable diseases and diseases resulting from exposure to environmental pollutants.

IV. THE "PERSON-PLACE-TIME" MODEL

A convenient way to describe the occurrence and distribution of disease within populations is in terms of person, place and time. These characteristics give clues that might explain differing exposure to the etiologic (causative) agent of the disease and the varying susceptibility of population subgroups to the disease when exposure occurs. While one particular characteristic of a person or his environment may lead that individual to have an increased risk, usually several characteristics of person, place, or time are involved in the development of a specific pattern of disease within a population. Determination of the risk of contracting a disease associated with specific characteristics of exposure and susceptibility permits hypotheses concerning the source, responsible agent, transmission, and spread of the disease to be formed and tested.

1. PERSON: This refers to the characteristics of individuals that may influence their exposure to and/or susceptibility to the disease in question. People can be described in terms of their genetic and acquired characteristics of age, sex, ethnic group or race, or their activities, occupations, habits, etc. Such characteristics of persons may determine or reflect their risk of exposure to or susceptibility to a particular disease and contribute to understanding of why persons or groups develop the disease.

Epidemiologists frequently describe the following characteristics of persons: age, race, sex, and social class. Consider the hypothetical illustration shown in Figure 1.

A. AGE

Question 1

a. How would you describe the pattern of risk shown in Figure 1?

Figure 1. Infection rate by age in the U.S., 1978.*

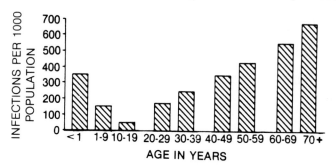

Note: Rates are calculated on the number of persons in each age group.

b.   Try to explain in different ways the distribution of infections in this
     population in terms of susceptibility and/or exposure.

Question 2

The J or U distribution illustrates one way in which the risk of disease might
vary with respect to age. Several other distributions may also be encountered. Try to explain why the distributions occur in these ways. The nota-
tion ↑ signifies "an increase."

Figure 2. Risk by age.

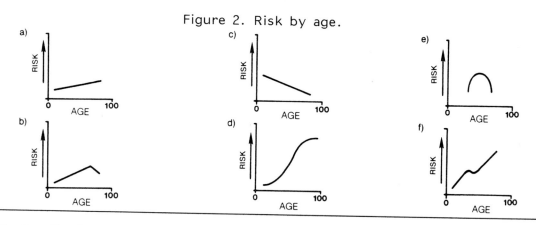

*Ordinarily frequency polygons, not bar graphs of the type depicted in Exer-
cise 1, are used to illustrate continuous variables such as age. The reasons
for this will be covered in Exercise 4.

Answer Question 2 in this space.

B.   SEX

Question 3

a.   How would you describe the pattern of risk shown in Figure 3?

b.   Try to explain the difference between rates of males and females.

C.   ETHNICITY, RACE OR COLOR

Question 4

a.   Describe the pattern of risk shown in Figure 4.

b.   Try to explain the pattern.

Figure 3.   Death rate by age and sex in the U.S., 1977.

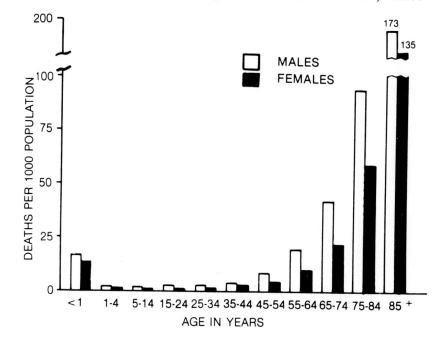

Source: U.S. Dept. HEW, Vital Statistics Report, Annual Summary, 1978.

Figure 4.   Death rate by age and color in the U.S., 1977.

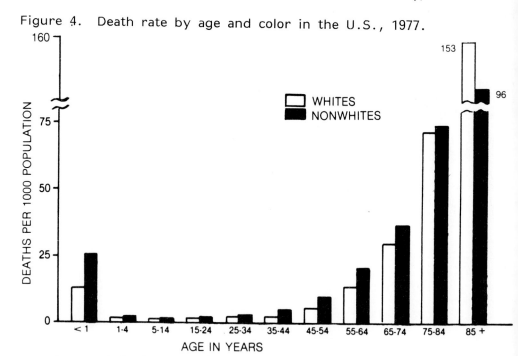

Source: U.S. Dept. HEW, Vital Statistics Report, Annual Summary, 1978.

D.   SOCIOECONOMIC STATUS   (SES)

Figure 5.   Severe illness by social class.

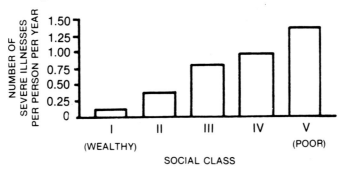

Source: Court, S.D.M., Epidemiology and Natural History of Respiratory Infections in Children.   J. Clin. Pathol. 21 (Supp 2): 31, 1968.

Question 5

A study of children in England found that the total number of respiratory
infections (colds, influenza, etc.) per person was similar in all social classes.
However, the rate of severe infections occurred as shown in Figure 5.

a.   Why are there differences in disease severity by social class?

b.   Epidemiologists most frequently use the characteristics of age, sex,
ethnicity and socioeconomic status to describe a disease pattern by the
characteristic of <u>person</u>.   Why do you think this is so?

E.   OTHER CHARACTERISTICS

Although the above characteristics are frequently used, ANY characteristics
may be used to describe the PERSON at risk of different health problems. A
few will be illustrated by the following examples.

Question 6

For each of the following examples suggest an explanation for the observed
pattern.

6a.   Marital Status

Figure 6a. Hysterectomy by marriage status.

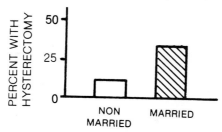

Source: Koepsell, T.D., et al., Prevalence of Prior Hysterectomy in the Seattle-Tacoma Area, Am. J. Pub. Health 70:40, 1980.

Explain the pattern shown in Figure 6a.

6b.   Smoking Status

Figure 6b. Respiratory symptoms by smoking status and sex.

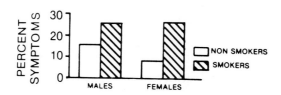

Source: Liard, R., et al., Chronic Respiratory Symptoms: Prevalence in Male and Female Smokers. Am. J. Pub. Health 70:271, 1980.

Explain the pattern shown in Figure 6b.

6c.   Tattoo Status

Figure 6c. Infection by tattoo status.

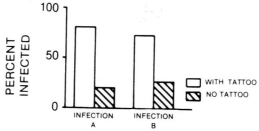

Source: James, J.J., and Smith, L., Serologic Markers for Hepatitis Types A and B Among US Army Soldiers, Germany. Am. J. Pub. Health 69:1216, 1979.

Explain the pattern shown in Figure 6c.

2.   PLACE: In addition to describing who (PERSON) is at risk of a disease or health problem, epidemiologists are interested in WHERE the problem occurs. The PLACE OF OCCURRENCE can refer to a specific geographic point or area. In looking at the distribution of disease in different locations, it is necessary to define what is meant by location. Boundaries for the area may be chosen in many different ways.   They may be determined by natural boundaries such as rivers and mountains or by political boundaries.   While natural boundaries define geographic areas that may be homogeneous in terms of climate and terrain, political boundaries are more convenient in terms of how frequencies of disease are reported and recorded. There can be great variation in the size of the areas compared (city blocks, neighborhoods, cities, counties, states, regions, or nations).

Place may also be classified in terms such as urban or rural, resident or nonresident, domestic or foreign, etc., or it might be thought of as a characteristic of person, e.g., place of residence or place of occupation.

The distribution of a disease by geographic area is one way in which the use of PLACE can illustrate a distinct pattern of disease.   For example, a certain disease of the nervous system of unknown etiology (cause), shows generally higher mortality rates in the colder areas.   This finding has been observed in several countries.   Figure 7 illustrates the distribution.

Question 7

How might the north-to-south pattern shown in Figure 7 be explained if disease X were caused by

a.   An infectious agent

b.   A genetically inherited defect

c.   Medical therapy

d.   Dietary factors

Figure 7. Death rates per 100,000 population in the U.S. and Canada.

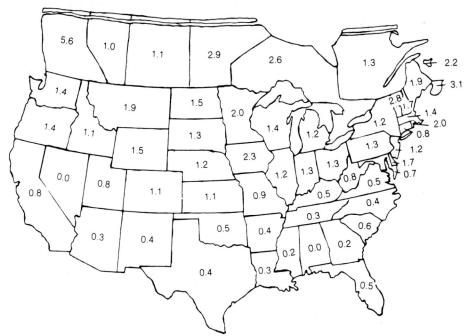

Source: Alter M. Etiologic consideration in the epidemiology of [disease x].
          Am. J. Epidem. 88:318, 1968.

URBAN VERSUS RURAL RESIDENCE

Question 8

For each of the following, describe the difference in the observed distribution and offer an explanation to account for it.

8a.   A viral infection contracted through direct contact with infected persons.

Figure 8a. Viral infection by urban-rural residence.

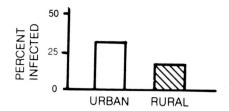

Describe and explain the observed finding from Figure 8a.

8b.   Infant mortality from all causes

Figure 8b. Infant deaths by urban-rural residence.

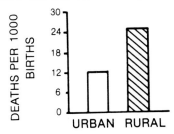

Describe and explain the observed finding from Figure 8b.

8c.   Death from lung cancer

Figure 8c. Lung cancer deaths by urban-rural residence.

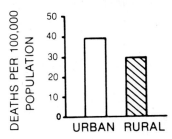

Describe and explain the observed finding from Figure 8c.

3.   TIME: This is the final component of the person-place-time model for describing the distribution of a health problem.   The occurrence of disease may
be grouped by week, month, year, the day of the week, hour of onset, etc.

Question 9

a.   Describe the distribution of deaths and births shown in Figure 9.
      What might account for seasonal variations?

Figure 9. Births and deaths by month in the U.S., 1978.

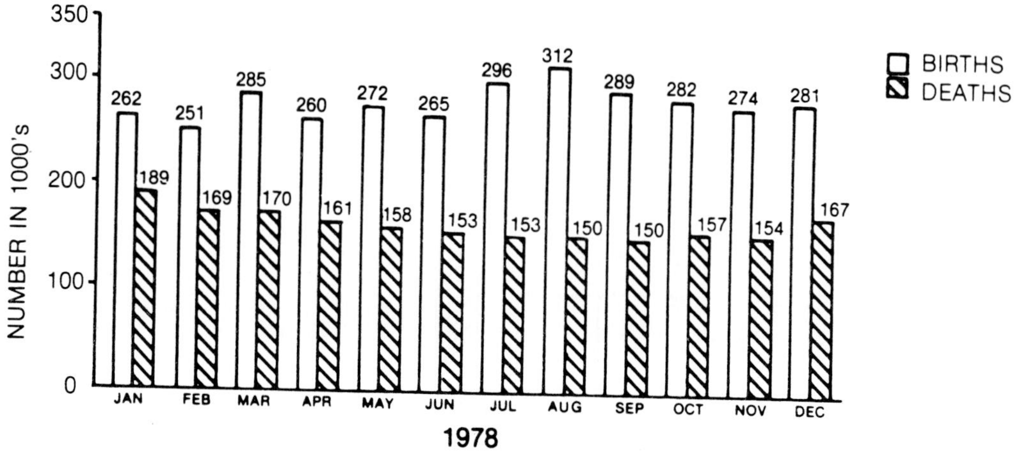

Source:　U.S. Dept. HEW.　Vital Statistics Report, Annual Summary 1978.

Question 9 (continued)

b.　The data for years prior to 1978 generally follows the same pattern, although the annual number of births and of deaths differs.　What factors might contribute to annual fluctuation in total births and deaths?

Question 10

Describe the distribution for suicide and homicide shown below.　What might account for the differences?

Figure 10. Average deaths per day from suicide and homicide, U.S., 1973.

Day	Suicide	Homicide
Sunday	66.6	68.0
Monday	75.0	51.2
Tuesday	68.8	47.2
Wednesday	68.3	43.1
Thursday	68.6	46.7
Friday	68.1	54.5
Saturday	66.4	82.4
Average	68.8	56.1

Source:　Lester, D.,　Temporal Variation in Suicide and Homicide. Am. J. Epidem. 109:571, 1979.

Describe and explain the observed finding in Figure 10.

The pattern of disease may also be described with respect to changes in the TREND of disease over long periods of time. A secular (long-term, worldly) trend is shown in Figure 11.

Figure 11. Deaths from lung cancer in New York State, 1960-1969.

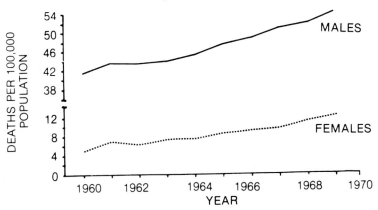

Source: Cancer Incidence and Mortality in New York State, Bureau of Cancer Control, New York State Dept of Health, 1976.

Question 11

a.   Describe the secular trend.

b.   What might account for the changes observed over time?

Question 12

In the blank graphs that follow, we would like you to visualize different ways in which a disease trend might occur. On the graphs place three or more dots to represent the rates of a disease occurring between 1960 and 1980. Try to place the dots in a variety of ways so that several different types of long-term trends are represented. Connect the dots to create trend lines.

Figure 12. Disease trends.

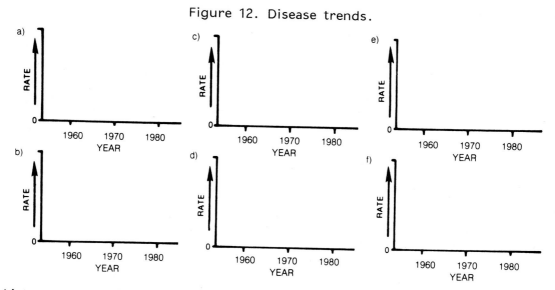

List as many reasons as you can to explain why the occurrence of a disease might seem to change over time. (Hint: a disease's frequency might vary for both biologic and nonbiologic reasons.)

Of special interest to epidemiologists are short-term changes in the trend of a disease. An example is shown below:

Figure 13. Measles in Greenland, 1940-1968.

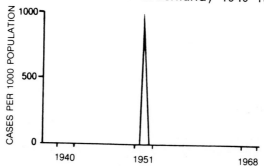

Source: Christensen, P., et al., An epidemic of measles in southern Greenland, 1951, Acta Medica Scand. 144:430, 1952.

Question 13

a.   Describe the trend of measles in Greenland between 1940 and 1968.

b.   What can you conclude about the susceptibility and exposure of this population to measles?

A different pattern of occurrence is more typical of measles.   Both long- and short-term variations are illustrated below.

Figure 14. Measles - reported cases by year, U.S., 1912-1977.

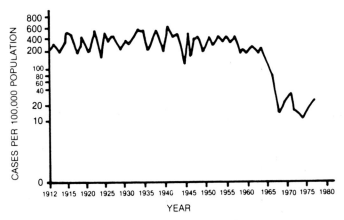

Source: Reported Morbidity and Mortality in the United States, 1977, Center for Disease Control, U.S. Dept. HEW, 1978.

Question 14

a.   Describe the trend.

b.   Suggest explanations for the shape of the curve before and after 1965.

V.   THE HOST-AGENT-ENVIRONMENT MODEL

We have seen how the characteristics of person-place-time can be useful in describing the pattern of disease or health problem and how the patterns stimulate speculation about possible reasons for the observed distribution.

A second model that epidemiologists use to explain variation in the frequency of disease in the community includes the components of HOST-AGENT-ENVI-RONMENT.

A.   THE HOST

The state of the host results from both environmental and genetic factors. Some host characteristics such as gender and certain enzyme deficiencies are genetic, while others such as acquired immunity to infection or nutritional status result from environmental exposure. However, many host characteristics such as personality, social behavior, and social class are combinations of genetic AND environmental influences. The distinction between the relative contributions to these characteristics of genetic inheritance and environmental exposure is quite important. Many social characteristics contribute to the etiology and distribution of disease. Illness caused by environmental factors should be amenable to prevention or control, whereas the genetic aspects of disease are more difficult to influence.

B.   THE AGENT

Agents of infectious diseases are the bacteria, fungi, rickettsiae and viruses as well as the insects, plants, and animals that transmit those diseases to man. Characteristics of the AGENT that are used by epidemiologists include its reservoir, mode of transmission, incubation period, pathogenicity, infectivity, and virulence. Definition of these terms may be found in Appendix 1 of this manual as well as the American Public Health Association Handbook of Communicable Diseases in Man. The Handbook also provides details of these characteristics of important infectious agents.

C.   THE ENVIRONMENT

The environment can be divided into three component parts: the BIOLOGICAL environment consists of the animals, plants, and living organisms external to the host; the SOCIAL environment consists of the economic, political, cultural, and social institutions comprising the host's society; the PHYSICAL environment consists of the temperature, altitude, water, air, chemicals and radiation to which the host is exposed. Many diseases and health problems are caused or influenced by environmental factors.

The model was originally used to explain patterns observed for infectious diseases, but because of its utility, the model has been used to explain non-infectious diseases, social behavior, diseases associated with environmental hazards, and other subjects.

As proposed, a susceptible HOST and an AGENT capable of causing a disease are subject to factors in the ENVIRONMENT which might affect the HOST's susceptibility and/or exposure to the disease AGENT, or the ability of the AGENT to cause disease. The amount of disease in the community results from the interaction of the three components.

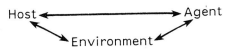

The three components are shown to be in a steady state (the usual condition) each affecting and being affected by the others. If any of the components change, sufficient to affect the steady state, changes would occur in one or both of the remaining components. This might result in:

1. a change in the frequency of disease in the community.
2. a change in the pattern of disease with respect to the characteristics of person, place, or time.

The model therefore can be seen to be a convenient way to try to explain the reasons underlying an observed change in a disease pattern.

A second way of presenting the model is

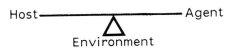

Any change in the steady state that favors the existence and proliferation of the agent or an increase in the pathogenicity (disease-producing power) of the agent would result in an increase of disease in the community. Conversely, any change that favors the host's biologic ability to resist the disease agent or reduces the host's possibility of exposure to the agent would result in a decrease of disease in the community. These situations can be depicted graphically as if this were a see-saw or set of scales; the heavier side sinks lower.

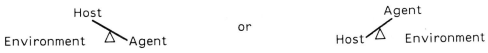

The steady state has tipped to favor the disease Agent, resulting in an increase of disease.

The steady state has tipped to favor the Host, resulting in a decrease of disease.

As seen with PERSON-PLACE-TIME, epidemiologists might easily use characteristics of HOST-AGENT-ENVIRONMENT interactions to describe a population and seek clues to explain differing risk patterns observed in the community. We shall not give detailed examples as the possibilities should be evident.

Until now we have given examples of disease or health problems illustrated by some of their major epidemiologic characteristics and asked you to describe the pattern and suggest explanations. Now, we shall try to apply some of these principles to some epidemiologic problems.

Question 15

You are a health officer whose task is to reduce deaths occurring from motor vehicle accidents. As a preliminary step you must discover whether or not a pattern exists with regard to this problem.

a.   List the items of information you will need to compile to investigate the distribution of motor vehicle accidents. Arrange these into PERSON-PLACE-TIME categories.

b.   How will you assess the information to determine the magnitude of the problem?

Question 16

Review your list of characteristics of PERSON-PLACE-TIME used to describe the pattern of motor vehicle accidents.

a.   Try to rearrange this list by putting each characteristic or type of information into the HOST-AGENT-ENVIRONMENT model.

b.   In what circumstances does the PERSON-PLACE-TIME model offer advantages over HOST-AGENT-ENVIRONMENT?

c. In what circumstances does the HOST-AGENT-ENVIRONMENT model offer advantages over PERSON-PLACE-TIME?

VI. EPIDEMICS

You have seen how patterns of disease may be studied by using the PERSON-PLACE-TIME and HOST-AGENT-ENVIRONMENT models. Let us now consider epidemics, a term that describes a special type of disease pattern.

The amount of a particular disease present in a specific population may remain stable for long periods or, as we have seen, it may alternately rise and fall due to fluctuation in the number of susceptible individuals and the nature and extent of their exposure to disease agents. Diseases continually present in populations are considered to be endemic to that population. The term endemic refers to the "usual" or expected frequency of the disease found in a population. An epidemic is an "unusual" frequency of disease above the endemic or expected occurrence, characteristically revealing itself in a relatively short period of time.

Question 17

In investigating an outbreak of disease an epidemiologist compares past and present disease frequencies. The amount of disease occurring in the past in the absence of an epidemic defines the EXPECTED frequency, whereas the present amount occurring in the suspected outbreak defines the OBSERVED frequency. Using the terms observed and expected suggest a mathematical relationship that defines an epidemic.

Question 18

a. How many cases of a disease are necessary for an epidemic?

b. How might you determine the presence of an epidemic of a common and endemic disease such as influenza?

Question 19

You are a health officer and you observe that a group of individuals has become ill with stomach pain, nausea, and vomiting.

a.   What information would you need to determine whether an epidemic is occurring or if a pattern is present?

b.   Indicate the sources from which you might obtain this information.   If those data do not already exist or if they are not readily obtainable, what would you do?

Question 20

Given the same group of cases with stomach pain, nausea, and vomiting, your preliminary conclusion is that the observed/expected greatly exceeds 1, therefore, you believe an epidemic is occurring.   Since the next step involves attempting to control the epidemic, you must now identify the cause.   Suggest some possible explanations (hypotheses) you might investigate.

Question 21

The distribution of events of epidemiologic interest according to age, sex and socioeconomic status can aid in identification of highly susceptible population subgroups and can sometimes lead to the identification of the responsible agent or agents.

Figures 15 and 16 describe a single and unusual event. See if you can discover the cause by analysis of the data.

Figure 15. Distribution by socioeconomic status and sex.

Socio-economic status	Population exposed to risk			Number of deaths			Deaths per 100 exposed to risk		
	Male	Female	Both	Male	Female	Both	Male	Female	Both
I (highest)	172	132	304	111	6	117	64.5	4.5	38.5
II (middle)	172	103	275	150	13	163	87.2	12.6	59.3
III (lowest)	504	208	712	419	107	526	83.1	51.4	73.9
Unknown	9	23	32	8	5	13	88.9	21.9	40.6
TOTAL	857	466	1,323	688	131	819	80.2	28.1	61.8

Source: Stallones, R.A. (unpublished).

Figure 16. Distribution by socioeconomic status and age.

Socio-economic status	Population exposed to risk			Number of deaths			Deaths per 100 exposed to risk		
	Adult	Child	Both	Adult	Child	Both	Adult	Child	Both
I & II (highest)	560	19	579	280	0	280	50.0	0.0	48.4
III (lowest)	645	67	712	477	49	526	73.9	73.1	73.9
Unknown	32	0	32	13	0	13	40.6	--	40.6
TOTAL	1,237	86	1,323	770	49	819	62.2	57.0	61.9

Source: Stallones, R.A. (unpublished).

a.   Describe the characteristics of the exposed population.

b.   What is unusual about the structure of this population?

c.   What subgroups have the highest and lowest death rates?

d.   What types of situations could have brought this population together in time and place?

e.   What do you think was responsible for this episode?   (Your explanation must account for all the facts.)

When investigating actual epidemics, the steps taken to compile preliminary information, discern disease patterns and develop working hypotheses to explain the observed distribution would be among the first actions performed by an epidemiologist.   Following that, you would attempt to prove the correctness (validity) of your hypotheses.   The strategy for achieving this will be demonstrated in later exercises.

SUGGESTED RESPONSES
Exercise 1--Patterns of Disease

1a.   There is a high rate of infection during infancy (less than 1 year of age), which decreases during childhood and adolescence. Thereafter, rates increase with age; the highest rates are observed in old age.

1b.   The distribution of infectious diseases may be explained in terms of two important factors, susceptibility and exposure. A given distribution may predominantly reflect either factor or it can be the resultant of the two acting together. Considering the factors one at a time, the distribution can be explained as follows:

Susceptibility.   Since this is an infectious disease infants probably have little immunity; therefore, there is a high rate of infection. During childhood and adolescence susceptibility decreases, thereafter, susceptibility to disease increases. This may reflect growth or development of an immune system reaching its peak before age 20; it then declines with age.

Exposure.   The degree of exposure to infectious agents might vary throughout life, being highest in infancy and old age and lowest during adolescence. This may be due to the kind of activities and contacts that people have at different ages.

A third factor that was not asked about is also important. This is the dose of the infectious agent. Dose refers to the number of or concentration of infecting organisms to which a person (or group) is exposed. If the dose of the infectious agent was high during infancy and old age, but low during adolescence, or if there were an effect due to the cumulated dose of exposure, a distribution similar to Figure 1 could occur.

While a given distribution can sometimes be explained in terms of these factors acting independently, this rarely is the case. Most distributions result from the influence of all the factors. The rate of infection would be the net effect of the degree of susceptibility that the group has as well as the likelihood of coming into contact with a sufficient dose of the infecting agent. Infection may occur when a susceptible individual is exposed to (comes in contact with) a sufficient dose of an infectious agent.

The factors of susceptibility and exposure determine the likelihood of individuals to contract an infection. For example, infants have low resistance to certain kinds of infections. They come in contact with older brothers or sisters and adults who have those infections. Old people may have diseases, which both lowers their resistance to infection and increases the possibility of going to a hospital where there are many patients who are hospitalized for infectious diseases.

The distribution of disease for the group as a whole also is an expression of the number of susceptible persons and exposure to persons already infected with the disease.

The distribution of infection by age illustrated in Figure 1 is termed a J- or U-shaped distribution and is seen for many infectious and noninfectious diseases.

2.   Virtually all diseases exhibit an association with age. The risk of disease will reflect the degree of susceptibility as well as the likelihood of contact with the disease agent. Infectious diseases, congenital illnesses, and most genetic disorders tend to occur at very high rates during infancy and childhood, while heart disease, cancer, and other diseases generally thought to be noninfectious occur later in life. Noninfectious diseases with insidious onset and extended duration are generally termed chronic diseases, and usually occur in older age groups. Another category of diseases is those due to exposure to chemicals, toxins, and pollutants in the environment. Diseases due to environmental exposure may occur at any stage of life. Because many of these diseases require prolonged exposure, or may have a long latent period, manifestation of disease might not occur until adulthood and middle age.

2a. A gradual increase in disease with age. Exposure or susceptibility may increase gradually and continually over time. Alternatively, there might be a cumulative effect of prolonged exposure. Many types of cancer show this kind of distribution.

2b. A decrease in disease among older persons suggests that they no longer are exposed to the cause of the disease. A marked decline in the curve also suggests that the number of susceptibles has diminished. A disease that confers protective immunity to survivors or that kills off susceptible individuals might show this distribution. Also, the likelihood of having a definitive diagnosis may decrease at advanced ages, for certain diseases.

2c. Declining risk with age might be seen if exposure or susceptibility decreased with age. A disease that confers immunity to survivors or kills off susceptibles would leave a gradually more resistant older population.

2d. Risk of disease is low in early life, shows a large increase in middle life, and levels off in old age. This is an S or sigmoid curve frequently encountered for diseases due to occupational exposures.

2e. Manifestation of disease is associated with a limited age group. Some genetic diseases would show this curve in early life. Diseases relating to pregnancy, reproduction, or menopause might show this unusual distribution. Both exposure and susceptibility are confined to a particular time of life.

2f. A disease with a double peak (a bimodal curve) implies that neither exposure nor susceptibility occurs uniformly, i.e., something unusual occurs that increases the risk for some relatively young people. The bimodal curve has been observed in female breast cancer. The first peak occurs before and the second peak after menopause. This implies that two distinct mechanisms may produce the same disease.

3a. This is a J-shaped distribution. For both sexes, there is a high rate in infancy, which decreases to a very low rate during childhood and early adolescence and increases steadily throughout the remainder of life. In all age groups males have a greater risk of death. The curve for mortality from all causes also looks like this.

3b. Males are either more exposed or more susceptible to the various causes of death at all ages. The excess male death rates suggest that being female might confer greater protection against death at any particular age. Perhaps there is some genetic or immune system mechanism that makes females less likely to die than males of similar ages. Or perhaps there is some relation to female sex hormones. However, if sex hormones played a protective role you might expect to see the death rates equalize for males and females after age 50, because females generally undergo menopause prior to that age; the hormones would either cease to play a role or decrease in importance. Nonbiologic reasons may play a role. For example, males in most societies are more aggressive and therefore might be exposed to risk of death through more accident or injury. Or they may engage in activities (smoking, drinking, or poor diet) or occupations that expose them to factors leading to illness and death at earlier ages than females.

4a. The age-death curve reveals the J-shaped distribution in both whites and nonwhites. Nonwhites have higher death rates at all ages except 85+.

4b. For those below age 85, nonwhites are more exposed or more susceptible to factors causing death than are whites. For those who are very old, nonwhites are "healthier" than whites, implying that all the sickly nonwhites died off, leaving a group of aged, relatively healthy people who will die off very slowly. This might be true; however, it is unlikely to be the reason since nonwhites as a group are known to have more diseases, lower income, and poorer nutrition and to receive less medical care than whites of similar age. A possible reason for the shift in risk is that the rate for older nonwhites might not be accurate. This could occur in two ways: the number of deaths (numerator of the death rate) might be underreported or the number still alive (the denominator) might be overestimated. If accurate ages of individuals were not known there might be an apparent increase in the number of old nonwhites "believed" to be 85+, thereby resulting in artifically low death rates.

5a. The children of poorer families might contract more severe infections by being exposed to more virulent types of infectious agents than children of wealthier families, e.g., pneumonia-producing organisms rather than the common cold.

However, it is more likely that children of wealthy families have access to and might obtain earlier diagnosis and better medical care, or perhaps they maintain better nutrition and have better infection-fighting defense mechanisms, which prevent an infection from progressing to a more serious illness than do children of poor families.

5b. These characteristics are related to all disease processes to a greater or lesser extent. Second, they are characteristics of a population or community that can be observed and measured in much the same way as a doctor will use an xray or blood test in evaluating a patient. Finally, they are the most readily available information easily obtained from birth or death certificates, medical and hospital records, or other sources of health information.

6a. Married women are exposed to factors that might lead to hysterectomy.

1.   Childbirth may damage the uterus or lead to problems for which surgery is necessary.

2.   Married women may have more frequent sexual intercourse. This might lead to infection or other conditions for which hysterectomy is necessary.

3.   Married women may visit the doctor more frequently than non-married women, increasing their risk of having uterine problems diagnosed and treated. In some cases, physicians may perform unnecessary operations due to mistaken diagnosis.

4.   Married women may have surgery as a permanent means of birth control.

6b. Smokers of both sexes report the same rate of symptoms. Non-smokers of both sexes have lower symptom rates; however, male nonsmokers have higher rates than female nonsmokers.

Male nonsmokers may be more exposed in their work to air or chemicals that cause respiratory symptoms than females. More male than female nonsmokers may spend more time in cars in heavy traffic traveling to work and spend more time in cities, both of which have air pollutants capable of producing respiratory symptoms.

6c. Those with tattoo have a higher percentage of both infection A and B. The needles or the ink used to draw tattoos may harbor the infectious agent. Or, there may be injury to the skin as a result of the presence of the ink. Injured skin may be more susceptible to the infecting organism.

A high rate of infection among those not having a tattoo suggests either that tattooed persons may transmit the infection to those who do not have a tattoo or that there may be one or more additional ways for persons to become infected with these diseases, besides tattooing. Finally, there may be something about the life style of tattooed individuals that make them more likely than the nontattooed persons to become exposed to the infectious agents. If this were true, then the needle and the ink might not be important factors in producing the diseases.

7a. Cold weather may promote the survival or transmission of the microorganism, e.g., influenza is a disease usually seen in colder months. People may congregate indoors more in cold weather. The respiratory mucous membranes may be less effective barriers to disease agents in cold weather or heated homes.

7b. People of similar genetic background may congregate in or migrate to certain geographic areas, e.g., Scandinavians in the Midwest, blacks and other ethnic groups in the industrial cities of the North. Any genetic disorders specific to these groups would result in geographic clusters of cases.

7c. Different modes of therapy may be more popular in certain areas than in others. For example, new diagnostic procedures or therapy may be confined to areas near medical schools or in wealthy communities where cost is not a deterrent to care. Disease caused by the therapy might reveal itself through higher disease rates in large cities or around medical centers.

7d. Differences in diet may result from climate variation, local custom, biochemical attributes of water and soil, and variation in the ethnic mixture of an area. These could affect the nutritional composition of foods as well as the types of food eaten and the manner of preparation. Dietary patterns would be expected to differ in cities and rural areas, mountain and seaside areas, cold and warm climates.

8a. Exposure to an infected person is more likely to occur in cities due to the crowding and greater number of persons encountered by urban residents.

8b. Rural areas are less likely to have access to doctors or hospitals. Deaths from infectious diseases and congenital or genetic diseases might contribute to higher death rates in rural areas. Although not shown in this example, some urban areas might have mortality rates higher than those seen in rural areas, if there are ghettos with large numbers of poor residents. In such areas, lack of medical care, poor nutrition, poor sanitation, and overcrowding may contribute to high infant mortality rates.

8c. Smoking, air pollution, and asbestos are known causes of primary lung cancer. Urban residents might have greater exposure to the first two causes. In certain rural areas, asbestos might be present in high concentrations, and in some urban areas, poor building practices might lead to exposure to asbestos particles. Smoking is the leading factor, however, and urban areas would be expected to have a higher proportion of smokers than rural areas. Chewing tobacco might be more commonly used in rural areas, however, leading to high cancer rates for the mouth and tongue. Better medical diagnosis may occur in urban than in rural areas.

9a. Births occur more frequently during the summer and fall. Counting back 9 months from birth suggests a large proportion of these were conceived during the fall and winter months. This suggests that sexual activity might be more frequent in the fall and winter or that females might be more fertile or males more potent in those months. Which do you think is likely?

Deaths occur more frequently in the colder months. We would expect respiratory infections to be more frequent at this time, also. Because infection may be a complication of illness in those with existing heart or lung disease the number of deaths might increase. Depression and suicide following the Christmas and New Year holidays might also increase the number of deaths noted in January.

9b. The number of births in a year reflects many factors, including the number of marriages and divorces, preferences for family size, economic conditions, migration of young fertile persons, and the availability of abortion or family planning services.

The number of deaths in a year reflects availability of medical care, implementation of more effective modes of therapy, fluctuation in exposure to the factors that cause disease, changes in factors relating to susceptibility, unusual events such as war or famine, etc.

While not necessarily true for the United States, birth and death data for other countries may also fluctuate because of the procedures for reporting these events.

Finally, any unusual in or out migration of large numbers of young or old persons might result in fluctuation of births or deaths.

10. Suicide occurs to excess on Mondays while homicides increase on the weekends. The different pattern suggests that the causal factors might differ. "Blue Monday" signifying loneliness and depression after the weekend might contribute to an excess of suicide. Homicide might be related to an increase in alcohol use on weekends coupled with an increase in contact between friends, family, and acquaintances. In a surprisingly large proportion of homicides the victim is either family, friend, or an acquaintance of the killer. Thus, weekend violence is associated with close contact.

11. There is an increase in the death rate in both sexes. The male rate is much higher than females, although the female rate shows a much greater percentage increase (4 to 12 or 300% vs. 41 to 53 or 29% in males). This probably reflects an increase in both exposure and dose, i.e., more smokers, heavier smokers, or change in the smoking habit (more inhaling), particularly for women.

It may also be possible that as the number of smokers increases, lung cancer might also result from the combined effects of carcinogens in tobacco smoke and potential cocarcinogens and mediator substances encountered in the workplace or general environment. Despite the strong evidence linking smoking and cancer, not all smokers develop lung cancer.

12. Each of the curves may be explained in terms of a change in the number of susceptibles, or a change in factors leading to or affecting the quality and quantity of exposure during the 20-year period. In or out migration of susceptibles or of resistant (immune) individuals in large numbers might produce an increase or a decrease in the disease rate. Changes in environmental quality (air or water pollution) and social customs (use of alcohol, tobacco, drugs) might produce increases or decreases of a disease rate over time.

Nonbiologic factors may also contribute to an apparent change of the disease. Legal requirements for reporting cases to health authorities may change over time. Improved diagnostic tests may be available to enable better case finding. Physician awareness of newer diseases may also result in more complete evaluation of patients and better case finding.

Figure 12. Disease trends

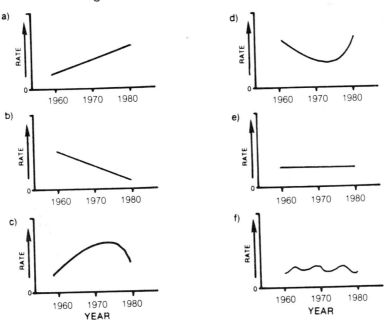

13a. 1940-1950, no disease occurred in the population. All persons were susceptible as shown by 100% of population getting the disease (1000 cases per 1000 population). Therefore, no one was exposed prior to 1951, a "virgin population."

13b. After 1951 everyone was immune to a second infection, the organism was not reintroduced into the community, or the organism lost its infectivity. Because Greenland is an island there would be no way for the disease to occur unless the organism entered the population from the outside, i.e., tourists, immigrants, etc. Theoretically it is possible that a nonpathogenic organism endemic to the island's human or animal populations could suddenly acquire pathogenic (disease producing) properties but that is not known to occur with measles.

14a. The U.S. is not an island; therefore, the measles virus is present in the community. The number of cases depends upon the number of susceptible persons (children) exposed to the virus. There is a cyclic pattern with peaks occurring at 2-3 year intervals. This suggests that every 2-3 years there is a sufficient number of new susceptibles, i.e., young children who contract the infection. As the number of cases increases, there are fewer susceptibles, and the curve dips.

14b. A major change in the frequency of cases occurred in the middle 1960s. The pattern of cyclic occurrence seems to still occur but at a much reduced rate. The reason is that a vaccine was developed, licensed, and came into widespread use at that time. The rate of illness will still reflect the number of susceptibles and exposures to the virus as it did prior to the vaccine. However, since most (but not all) children are immunized, the probability of infected and susceptible persons coming in contact with each other is reduced.

15a. You may not be able to categorize some of the pertinent information conveniently by PERSON-PLACE-TIME, for example, number of deaths.

Distribution of deaths by month, day of the week, time of day. (TIME)

Age, sex of person killed and driver who caused the accident. (PERSON)

Location of accident. (PLACE)

Status of person killed--driver, front seat or back seat passenger. (PERSON)

Driving conditions on day of accident, type of vehicle--motorcycle, foreign or domestic; type of accident, car/car, car/person, motorcycle/car, speed of the vehicles, mechanical condition of the motor vehicles involved.

Was emergency medical vehicle or police rescue squad called to the accident site? Other pertinent data pertaining to PERSON-PLACE-TIME.

15b. In order to assess the risk some measure of population at risk is necessary to calculate rates. Frequently used denominators are the number of
licensed drivers, number of registered vehicles, and an estimate of the
miles driven.

In judging the importance of a problem epidemiologists must assess the
actual number and also the rate of that problem relative to the population. Thus, 50 deaths in a small town may be judged more of a public
health problem requiring action than 50,000 deaths involving automobiles
for the entire country.

16a. Characteristics of person can readily be assigned to the host. Some
characteristics of place and time can readily be assigned to the environment. Some characteristics of place may be assigned to either the agent
or the environment depending upon how the terms are defined. There
might be overlap in definitions of agent and environment. You may have
difficulty in assigning some of the person-place-time characteristics to an
appropriate category of the other model.

16b. Both person-place-time and host-agent-environment models are useful and
may be used whenever appropriate.

In diseases of unknown cause, the person-place-time model may be very
useful as it permits a convenient framework for describing the disease in
terms of who, what, when, and where. In diseases of unknown cause,
we could describe host and environment characteristics, but we would not
know the agent.

16c. In diseases of known cause, particularly the infectious or communicable
diseases, the host-agent-environment model is convenient and useful.
The advantage of this model is that it permits characteristics of the
disease agent to be included, whereas it may be difficult to put those
characteristics into the person-place-time model.

17. Observed/expected >> 1.0   The sign >> signifies "greatly in excess of."

Or endemic frequency: observed = expected; epidemic frequency: observed > expected.

18a. The number of cases that constitutes an epidemic will vary with the
disease, the population, and its previous experience with that disease.
The outbreak of an "epidemic" cannot be determined strictly in absolute
terms. Rather, it is a relative concept.

In the United States a disease such as cholera is not normally present in
the population and many persons would be susceptible if exposed to the
cholera organism. If the disease reappeared, the source of the outbreak
would be investigated in order to prevent rapid and serious spread of the
disease. Therefore, even one case of cholera would constitute an epidemic in the U.S. But in a country like India where cholera is always

present in some population subgroups, a few hundred cases a year may be the usual or expected incidence. For cholera to be considered an epidemic in India several hundred or thousands of cases (i.e., cases above the endemic frequency) would have to occur.

As new control and preventive measures are developed, the endemic rate of a disease may change. Measles was once a disease that almost all children would contract, and therefore large numbers of cases occurred each year. Now that an effective vaccine has been developed, most cases of measles can be prevented. Thus, a few cases of measles clustered in one area in a short period of time may constitute an epidemic, whereas a much larger number of cases in previous years might have been the usual endemic frequency.

18b. An epidemic is determined by comparison of the observed number of cases to the usual pattern of the disease. Due to the fact that disease occurrence is dependent upon many factors, the expected incidence may vary over time. The actual number of cases of a disease will usually fluctuate about the predicted level. An arbitrary limit of 2 standard errors from the endemic occurrence is used to define the <u>epidemic threshold for common diseases</u> such as influenza, as shown in the Figure below. Standard error is a type of statistical measurement that enables us to describe the amount of fluctuation observed in a set of data.

Pneumonia-Influenza - reported deaths in 121 cities compared with deaths from all causes by age group and by week, U.S., 1971-1974.

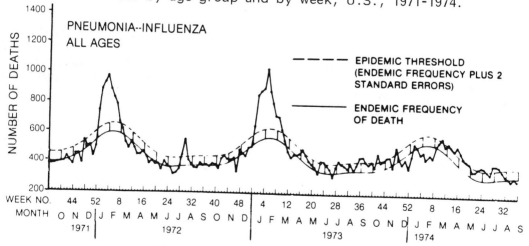

SOURCE: REPORTED MORBIDITY AND MORTALITY IN THE U.S.
1974 DEPT. HEW PUBLIC HEALTH SERVICE

The periodicity of the disease can be used to identify an epidemic. Many diseases recur with predictable patterns. For example, influenza (a viral respiratory disease) recurs in cycles with worldwide epidemics (pandemics) approximately every 10 years. Moreover, the disease is associated with

cold weather and within any given year would also show seasonal variation. Completeness of reporting is an important element in defining the
presence and magnitude of epidemics.

19a. The information you will need includes:

1.   The number of cases and characteristics of those becoming ill including the age, sex, onset of disease by day, date, time, and place. Complete list of symptoms.

2.   Activities of cases preceding the disease onset varying from several
hours to several weeks or longer, depending upon the disease in question.
This may include foods and liquids ingested, social and business activities, and persons contacted during the period.

3.   Knowledge of the expected number of cases for the area. In some
cases you may need to calculate the rate of infection, thus, a denominator
(y term of a rate) will be necessary. You may need to determine the
disease trend for months or years, as well as seasonal or cyclic variation
in the area.

4.   Presence of similar illness among family, friends, or business contacts.

5.   Determination and comparison of illness rates among persons ill and
thought to be exposed to potential disease agents vs. those persons not
ill or who were not exposed.

19b. The above information might be obtained from any of the following:

1.   Local doctors, county medical society, city or county health department, school nurses, hospitals, clinics, other health agencies, company
medical department, clinical laboratories.

2.   Supplementary information from library, census records, maps,
postal service, etc.

3.   Special surveys of known ill persons and their contacts.

4.   Special community surveys of ill and nonill persons. Special studies
obviously require going to the field site where illness has been reported
IF PRELIMINARY ASSESSMENT SUGGESTS AN EPIDEMIC.

20.   Because symptoms are referable to the gastrointestinal system, a potential
source of the problem might be exposure to a common source of foods or
liquids: (a)   contaminated containers due to improper manufacture,
storage, or transport of processed foods or liquids, (b) improper preparation or storage of freshly prepared (home-cooked) foods, (c) contamination of surface or underground water supply.

A second general area for consideration would be insect-borne infections. A third area would be environmental toxins due to hazards such as cleaning solutions.

A complete list of the different disease categories and means of transmission to humans will be found in Exercises 6 and 7.

21a. This is a population of 1323 individuals that includes males, females, and children of all three socioeconomic classes.

21b. The number of males greatly exceeds females and very few children are present. The number of persons of the lowest social class greatly exceeds that of the upper classes.

21c. Deaths occur in all three classes. Men have the highest death rates particularly in classes II and III. Among women, the upper social class has the lowest death rate and women of class II have an intermediate rate. Children of classes I and II were spared but lower-class children had a very high death rate; in fact, it is nearly equal to the rate among class III adults.

21d. The event must bring together 1323 individuals in the proportions noted. Several possibilities exist: a small town, a factory, a group of people traveling together.

21e. Your answer must explain all the data. An infectious disease is not likely because it is rare to see such high mortality. Moreover, most infectious diseases affect children more than adults.

An accident in or near a factory is a possibility. This explanation would require specific details concerning how the children were involved.

A chemical or environmental pollutant in or near a small town is also a reasonable guess, although the death rates seem unusually high. Perhaps the upper-class children were located much further from the highest exposure area and were not killed.

A group of people traveling together is a good possibility. Perhaps a mass transit system such as a train or a subway at certain hours of the day might bring together 1323 people in this way. But it is not clear why the upper socioeconomic class women and children would be spared.

Finally, we have the answer. This is the distribution of the exposed population and mortality of the luxury ship Titanic, which sank at sea. Women and children (and some men) of the upper classes escaped the ship. Passengers and crew of the lowest class could not get away.

EXERCISE 2.   POPULATION AT RISK

Epidemiologic work constantly emphasizes the population at risk (the denominator in the calculation of rates). The population at risk is one of the most important concepts in epidemiology because it focuses your attention on groups at risk of disease, rather than on individuals. The population at risk is important because it enables diseased individuals (cases) to be referred back to the population from which they came. Epidemiologists can then concentrate their attention on identifying those shared characteristics of the group's members that might lead to better understanding of the causal factors of disease and the mechanisms through which they affect health.

Goals

Upon completion of this exercise: (1) you should understand the term population at risk and its relation to identifying disease patterns and health problems in the community; (2) you should also understand the ways in which particular populations can be utilized for epidemiologic study.

Methods

In order to achieve these goals you will need to understand:

I.   AGE- AND CAUSE-SPECIFIC RATES
II.   DEFINITION OF THE TERM POPULATION AT RISK
III. POPULATIONS USEFUL IN IDENTIFYING EPIDEMIOLOGIC PROBLEMS
      A.   Populations with exposure characteristics of interest
      B.   Populations with biologic characteristics of interest
      C.   Populations involved in natural experiments
IV.   COHORT ANALYSIS

Terms

Age- and cause-specific rates, population at risk, attack rates, secondary attack rates, person-years, primary case, index case, incubation period.

Suggested Readings

The readings listed are for review, since you have read them previously. The references do not emphasize population at risk.

Lilienfeld and Lilienfeld, Foundations of Epidemiology, Chapter 7.
Fox, Hall, and Elvebach, Epidemiology, Man and Disease, Chapters 5, 7.
MacMahon and Pugh, Epidemiology, Principles and Methods, Chapters 6-10.
Mausner and Bahn, Epidemiology, Appendix 4-1.
Friedman, Primer of Epidemiology, Chapter 5.

I.   AGE- AND CAUSE-SPECIFIC RATES

In the previous exercise you became familiar with the way RATES are defined and how they can be used to describe or discover disease patterns. Before beginning more detailed study of the concept of POPULATION AT RISK, it will be helpful to understand the notion of SPECIFIC RATES. This term denotes a rate that describes the frequency of death, illness, or some other health problem in a particular subset of the population. In a sense, many rates used in epidemiology are specific rates, however, in some situations the word SPECIFIC appears in the title of the rate being presented.

SPECIFIC RATES are expressed in the same form as defined in Exercise 1. They include the name of the disease or problem to be described, the place and population to which the findings refer, the time during which the count of events was made, and a convenient number to indicate the magnitude of the population to which the rate is applied. The specificity of the rate may be used to qualify either the numerator or the denominator of the rate.

A common type of specific rate is the AGE-SPECIFIC RATE. This rate refers to the risk of the disease or health problem in persons of a given age group. You have already had some experience in interpreting age-specific rates, which were presented graphically, e.g., Exercise 1, Figure 1. Hereafter, you will encounter both graphic and tabular presentation of data, as shown in Figures 1a and 1b.

You may see the term CAUSE-SPECIFIC rate in discussions of death or illness in a population. It refers to the death (mortality) or illness (morbidity) rate of particular diseases. This method of presentation may also be used for important characteristics, such as sex-, race-, or occupation-specific death or illness rates. The most commonly seen examples are death rates specific for age and cause simultaneously, as shown in Figure 2.

Figure 1a. Age-specific death rates from all causes per 1000 population, U.S., 1978.*

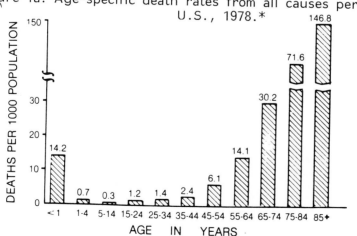

*As in Exercise 1, the bar graph is used for ease of illustrating the age distribution.

Figure 1b. Age-specific death rates from all causes per 1000 population, U.S., 1978.

Age in years	Midyear population by age group	Number of deaths	Age-specific deaths per 1000
< 1	3,196,900	45,300	14.2
1-4	11,628,600	8,140	0.7
5-14	41,066,700	12,320	0.3
15-24	41,333,300	49,600	1.2
25-34	33,722,600	46,200	1.4
35-44	24,343,100	58,180	2.4
45-54	23,186,900	141,440	6.1
55-64	20,673,300	292,320	14.1
65-74	14,935,400	450,750	30.2
75-84	6,914,300	495,130	71.6
85+	2,206,000	323,820	146.8

Source: Dept. of HEW, Vital Statistics Report, Annual Summary for the U.S., 1978.

Figure 2. Death rate per 10,000 population by age and cause in the U.S. in 1968 and 1978.

Causes of Death	Year	All ages	< 1	1-14	15-24	25-34	35-44	45-54	55-64	65-74	75-84	85+
All causes	1978	88.2	141.7	4.3	12.0	13.7	23.9	61.0	141.4	301.8	716.1	1467.9
	1968	96.8	226.6	5.5	12.4	15.7	32.0	75.1	170.4	372.4	829.4	1958.3
Diseases of the heart	1978	33.4	1.85	0.10	0.25	0.73	4.6	19.4	52.0	122.6	319.1	708.8
	1968	37.4	1.23	0.12	0.28	1.19	7.1	25.2	68.7	163.3	382.5	927.8
Cancer	1978	18.2	0.25	0.47	0.64	1.36	4.7	18.1	43.9	80.3	130.3	146.2
	1968	16.0	0.49	0.68	0.82	1.73	6.1	18.3	41.4	74.9	113.4	147.5
Cerebrovascular diseases	1978	7.9	0.28	0.40	0.10	0.26	1.0	2.6	7.2	24.1	89.7	224.7
	1968	10.6	0.53	0.70	0.17	0.49	1.7	4.5	12.2	41.0	131.8	360.6
Accidents	1978	4.9	3.9	2.1	6.8	4.5	4.0	4.0	4.6	6.5	13.2	27.8
	1968	5.7	7.5	2.4	6.9	5.3	4.8	5.4	6.5	9.0	18.9	51.4
All other causes	1978	23.8	135.4	1.2	4.2	6.9	9.6	16.9	33.7	68.3	163.8	360.4
	1968	27.1	216.9	1.6	4.2	7.0	12.3	21.7	41.6	84.2	182.8	471.0

Source: Dept. of HEW, Vital Statistics Reports, Annual Summary for the USA, 1978.

Question 1

a. What do the data show with regard to the importance of these cause of death categories?

b.   What changes have occurred in the pattern of deaths in the US population between 1968 and 1978?

II.   DEFINITION OF THE TERM POPULATION AT RISK*

The term POPULATION AT RISK is usually used for two general purposes:

1.   When describing the rate of death, disease, or health problem FOR A COMMUNITY. By convention, the population to which the risk refers is the average population of the community exposed, for the given period of time. The average population represents an estimate of the population of that community thought to be alive on July 1 of a calendar year. If more than one year is used as the period of observation, the average of the midyear estimates is commonly used to denote the population at risk.

2.   When describing the rate of death, disease, or health problem for a particular group of persons, A SUBGROUP OF THE ENTIRE COMMUNITY. The subgroup should be confined to persons who are KNOWN OR THOUGHT TO BE SUSCEPTIBLE to the disease or health problem during a given period of time. A subgroup may be preferable for study rather than the entire population of that community, if a significant proportion of the community is known to be unexposed or is not at risk of the disease or health problem. In such situations, the population at risk would be defined as the number of persons who were present, susceptible to and free of disease AT THE START OF THE PERIOD rather than the midyear estimate of that population.

Question 2

Suggest a suitable population at risk (one for each of the two above categories) if you wanted to investigate the following in any given year:

a.   deaths due to lung cancer

---

*Note: The population at risk is also referred to as "the denominator" since it is the denominator or "y" term of rates. One frequently hears an epidemiologist ask the questions, "what is the population at risk?" or "what is the denominator?" These phrases are used interchangeably and are of extreme importance from both qualitative and quantitative points of view.

b.   births

c.   the occupancy of hospital beds

Question 3

You have been requested to evaluate the impact of a county family planning program and to make suggestions for possible improvement. The county program's objectives include providing services to certain age groups and economic groups. You have decided to start your evaluation by investigating the birth rate among women less than 19 years of age. (Success would be reflected by a rate close to zero.)

a.   How would you define the population at risk?

b.   What group(s) would you consider appropriate for study (i.e., where would you obtain a suitable population)?

c.   What factors of importance might influence the observed birth rate?

Question 4

What are the major decisions to be made in selecting a population to be used for study?

Question 5

What differences are evident in the data shown in Figures 3a and 3b? What questions are raised by these data?

Figure 3a.   Death rates for stomach cancer, 1966-1967.

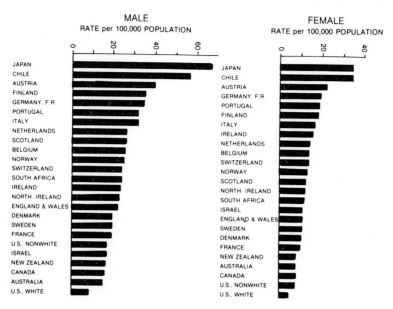

Figure 3b.   Death rates for skin cancer, 1966-1967.

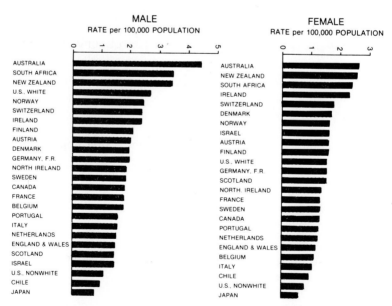

Source: Segi, M. and Kurihara, M. Cancer mortality for selected sites in 24
          countries, No. 6, 1966-1967; Japan Cancer Society, 1972.

Figure 4. Death rates from major cancers for U.S. White and Japanese, 1964-65.

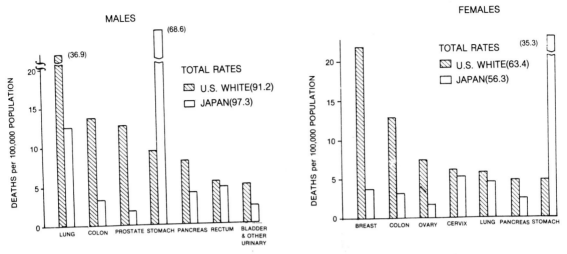

Source: Nakahara, W., et al., Analytic and experimental epidemiology of cancer, University of Tokyo Press, 1973.

Question 6

a. Describe the pattern from Figure 4 of cancer deaths by sex in the two countries.

b. What might explain these differences?

Exercise 2-8

Let us return to some infectious disease examples to examine a way in which the population at risk affects the pattern of disease.

Figure 5.   Measles in Greenland, 1940-1968.

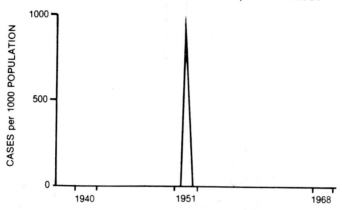

Source: Christensen, P., et al., An epidemic of measles in southern Greenland, 1951, Acta Medica Scand. 144:430, 1952.

Question 7

a.   What might you conclude about the population at risk, in terms of sus-
ceptibility and immunity to measles, before and after 1951?   Review
Exercise 1, Figure 14, and compare the problem of measles in Greenland
(Figure 5) with that of the U.S.

In populations in which the infectious agents are endemic, the data in Figure
6a and 6b were observed.

b.   What do the data suggest about the relationship between the disease
agents and susceptibility to infectious diseases?

Figure 6a. Percent of school children affected by measles in Iowa, 1978.

	Number surveyed	Percent affected		
		Measles[a]	Measles-associated illness[b]	No illness
History of measles	56	0	0	100
Immunized[c]	690	13.3	28.4	58.3
Unimmunized[c]	167	36.5	16.8	46.7

[a]Symptomatic with fever, cough, rash, and conjunctivitis.

[b]Symptomatic with fever, cough, rash, or conjunctivitis (excludes 'a').

[c]Excludes children with a previous history of measles.

Source: Wintermyer, L. and Myers, M.G., Measles in a partially immunized community. Am. J. Pub. Health 69:923, 1979.

Figure 6b. Estimated percent of school children affected by influenza in Iowa, 1978.

	Number surveyed	Percent affected	
		Influenza	No illness
History of influenza	100	21	79
Immunized	100	26	74
Unimmunized	100	32	68

Source: Hypothetical data estimated for Iowa, based upon data from Center for Disease Control Influenza surveillance reports.

c. Suppose you want to calculate the rates of newly occurring cases of measles and influenza for a survey of diseases in your community during the last calendar year. How would immunity to each of these diseases affect your definition of the population at risk for each disease?

d. For what purpose might an epidemiologist use:

(1) The community population rather than the number of susceptibles.

(2) The number of susceptibles rather than the community population.

Question 8

What sources of information could be used to determine who is susceptible to a disease? What problems are associated with these sources?

Epidemiologists strive to identify a population at risk that is biologically "susceptible" to the disease and exposed to the causative agent. In most situations, however, it is not possible to define the denominator to include only those individuals because we do not know enough about the actual exposure or the factors that influence susceptibility. Study of the entire community may therefore be necessary, but it is expensive, time consuming, and wasteful of your limited resources, particularly if many individuals in the community are either not susceptible or not likely to be exposed to the disease agent.

It is very important for epidemiologists to determine the factors affecting the biologic susceptibility of the host with as much precision as possible. The more precisely this can be done, the greater the chance that the disease or health problem can be studied effectively and that it can be prevented or controlled.

III. POPULATIONS USEFUL IN IDENTIFYING EPIDEMIOLOGIC PROBLEMS

The remainder of this exercise will look at several categories of population at risk to familiarize you with some of the population subgroups that help epidemiologists identify community health problems. Sections A-C are convenient for illustrating some of these groups. Space does not permit a complete list of all appropriate subgroups, given the variety of subjects with which epidemiology is concerned.

A.   POPULATIONS WITH EXPOSURE CHARACTERISTICS OF INTEREST

1.   Location

1a.   Census tract of residence

Figure 7. Survival of patients with colon-rectal cancer residing in the highest and lowest income areas of a community.

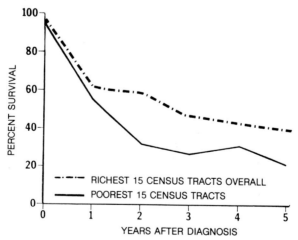

Source: Lynch, H.T., et al.   Cancer of the colon: socioeconomic variables in a community.   Am. J. Epidemiol. 102:119, 1975.

Question 9.

a.   Why are comparisons of census tracts of interest?

b.   Can you indicate a population at risk, other than census tracts, that
     would be a suitable alternative for this study?

1b. State or regional residence

Figure 8. Percentage of white navy recruits ages 17-21 with positive tubercu-
          losis skin tests between 1958 and 1964, by state economic area and
          home of residence.

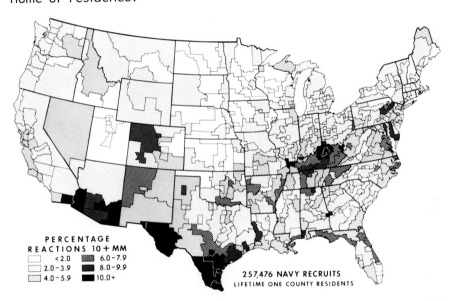

PERCENTAGE
REACTIONS 10+MM
    □ <2.0   ▨ 6.0-7.9
    ▢ 2.0-3.9   ▨ 8.0-9.9
    ▨ 4.0-5.9   ■ 10.0+

257,476 NAVY RECRUITS
LIFETIME ONE COUNTY RESIDENTS

     Source: Lowell, A.M., et al., Tuberculosis, Harvard University Press, 1969.

Question 10

a.   What factors of PLACE might explain this distribution?

b.   Can you suggest an alternative population suitable for studying tubercu-
     losis prevalence?

2. Exposure to a common experience or event

2a. Persons admitted to the same hospital or clinic

Figure 9. Infections acquired in a university hospital, Sept. 1972 - Aug. 1975.

Service	Total No. of admissions	Total No. of infections	Rate per 100 admissions	Rate of infections by site/100 admissions by service					
				Post-operative wounds	Blood	Pulmonary	Urinary tract infection		Other
							Catheterized	Not catheterized	
Newborn Intensive Care Unit	344	82	23.8	0.29	3.78	1.74		5.23	12.79
General Surgery	5,827	609	10.5	4.55	1.03	1.84	1.20	1.25	.58
Neuro-Surgery	3,203	331	10.3	1.53	.56	1.44	2.56	1.84	2.40
Thoracic Cardio-vascular Surgery	3,038	301	10.0	2.96	.53	3.69	1.12	.72	.89
Plastic Surgery	3,084	306	10.0	3.73	.55	.62	1.33	1.39	2.30
Urology	2,807	281	10.0	2.00	.57	.68	3.63	2.57	.57
Orthopedics	4,368	327	7.5	2.08	.21	.73	2.34	1.60	.53
Medicine	13,275	667	5.0	0.03	.67	.96	.64	1.45	1.27
Pediatrics	5,050	216	4.3	0.04	.73	.38	.22	.89	2.02
Neurology	2,676	112	4.2	0.07	.30	.67	1.38	1.08	.67
Gynecology	2,812	99	3.5	1.53	.14	.14	.50	.75	.46
Otolaryngology	3,012	60	2.0	.70	9.10	.50	.06	.20	.40
Obstetrics	4,673	39	0.8	.24	.02		.04	.15	.40
Ophthalmology	1,307	2	0.2					.15	.39
								.15	
TOTAL	55,476	3,432	6.2	1.35	0.52	0.94	1.05	1.19	1.12
% of 3,432 infections				21.9	8.5	15.3	16.9	19.2	18.2

Source: Wenzel, R.P., et al., Hospital acquired infections: infection rates by site, service and common procedures in a university hospital, Am. J. Epidemiol. 104:645, 1976.

Question 11

Hospital or clinic data provide much useful epidemiologic information. However, data from different sources may not be appropriate for comparison.

What factors influence the rate of infection in a hospital and how can they affect the comparison of data from different hospitals?

2b. Persons of similar diagnostic or treatment categories

Figure 10. Adverse reaction rates to drugs received by at least 50 hospital-ized children, Boston Children's Hospital, 1974-1977.

Drug	Use	Reported adverse reactions	Number exposed	Percentage (%)
Vincristine	anticancer agent	31	85	36.5
Phenytoin	anticonvulsant	8	69	11.6
Chlorpromazine	tranquilizer	7	67	10.4
Furosemide	diuretic	8	78	10.3
Phenobarbital	barbiturate	10	102	9.8
Prednisone	cortisone	15	169	8.9
Packed red blood cells	transfusion	14	179	7.8
Theophylline	asthma	12	163	7.4
Ampicillin	antibiotic	28	394	7.1
Penicillin	antibiotic	17	268	6.3
Morphine	pain relief	6	113	5.3
Carbenicillin	antibiotic	4	80	5.0

Source: Mitchell, A.A., et al., Drug utilization and reported adverse reac-tions in [1669] hospitalized children, Am. J. Epidemiol. 110:196, 1979.

Question 12

What are some characteristics of the population at risk that influence the rate of adverse reactions to treatment?

2c. Persons exposed at the same time or place

Among 53 passengers and crew of an airplane whose flight was delayed due to engine trouble, 37 persons (72%) became ill with severe influenza. A young woman (the index case or first person ill) became ill within 15 minutes after boarding the aircraft, causing the flight to be delayed for 4½ hours. During the delay most of the passengers remained on board and mixed freely with each other. Onset of illness began within a few days.

Question 13

Figure 11 shows an unusual occurrence of a disease in a unique population. How would you determine the expected rate of illness in this population to help you to decide if an epidemic had occurred, i.e., does the observed rate ex-ceed the expected rate of illness?

Answer to Question 13 in this space.

Figure 11.   Onset of illness following exposure, Alaska, 1977.

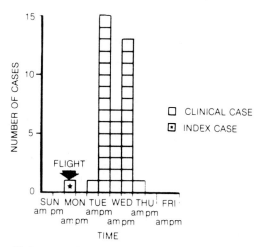

Source: Moser, M.R., et al., An outbreak of influenza aboard a commercial
          airliner, Am. J. Epidemiol. 110:1, 1979.

3.   Vital records

The study of vital events--births and deaths--is an important area of epidemiologic interest because it helps to identify a variety of health problems among
segments of the population.   Standard birth, death, and fetal death certificates used by the U.S. National Center for Health Statistics are shown in
Figures 12a, 12b, and 12c.

Question 14

Examine the data routinely collected on vital registration certificates.   What are
the useful features and the limitations of these certificates?

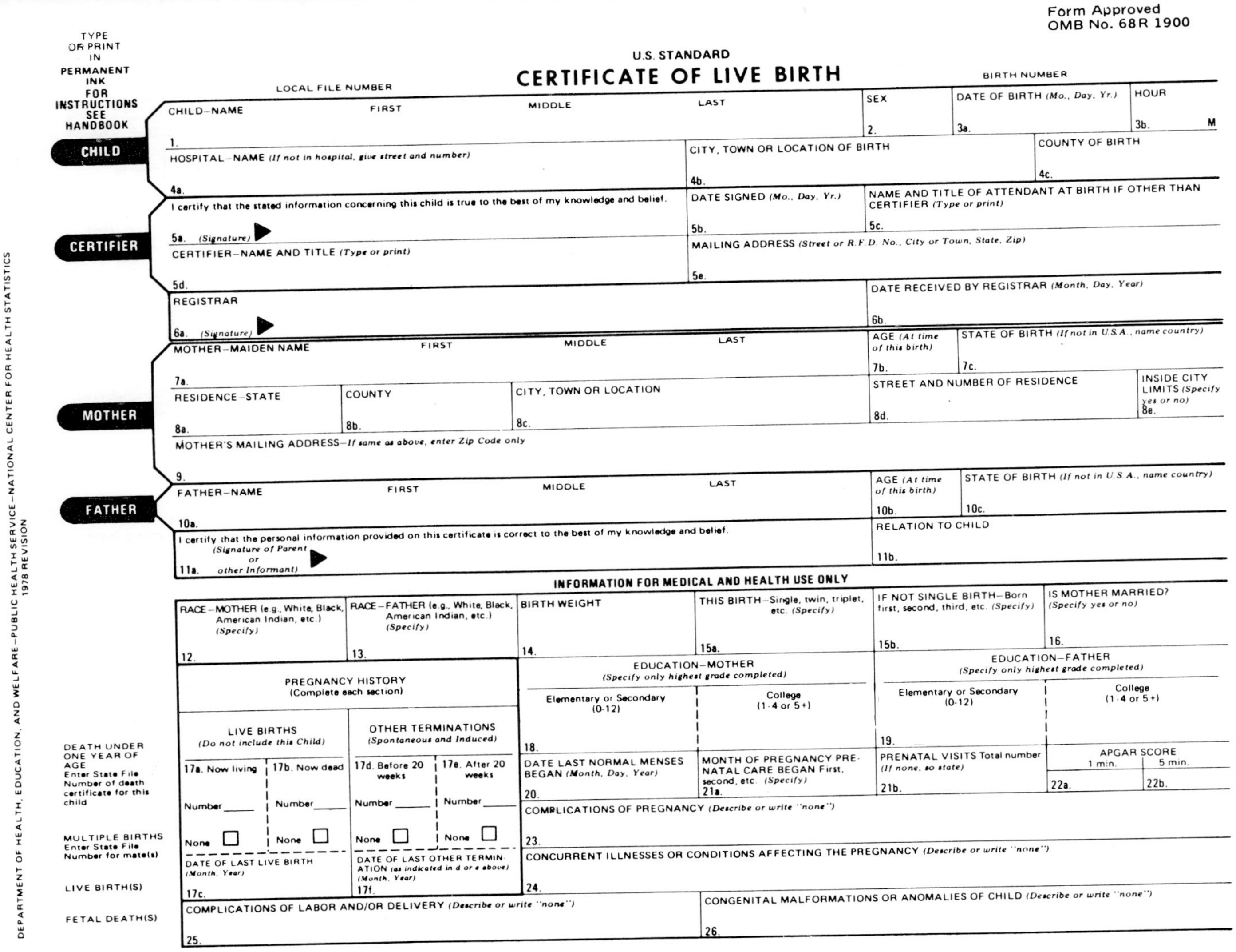

Form Approved
OMB No. 68R 1900

TYPE OR PRINT IN PERMANENT INK
FOR INSTRUCTIONS SEE HANDBOOK

U.S. STANDARD
CERTIFICATE OF LIVE BIRTH

LOCAL FILE NUMBER
BIRTH NUMBER

CHILD

CHILD–NAME FIRST MIDDLE LAST 1.
SEX 2.
DATE OF BIRTH *(Mo., Day, Yr.)* 3a.
HOUR 3b. M
HOSPITAL–NAME *(If not in hospital, give street and number)* 4a.
CITY, TOWN OR LOCATION OF BIRTH 4b.
COUNTY OF BIRTH 4c.

CERTIFIER

I certify that the stated information concerning this child is true to the best of my knowledge and belief.
5a. *(Signature)* ▶
DATE SIGNED *(Mo., Day, Yr.)* 5b.
NAME AND TITLE OF ATTENDANT AT BIRTH IF OTHER THAN CERTIFIER *(Type or print)* 5c.
CERTIFIER–NAME AND TITLE *(Type or print)* 5d.
MAILING ADDRESS *(Street or R.F.D. No., City or Town, State, Zip)* 5e.
REGISTRAR
6a. *(Signature)* ▶
DATE RECEIVED BY REGISTRAR *(Month, Day, Year)* 6b.

MOTHER

MOTHER–MAIDEN NAME FIRST MIDDLE LAST 7a.
AGE *(At time of this birth)* 7b.
STATE OF BIRTH *(If not in U.S.A., name country)* 7c.
RESIDENCE–STATE 8a.
COUNTY 8b.
CITY, TOWN OR LOCATION 8c.
STREET AND NUMBER OF RESIDENCE 8d.
INSIDE CITY LIMITS *(Specify yes or no)* 8e.
MOTHER'S MAILING ADDRESS–*If same as above, enter Zip Code only* 9.

FATHER

FATHER–NAME FIRST MIDDLE LAST 10a.
AGE *(At time of this birth)* 10b.
STATE OF BIRTH *(If not in U.S.A., name country)* 10c.
I certify that the personal information provided on this certificate is correct to the best of my knowledge and belief.
11a. *(Signature of Parent or other Informant)* ▶
RELATION TO CHILD 11b.

INFORMATION FOR MEDICAL AND HEALTH USE ONLY

RACE–MOTHER (e.g., White, Black, American Indian, etc.) *(Specify)* 12.
RACE–FATHER (e.g., White, Black, American Indian, etc.) *(Specify)* 13.
BIRTH WEIGHT 14.
THIS BIRTH–Single, twin, triplet, etc. *(Specify)* 15a.
IF NOT SINGLE BIRTH–Born first, second, third, etc. *(Specify)* 15b.
IS MOTHER MARRIED? *(Specify yes or no)* 16.

PREGNANCY HISTORY (Complete each section)
LIVE BIRTHS *(Do not include this Child)*
17a. Now living Number ___ None ☐
17b. Now dead Number ___ None ☐
DATE OF LAST LIVE BIRTH *(Month, Year)* 17c.
OTHER TERMINATIONS *(Spontaneous and Induced)*
17d. Before 20 weeks Number ___ None ☐
17e. After 20 weeks Number ___ None ☐
DATE OF LAST OTHER TERMINATION *(as indicated in d or e above)* *(Month, Year)* 17f.

EDUCATION–MOTHER *(Specify only highest grade completed)*
Elementary or Secondary (0-12) College (1-4 or 5+) 18.
EDUCATION–FATHER *(Specify only highest grade completed)*
Elementary or Secondary (0-12) College (1-4 or 5+) 19.
DATE LAST NORMAL MENSES BEGAN *(Month, Day, Year)* 20.
MONTH OF PREGNANCY PRENATAL CARE BEGAN First, second, etc. *(Specify)* 21a.
PRENATAL VISITS Total number *(If none, so state)* 21b.
APGAR SCORE 1 min. 22a. 5 min. 22b.
COMPLICATIONS OF PREGNANCY *(Describe or write "none")* 23.
CONCURRENT ILLNESSES OR CONDITIONS AFFECTING THE PREGNANCY *(Describe or write "none")* 24.
COMPLICATIONS OF LABOR AND/OR DELIVERY *(Describe or write "none")* 25.
CONGENITAL MALFORMATIONS OR ANOMALIES OF CHILD *(Describe or write "none")* 26.

DEATH UNDER ONE YEAR OF AGE Enter State File Number of death certificate for this child
MULTIPLE BIRTHS Enter State File Number for mate(s)
LIVE BIRTH(S)
FETAL DEATH(S)

DEPARTMENT OF HEALTH, EDUCATION, AND WELFARE–PUBLIC HEALTH SERVICE–NATIONAL CENTER FOR HEALTH STATISTICS
1978 REVISION

Figure 14. Certificate of live birth

Figure 15. Certificate of death

(PHYSICIAN, MEDICAL EXAMINER OR CORONER)
U.S. STANDARD
CERTIFICATE OF DEATH

Form Approved
OMB No. 68R 1901

LOCAL FILE NUMBER
STATE FILE NUMBER

TYPE OR PRINT IN PERMANENT INK FOR INSTRUCTIONS SEE HANDBOOK

DECEDENT

DECEDENT–NAME FIRST MIDDLE LAST 1. | SEX 2. | DATE OF DEATH (Mo., Day, Yr.) 3.

RACE–(e.g., White, Black, American Indian, etc.) (Specify) 4 | AGE–Last Birthday (Yrs.) 5a. | UNDER 1 YEAR MOS. DAYS 5b. | UNDER 1 DAY HOURS MINS. 5c. | DATE OF BIRTH (Mo., Day, Yr.) 6. | COUNTY OF DEATH 7a.

CITY, TOWN OR LOCATION OF DEATH 7b. | HOSPITAL OR OTHER INSTITUTION–Name (If not in either, give street and number) 7c. | IF HOSP. OR INST. Indicate DOA, OP/Emer. Rm., Inpatient (Specify) 7d.

STATE OF BIRTH (If not in U.S.A., name country) 8. | CITIZEN OF WHAT COUNTRY 9. | MARRIED, NEVER MARRIED, WIDOWED, DIVORCED (Specify) 10. | SURVIVING SPOUSE (If wife, give maiden name) 11. | WAS DECEDENT EVER IN U.S. ARMED FORCES? (Specify Yes or No) 12.

SOCIAL SECURITY NUMBER 13. | USUAL OCCUPATION (Give kind of work done during most of working life, even if retired) 14a. | KIND OF BUSINESS OR INDUSTRY 14b.

IF DEATH OCCURRED IN INSTITUTION, SEE HANDBOOK REGARDING COMPLETION OF RESIDENCE ITEMS

RESIDENCE–STATE 15a. | COUNTY 15b. | CITY, TOWN OR LOCATION 15c. | STREET AND NUMBER 15d. | INSIDE CITY LIMITS (Specify Yes or No) 15e.

PARENTS

FATHER–NAME FIRST MIDDLE LAST 16. | MOTHER–MAIDEN NAME FIRST MIDDLE LAST 17.

INFORMANT–NAME (Type or Print) 18a. | MAILING ADDRESS STREET OR R.F.D. NO. CITY OR TOWN STATE ZIP 18b.

DISPOSITION

BURIAL, CREMATION, REMOVAL, OTHER (Specify) 19a. | CEMETERY OR CREMATORY–NAME 19b. | LOCATION CITY OR TOWN STATE 19c.

FUNERAL SERVICE LICENSEE Or Person Acting As Such (Signature) 20a. ▶ | NAME OF FACILITY 20b. | ADDRESS OF FACILITY 20c.

CERTIFIER

To be Completed by CERTIFYING PHYSICIAN Only

21a. To the best of my knowledge, death occurred at the time, date and place and due to the cause(s) stated.
(Signature and Title) ▶

DATE SIGNED (Mo., Day, Yr.) 21b. | HOUR OF DEATH 21c. M

NAME OF ATTENDING PHYSICIAN IF OTHER THAN CERTIFIER (Type or Print) 21d.

To be Completed by MEDICAL EXAMINER or CORONER Only

22a. On the basis of examination and/or investigation, in my opinion death occurred at the time, date and place and due to the cause(s) stated.
(Signature and Title) ▶

DATE SIGNED (Mo., Day, Yr.) 22b. | HOUR OF DEATH 22c. M

PRONOUNCED DEAD (Mo., Day, Yr.) 22d. ON | PRONOUNCED DEAD (Hour) 22e. AT M

NAME AND ADDRESS OF CERTIFIER (PHYSICIAN, MEDICAL EXAMINER OR CORONER) (Type or Print) 23.

REGISTRAR 24a. (Signature) ▶ | DATE RECEIVED BY REGISTRAR (Mo., Day, Yr.) 24b.

CAUSE OF DEATH

CONDITIONS IF ANY WHICH GAVE RISE TO IMMEDIATE CAUSE STATING THE UNDERLYING CAUSE LAST

25. IMMEDIATE CAUSE [ENTER ONLY ONE CAUSE PER LINE FOR (a), (b), AND (c).]

PART I
(a) | Interval between onset and death
DUE TO, OR AS A CONSEQUENCE OF:
(b) | Interval between onset and death
DUE TO, OR AS A CONSEQUENCE OF:
(c) | Interval between onset and death

PART II OTHER SIGNIFICANT CONDITIONS–Conditions contributing to death but not related to cause given in PART I (a) | AUTOPSY (Specify Yes or No) 26. | WAS CASE REFERRED TO MEDICAL EXAMINER OR CORONER (Specify Yes or No) 27.

ACC., SUICIDE, HOM., UNDET., OR PENDING INVEST. (Specify) 28a. | DATE OF INJURY (Mo., Day, Yr.) 28b. | HOUR OF INJURY 28c. M | DESCRIBE HOW INJURY OCCURRED 28d.

INJURY AT WORK (Specify Yes or No) | PLACE OF INJURY–At home, farm, street, factory, office building, etc. (Specify) | LOCATION STREET OR R.F.D. No. CITY OR TOWN STATE

DEPARTMENT OF HEALTH, EDUCATION, AND WELFARE–PUBLIC HEALTH SERVICE–NATIONAL CENTER FOR HEALTH STATISTICS
1978 REVISION

Figure 16. Certificate of fetal death

U. S. STANDARD

REPORT OF FETAL DEATH

STATE FILE NUMBER

TYPE OR PRINT IN PERMANENT INK
SEE HANDBOOK FOR INSTRUCTIONS

1a. HOSPITAL–NAME *(If not in hospital, give street and number)*
1b. CITY, TOWN OR LOCATION OF DELIVERY
1c. COUNTY OF DELIVERY
2a. DATE OF DELIVERY *(Month, Day, Year)*
2b. HOUR OF DELIVERY M
3. SEX OF FETUS
4. WEIGHT OF FETUS

MOTHER

5a. MOTHER–MAIDEN NAME FIRST MIDDLE LAST
5b. AGE *(At time of this delivery)*
6a. RESIDENCE–STATE
6b. COUNTY
6c. CITY, TOWN OR LOCATION
6d. STREET AND NUMBER
6e. INSIDE CITY LIMITS *(Specify yes or no)*
7. RACE–(e.g., White, Black, American Indian, etc.) *(Specify)*
8. EDUCATION *(Specify only highest grade completed)* (Elementary or Secondary (0-12)) College (1-4 or 5+)
9. DATE LAST NORMAL MENSES BEGAN *(Month, Day, Year)*
10. IS MOTHER MARRIED? *(Specify yes or no)*

PREGNANCY HISTORY *(Complete each section)*

LIVE BIRTHS
11a. Now living Number____ None ☐
11b. Now dead Number____ None ☐
11c. DATE OF LAST LIVE BIRTH *(Month, Year)*

OTHER TERMINATIONS *(Spontaneous and Induced)*
11d. Before 20 weeks Number____ None ☐
11e. After 20 weeks Number____ *(Do not include this fetus)* None ☐
11f. DATE OF LAST OTHER TERMINATION *(as indicated in d or e above)* *(Month, Year)*

12a. MONTH OF PREGNANCY PRENATAL CARE BEGAN First, second, etc. *(Specify)*
12b. PRENATAL VISITS–Total number *(If none, so state)*
13a. THIS BIRTH–Single, twin, triplet, etc. *(Specify)*
13b. IF NOT SINGLE BIRTH–Born first, second, third, etc. *(Specify)*

FATHER

14a. FATHER–NAME FIRST MIDDLE LAST
14b. AGE *(At time of this delivery)*
14c. RACE–(e.g., White, Black, American Indian, etc.) *(Specify)*
14d. EDUCATION *(Specify only highest grade completed)* Elementary or Secondary (0-12) College (1-4 or 5+)

CAUSE OF FETAL DEATH

15. PART I
[ENTER ONLY ONE CAUSE PER LINE FOR (a), (b), AND (c).]

Fetal or maternal condition directly causing fetal death. IMMEDIATE CAUSE
(a) ____ Specify Fetal or Maternal

Fetal and/or maternal conditions, if any giving rise to the immediate cause (a), stating the underlying cause last.
DUE TO, OR AS A CONSEQUENCE OF:
(b) ____ Specify Fetal or Maternal
DUE TO, OR AS A CONSEQUENCE OF:
(c) ____ Specify Fetal or Maternal

PART II OTHER SIGNIFICANT CONDITIONS OF FETUS OR MOTHER: Conditions contributing to fetal death but not related to cause given in (a)
16. FETUS DIED BEFORE LABOR, DURING LABOR OR DELIVERY, UNKNOWN *(Specify)*
17. PHYSICIAN'S ESTIMATE OF GESTATION Weeks
18. AUTOPSY *(Specify yes or no)*

MULTIPLE BIRTHS
Enter State File Number for mate(s)
LIVE BIRTH(S)
FETAL DEATH(S)

19. COMPLICATIONS OF PREGNANCY *(Describe or write "none")*
20. COMPLICATIONS OF LABOR AND/OR DELIVERY *(Describe or write "none")*
21. CONCURRENT ILLNESSES OR CONDITIONS AFFECTING THE PREGNANCY *(Describe or write "none")*
22. CONGENITAL MALFORMATIONS OR ANOMALIES OF FETUS *(Describe or write "none")*
23. NAME OF PHYSICIAN OR ATTENDANT *(Type or print)*
24. NAME OF PERSON COMPLETING REPORT *(Type or print)* TITLE

DEPARTMENT OF HEALTH, EDUCATION, AND WELFARE–PUBLIC HEALTH SERVICE–NATIONAL CENTER FOR HEALTH STATISTICS
1978 REVISION

HRA-163
Rev. 1/78

The next few problems illustrate some uses of birth and death records.

3a. Vital records--births

The data in Figure 13 were obtained in a study of selected variables from all birth certificates reported in the U.S. in 1974.

Figure 13. Number of births and percent low birthweight (< 2501 g or 5½ lbs) for selected variables by race for single live births, U.S., 1974.

Variable	Number of births				Percent less than 2501 grams			
	Total	White	Black	Other	Total	White	Black	Other
TOTAL	3,101,117	2,529,411	495,950	75,756	6.5	5.4	12.0	6.5
Maternal Age (years)								
Less than 15	12,436	5,010	7,241	185	15.3	12.2	17.5	9.2
15-17	231,691	150,777	76,987	3,927	10.5	8.5	14.5	8.3
18-19	356,461	264,655	85,009	6,797	8.4	6.9	13.3	8.0
20-29	1,992,622	1,683,234	262,392	46,996	5.7	4.9	10.9	6.1
30-39	478,952	402,831	59,179	16,942	6.1	5.5	10.9	6.5
40 and over	28,955	22,904	5,142	909	8.5	7.6	12.1	10.0
Prenatal care[1]								
First trimester	1,852,701	1,592,762	217,871	42,068	5.7	4.9	11.0	6.2
Second trimester	557,092	400,029	140,049	17,014	7.7	6.2	12.1	6.8
Third trimester	123,935	84,397	34,324	5,214	7.8	6.4	11.5	5.7
No prenatal care	35,871	22,070	12,412	1,389	18.9	15.3	25.7	14.5
Maternal education (years)[1]								
0-11	643,257	453,956	172,894	16,407	9.4	7.8	13.7	7.3
12	994,045	829,566	147,812	16,667	5.9	5.0	11.0	6.5
13-15	325,635	282,314	36,187	7,134	5.0	4.3	10.1	5.9
16 and over	239,482	214,412	15,430	9,640	4.2	3.8	8.7	6.0
Reproductive history[2]								
No previous losses	1,311,558	1,083,255	195,368	32,935	5.4	4.5	10.4	5.5
One or more previous losses	405,902	324,500	70,707	10,695	9.0	7.6	15.2	8.7
No previous pregnancy	1,146,894	940,840	177,671	28,383	6.9	5.9	12.5	7.0
Interpregnancy interval[1]								
Less than 6 months	116,514	92,979	19,341	4,194	7.8	6.4	14.5	8.1
6-11 months	133,685	108,287	20,832	4,566	6.3	5.2	12.1	6.7
12-23 months	263,377	223,994	32,102	7,281	5.1	4.3	10.7	5.7
24 months and over	605,387	502,851	88,961	13,575	5.2	4.4	9.7	4.7
No previous pregnancy	964,762	793,079	145,003	26,680	6.8	5.8	12.5	6.9

[1]This item not reported or not stated on birth certificates in a number of states.   [2]Excludes those with history unstated.

Source: Eisner, V., et al. The risk of low birthweight, Am. J. Pub. Health 69:887, 1979.

Question 15

If you wished to study possible determinants of low birthweight, indicate a subject and the population or data source you would select.

3b.   Vital records--deaths

In a study of death certificates for Nebraska, 1957-1974, a number of cases of leukemia were observed among farmers.

Figure 14.   Distribution of occupations of cases among Nebraska decedents, 1957-1974.

Occupational group	Cases	
	No.	%
Teachers	9	0.8
Engineers, scientists	25	2.3
Farmers	433	39.9
Clerks and salespersons	84	7.7
Carpenters, woodworkers	31	2.9
Printers	3	0.3
Machinists, mechanics	33	3.0
Laborers	49	4.5
No occupation listed	65	6.0
Other	352	32.5
TOTAL	1084	100.0

Question 16

a.   From Figure 14 would you be correct to conclude that farmers are at increased risk of death from leukemia?

b.   Having identified farmers (PERSON) as a group in which leukemia occurs, the investigators began to look at other factors related to PLACE and ENVIRONMENT.   They found the data shown in Figures 15a and 15b. Based on these data, what conclusions can be drawn about the risk of death from leukemia among Nebraska farmers?

Figure 15a. Geographic distribution of Nebraska counties having high levels of agricultural activities (shown as shaded areas).

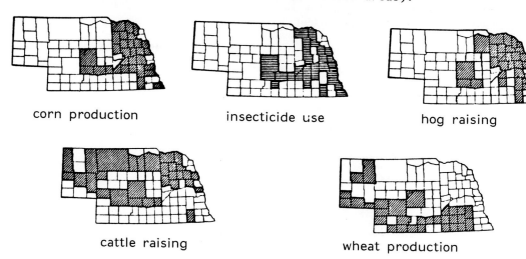

corn production   insecticide use   hog raising

cattle raising   wheat production

Figure 15b. Observed to expected ratio of leukemia deaths by type of agricultural activity, Nebraska 1957-1974.

Agricultural activity	Observed to expected ratio of leukemia deaths
corn production	1.85
insecticide use	1.95
hog raising	2.04
cattle raising	1.72
wheat production	1.06

Source: Blair, A., Thomas, T.L. Leukemia among Nebraska farmers: a death certificate study. Am. J. Epidemiol. 110:264, 1979.

4.   Nonvital records

Potential health problems and their possible determinants may be studied from data sources other than vital records. All departments of health collect information on a variety of legally reportable communicable diseases. The data in Figure 16 were reported from Minnesota, for the three varieties of viral hepatitis: type A, type B, and type non-A non-B. Detection of virus particles is one of the criteria used to establish the diagnosis of hepatitis.

Question 17

Select 2 or 3 categories of potential sources of hepatitis exposure and suggest where or how you might obtain data to study hepatitis in that population.

Figure 16.   Percentages of patients who were positive for hepatitis B infection by reported history of potential exposure.

Patient history of potential hepatitis exposure during previous 6 months*†	Virus particles detected
Contact with hepatitis patient‡	31.9
Consumption of shellfish	2.8
Drug abuse	17.9
Receipt of transfusion	2.7
Dental visit§	29.6
Hemodialysis	3.5
Contact with hemodialysis patientψ	14.3
Surgery	6.7
Contact with surgery patient	14.3
Ear piercing	0.9
Tattooing	0.4
Blood or blood product donation	4.0
Razor sharing with another person	13.0
Foreign travel	4.8

*Exposure categories are not mutually exclusive (i.e., some patients may have more than 1 kind of exposure.

†No patient reported having had acupuncture, electrolysis, or a hair transplant in the 6 months before onset.

‡21.9% of all contacts were household contacts.

§70.7% of all dental visits were for prophylaxis only.

ψ54.1% of hemodialysis patient contacts were work-related.

Source: Levy, B.S., Mature, J., Washburn, J.W. Intensive hepatitis surveillance: methods and results. Am. J. Epidemiol. 105:127, 1977.

5.   Occupation

A relationship exists between occupational exposure and a variety of diseases. Figures 17a, 17b, and 18a-18d illustrate an acute infectious disease hepatitis B reported among certain workers.

Figure 17a. Percentage of hepatitis B antibody and virus particles in prostitutes, age-matched female blood donors, and nuns.

Population	Total no. of sera	Number positive for virus particle	Positive for antibody No.	%
Female prostitutes				
In a brothel	67	0	16	24
Living independently	191	6	64	34
Total	258	6	80	31
Female blood donors	258	0	27	10
Nuns				
Living in a convent	48	1	5	10
Working as teachers	94	0	14	15
Total	142	1	19	13

Figure 17b. Age distribution of hepatitis B antibody in prostitutes and female blood donors.

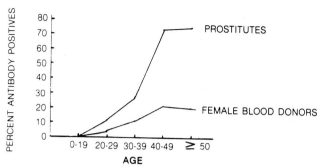

Source: Frösner, G.C. et al., Prevalence of Hepatitis B antibody in prostitutes, Am. J. Epidemiol., 102:241, 1975.

Question 18

Comment on the assertion that prostitutes have an unusually high risk of developing hepatitis B and that the infection may be sexually transmitted.

Figure 18a. Percentage of persons positive for hepatitis B virus particles or antibody among hospital personnel for selected characteristics.

Characteristics	No. tested	No. positive	Percent
Age			
19-29	139	10	7.2
30-39	83	11	13.2
40-49	129	22	17.0
≥50	162	31	19.1
Duration of employment (years)			
< 3	189	20	10.6
3-5	180	19	10.6
> 5	144	35	24.3
Socioeconomic level			
1-2 (highest)	167	20	12.0
3-4	227	29	12.8
5 (lowest	119	25	21.0
All individuals	513	74	14.4

Question 19

The above data may be examined by categorizing the personnel differently as shown in Figures 18b-18d. Comment on the relationship between employment in a hospital and the risk of infection based on the data from Figures 18a-18d.

Figure 18b

Job category	No. tested	Percent positive
Technician	63	22
Practical nurse	41	22
Physician	52	12
Registered nurse	77	12
Nursing aide	60	20
Food services	28	21
Clerical	84	8
Housekeeping	56	13
Other	52	8

Figure 18c

Job exposures	No. tested	Percent positive
Patient contact		
None	201	13.9
Occasional	75	13.3
Frequent	237	15.2
Contact with blood or blood products		
None	211	11.4
Occasional	127	13.4
Frequent	175	18.9

Figure 18d

Job location	No. tested	Percent positive
Operating room	21	29
Laboratories	47	21
Wards		
Ob-Gyn	41	20
Medicine	46	20
Pediatrics	18	17
Surgery	51	12
Kitchen	28	21
Administration	78	9
Radiology	14	7
Emergency room	20	5
Pharmacy	11	0
Other	86	13

Source: Pattison, C.P, et al. Epidemiology of Hepatitis B in hospital personnel, Am. J. Epidemiol. 101:59, 1975.

Figures 19-21 illustrate noninfectious diseases among working populations. In the first example, a study was made to determine the risk of cancer among physicians who became specialists in the three decades of the 1920s, 1930s, and 1940s. Since the physicians in each specialty were at risk of developing the disease for differing lengths of time, a modification in the denominator of the rate defining the population at risk is necessary. Rather than persons at risk, PERSON-YEARS is used. A person-year represents 1 year of risk per person. Thus if a physician became a specialist in 1920 and survived until his death in 1950 he would contribute 30 person-years to the denominator of the

cancer rate. Rates using person-years are advantageous because their denominators reflect the group's period of exposure more appropriately. The subject
of person-years will be discussed further in Exercise 3.

Figure 19.   Cancer deaths by age at death and year of medical specialty,
             1920-1949. Radiologist (RSNA), General Practice (ACP), Eye (E),
             and Ear-Nose-Throat (ENT) Specialties.

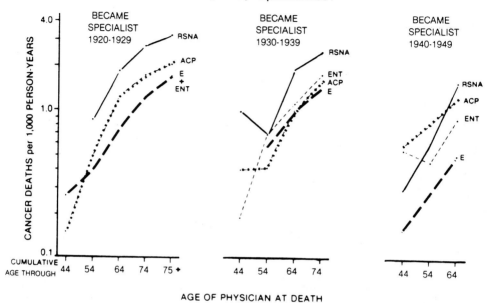

AGE OF PHYSICIAN AT DEATH

Figure 20.   Deaths per 1000 person-years by cause and year of medical spe-
             cialty. Radiologists, General Practice, Eye, and Ear-Nose-Throat
             specialties.

Cause of death	Began specialty in years	Cancer deaths per 1000 person-years			
		Radiologist	General practice	Eye	Ear-nose-throat
Skin cancer	1920-29	0.31	0.01	0.03	0.03
	1930-39	0.12	0.02	0.04	0
	1940-49	0.05	0	0.06	0
Leukemia	1920-29	0.44	0.17	0.05	0.05
	1930-39	0.44	0.12	0.13	0.09
	1940-49	0.05	0.06	0	0.08

Source: Matanoski, G.M., et al. The current mortality rates of radiolo-
          gists and other physician specialists: deaths from all causes
          and from cancer, Am. J. Epidemiol. 101:188, 1975.

Radiologists are not the only occupational group at excess risk of developing
cancer, as shown in Figure 21.

Figure 21.   Selected causes of death by dose, among women employed in the U.S. radium dial-painting industry between 1915-1929, who were alive in 1954.

use	<50 µCi (N = 302)			≥50 µCi (N = 58)		
	Observed no.	Expected no.	Observed/ expected	Observed no.	Expected no.	Observed/ expected
causes	46	53.29	0.86	23	12.04	1.91
lignant cancers	16	13.33	1.20	12	3.02	3.97
lignant cancers by site:						
Digestive organs	7	4.13	1.69	0	0.95	-
Large intestine	5	1.72	2.90	0	0.39	-
Lung	0	0.84	-	1	0.18	5.61
Breast	3	2.79	1.07	1	0.62	1.62
Brain and central nervous system	1	0.29	3.47	0	0.06	-
Bone	0	0.06	-	3	0.01	225.41
Other and unspecified	1	0.85	1.18	5	0.18	22.73
Leukemia	0	0.44	-	1	0.10	9.95
ood and blood-forming organs	1	0.17	5.72	0	0.04	-
ascular lesions of CNS	3	5.75	0.52	1	1.31	0.76
seases of circulatory system	18	22.11	0.81	7	5.00	1.40
rteriosclerotic heart disease	13	15.59	0.83	6	3.54	1.70
xternal causes	1	1.94	0.52	2	0.42	4.75
mber of person-years	3542			790		
ath rate/1000 person-years	13.0			29.1		

Source: Polednak, A.P. Stehney, A.F. and Rowland, R.E.   Mortality among women first employed before 1930 in the U.S. radium dial-painting industry, Am. J. Epidemiol. 107:179, 1978.

Question 20

a.   If you were to study health hazards due to radiation exposure, how would you determine the "expected" number of deaths?

b.   Can you suggest any additional populations that are at excess risk of radiation-induced cancer?

6.   Environment

Recent years have witnessed a tremendous increase in interest and awareness of the ways in which the environment can affect human health.   Among the earliest documented incidents suggesting a relationship between air pollution and health were the 1930 fog episode in the Meuse Valley of Europe, which caused 64 deaths, and the 1948 smog episode in Donora, Pennsylvania, which caused 20 deaths.   In December 1952, London, England, experienced an extremely heavy fog lasting for four days, which was accompanied by an increase in air pollution.   The effects on the community's health were surprising.

Figure 22a. Deaths registered in Greater London from week ended November 15, 1952, to Jan. 10, 1953, compared to the annual average for the corresponding period, 1947-1951, and atmospheric pollution in December, 1952.

Figure 22b. Deaths from selected causes, London, November 1952 to January 1953.

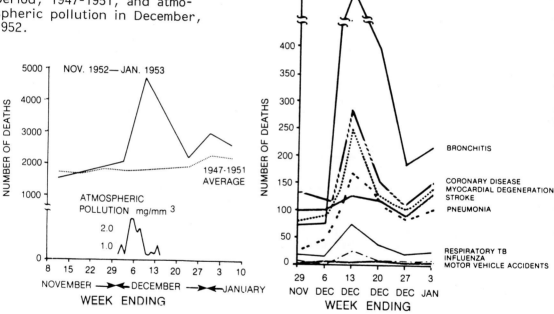

Source: Logan, W.P.D., Mortality in the London fog incident, 1952, The Lancet 244:336, 1953.

Question 21

What was learned from this incident? What was the effect of this event on the population? What subgroups of the population may have been at increased risk of death?

B.   POPULATION GROUPS WITH BIOLOGIC CHARACTERISTICS OF INTEREST

1.   Ethnic groups

Figure 23a. Percentage of diabetes according to age and degree of Indian inheritance at Fort Berthold.

Age (years)	Full-inheritance* Indians (8/8)		Indian inheritance less than 8/8, more than 4/8		Indian inheritance 4/8 or less		Non-Indians	
	No.	% diabetic	No.	% diabetic	No.	% diabetic	No.	% diabetic
0-9	346	0.0	193	1.0	293	0.0	148	0.0
10-19	365	0.0	353	0.8	301	0.3	74	0.0
20-29	321	0.9	284	0.0	163	1.2	97	1.0
30-39	213	4.7	112	4.5	82	4.9	42	0.0
40-49	160	11.9	75	10.7	55	0.0	32	0.0
50-59	140	29.3	33	15.2	26	7.7	21	0.0
60-69	72	40.3	19	36.8	25	8.0	21	14.3
70-79	47	46.8	8	62.5	9	0.0	7	14.3
and over	18	22.2	2	0.0	4	25.0	0	0.0
TOTAL	1682	7.6	1079	3.2	958	1.3	442	1.6

andan tribe: 134 persons;   Arickara tribe: 323 persons;   Hidatsa tribe: 468;   mixed 3 tribes: 570 per-
ns;   other Indian: 187;   total: 1682 persons.

Source: Brosseau, J.D., et al.   Diabetes among the three affili-
ated tribes: Correlation with degree of Indian inheritance.   Am. J. Pub. Health 69:12:1277, 1979.

Figure 23b. Diabetes rate per 1000 person-years in males and females, Pima Indians and Rochester, Minnesota Whites, 1970.

	Pima	Rochester	Ratio:Pima/ Rochester
Males	23.6	1.58	14.9
Females	29.0	1.13	25.7
Both	26.5	1.34	19.8

Source: Knowler W.C., et al.   Diabetes incidence and prevalence in Pima
Indians: a 19 fold greater incidence than in Rochester, Minnesota.
Am. J. Epi. 108:6:497, 1978.

Question 22

What do these data suggest regarding the risk of diabetes in these populations?

Exercise 2-28

2.   Families

Figure 24a. Observed/expected risk of breast cancer in a 1976 sample of U.S. nurses having a positive family history of breast cancer.

Family member with breast cancer	Number with cancer	observed/ expected risk
Mother	106	1.8
Sister	65	2.5
Both mother and sister	10	5.6

Figure 24b. Age-specific observed/expected risk of breast cancer in a 1976 sample of U.S. nurses having a positive family history of breast cancer.

Family member with breast cancer	Nurses age in 1976	No. with Cancer	Risk observed/ expected
Mother	30-39	9	3.2
	40-44	12	1.6
	45-49	25	1.5
	50-54	60	1.9
Sister	30-39	4	8.4
	40-44	6	3.1
	45-49	14	2.5
	50-54	41	2.2

Source: Bain, C. et al.,   Family history of breast cancer as a risk indicator for the disease, Am. J. Epidemiol. 111:301, 1980.

Question 23

a.   What can be learned from the study of noninfectious diseases in families?

b.   Assuming the above findings can be duplicated in the general population, of what importance would they be to someone responsible for a health program to discover breast cancer in women?

Studies of acute infectious diseases in families are frequently performed by epidemiologists. Two terms that are useful in discussions of infectious diseases are the <u>attack</u> <u>rate</u> and <u>secondary</u> <u>attack</u> <u>rate</u>. The term <u>attack</u> <u>rate</u> refers to the proportion of ill individuals among the population at risk. The term <u>secondary</u> <u>attack</u> <u>rate</u> refers to the percentage of cases, within the <u>incu</u>-<u>bation</u> <u>period</u> of the disease, among household or family contacts of the first person (<u>primary</u> or <u>index</u> <u>case</u>) in that household who becomes ill.

Figure 25. Household secondary attack rates of mumps by age. Selected elementary schools, Baltimore, 1958-61.

Age at time of exposure (years)	Total	Suscep- tible*	Primary and coprimary[†]	Secondary and tertiary	Secondary attack rate among susceptibles	
					Number	Percent
Under 2	54	54	0	12	12/54	22
2-4	168	168	69	67	67/99	68
5-9	253	236‡	154	44	44/82	54
10-19	113	55	21	6	6/34	18
Total under 20	588	513	244[†]	129[§]	129/269	48
Adults (1959-1960)	327	99‡	2	18	18/97	19

*Persons with no previous history of mumps.

[†]Includes 16 coprimary cases.

‡Five children age 5-9 and one adult who had second attacks are included as susceptibles.

[§]Nine cases were tertiary.

Source: Meyer, M.B. An epidemiologic study of mumps; its spread in schools and families, Am. J. Hygiene 75:259, 1962.

Question 24

What can be learned from the study of infectious diseases in families?

3.   Twin Studies

In a study of identical twins in Sweden, where one twin was a smoker and the other a nonsmoker, the deaths were observed as shown in Figures 26a and 26b.

Question 25

a.   Describe the findings shown in Figures 26a and 26b. Suggest some reasons why an association between smoking and death is not demonstrated.

b.   Of what value are findings derived from twin studies?

c.   What do these data suggest about the role played by genetic and environ-
      mental factors?

Figure 26a.   Deaths among identical (monozygous) twins identified from the
              Swedish national twin registry, by smoking status and age.

Age in years	No. of pairs	Deaths among males		No. of pairs	Deaths among females	
		Smokers	Non-smokers		Smokers	Non-smokers
45-59	115	6	2	213	10	8
60-69	46	4	4	59	3	5
Total	161	10*	6*	272	13	13

*Statistical tests indicated that the difference in the number of male deaths
is not large enough to be "statistically significant." Therefore, one should
not infer that the observed difference is necessarily due to the biologic or
physiologic effects of the factors under study.

A second analysis that included some additional data was performed.

Figure 26b.   Deaths among identical (monozygous) twins, by smoking status
              and age.

Age in years	No. of pairs	Deaths among males		No. of pairs	Deaths among females	
		Non/light smokers	Moderate/ heavy smokers		Non/light smokers	Moderate/ heavy smokers
45-59	177	6	11	262	10	9
60-69	69	12	7	64	3	5
Total	246	18	18	226	13	14

Source: Friberg, L., Mortality in twins in relation to smoking habits
          and alcohol problems, Arch. Environ. Health, 27:294, 1973.

C.   POPULATIONS INVOLVED IN NATURAL EXPERIMENTS

Political actions, acts of war, natural phenomena relating to geographic location, catastrophes, etc., may create populations at risk or population subgroups that offer an epidemiologist interesting opportunities for studying possible causes of disease or examining the effects on human health, of prior
events connected with "natural" experiments.

1. Migrants

The scientific literature often reveals disagreement about the relative importance of genetic and environmental factors in causing disease.

Coronary heart disease (CHD), a disease of the coronary arteries that may lead to a "heart attack" (myocardial infarction), was studied among the offspring of Japanese migrants and native Japanese and revealed the following:

Figure 27. Age- and cause-specific mortality among Japanese men living in Japan, Hawaii, and San Francisco, California.

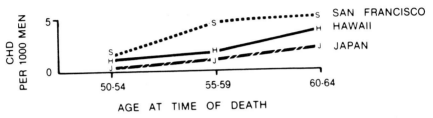

Source: Worth, R.M., Epidemiologic studies of coronary heart disease and stroke in Japanese men living in Japan, Hawaii, and California: Mortality, Am. J. Epidemiol. 102:481, 1975.

Question 26

a. In what ways can studies such as this be of value in discovering the causes of a disease?

b. Suggest some reasons that might contribute to the higher CHD rate of those not living in Japan.

2. Special Religious or Social Groups.

Although not necessarily biologically distinct, various religious and cultural groups may, by virtue of their habits, beliefs, and customs, provide unique opportunities to study disease processes.

For example, the state of Utah is comprised of a large number of Mormons (Church of Jesus Christ of Latter-Day Saints). Approximately 72% of the state population is Mormon. Church doctrine prohibits its members from using tobacco (all forms), alcohol, coffee, and tea, although not all members conform to these requirements. In the United States, Utah has the lowest per capita cigarette and alcohol consumption, and very low death rates from lung cancer and heart disease.

The association between heart disease and factors such as cigarette smoking, high blood pressure, high blood cholesterol, and family history of heart disease has been shown in many studies.

Figure 28.   Cardiovascular death rates by age per 10,000 population for Mormons and non-Mormons, Utah, 1969-1971.

Heart disease type	Sex	Age < 65 years			Age > 65 years		
		Mormon	Non-Mormon	Ratio M/nM	Mormon	Non-Mormon	Ratio M/nM
Rheumatic	Male	14.9	14.5	1.03	59.8	65.4	0.91
	Female	13.6	22.1	0.62	59.3	91.0	0.65
Hypertensive	Males	1.4	3.9	0.36	31.9	65.9	0.48
	Females	1.2	0.0	∞	43.9	71.4	0.61
Acute Ischemic	Males	167.0	206.6	0.81	1253.6	1722.0	0.73
	Females	32.8	47.6	0.69	571.3	976.2	0.59
Chronic Ischemic	Males	47.6	65.6	0.73	773.8	1602.2	0.48
	Females	19.9	25.5	0.78	821.8	1266.0	0.65

Source: Lyon, J.L., et al., Cardiovascular mortality in Mormons and non-Mormons in Utah, 1969-1971. Am. J. Epidemiol. 108:357, 1978.

Question 27

How is the comparison of heart disease in Mormons and non-Mormons useful or not useful in studying heart disease and its possible causes?

3.   The Swine influenza vaccine program

During the mid-1970s, reports of human cases associated with a variety of influenza virus (type A swine influenza) together with the knowledge that this serotype of the virus was responsible for one or more earlier worldwide epidemics (pandemics) of a very severe form of influenza, led the U.S. Dept. of Health, Education and Welfare to recommend that a national vaccination program be started to immunize the population. Hoping to prevent a potential epidemic from occurring, the U.S. Congress voted an emergency fund of $135 million for the campaign. Shortly after the start of the vaccination program, physicians and health agencies began reporting cases of the GUILLAIN-BARRE syndrome as shown below.

The Guillain-Barre syndrome is an acute, progressive disease characterized by numbness, tingling, tenderness, weakness, and sensory loss due to involvement of the nerves of the legs and arms. The face and central nervous system may also be affected occasionally. Paralysis of the nerves controlling respiration and other vital functions may result in death. Prior to the vaccination campaign it had been known that some cases of the disease occurred concurrent with or shortly after viral infections.

Figure 29. Guillain-Barre syndrome attack rates for population over 17 years of age, by week of onset after A/New Jersey influenza vaccination, U.S., Oct. 3, 1976 - Jan. 29, 1977.

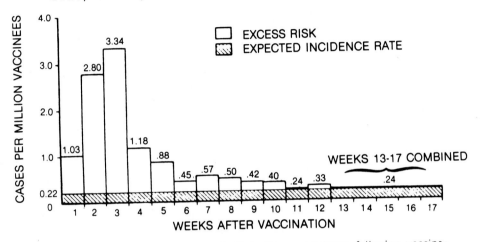

Source: Schonberger, L.B. et al., Guillain-Barre syndrome following vaccination in the national influenza immunization program, United States, 1976-1977. Am. J. Epidemiol. 110:105, 1979.

Question 28
_____

What do the data from Figure 29 suggest about the relation between vaccination and illness? What might explain the shape of the distribution?

4.   Atomic Bombing of Japan
     _____

Just prior to the conclusion of World War II, for both political and military reasons, President Harry S. Truman ordered the U.S. Army Air Corps to detonate atomic bombs over the cities of Hiroshima and Nagasaki, Japan, on August 6 and August 9, 1945, respectively. Both cities were virtually destroyed and over 80,000 persons are believed to have died in each city. Japan surrendered on August 15, 1945.

After the war, the U.S. Atomic Energy Commission created the Atomic Bomb Casualty Commission (ABCC) to monitor the effects of radiation exposure in survivors of the blasts and in persons known to have entered the cities shortly after the bombings. The ABCC has since been renamed the Radiation Effects Research Foundation (RERF) and is currently continuing study of the remaining survivors, and their children and grandchildren. RERF is now jointly sponsored by the U.S. and Japanese governments, and is staffed by scientists from both countries.

Results of the RERF studies indicate a variety of conditions that may be associated with high-level radiation exposure. Additional information on the dangers of radiation may be obtained from the Annual Reports of the ABCC or RERF (1952-1980) and the book Death in Life, Survivors of Hiroshima by R.J. Lifton (Random House, 1967). The occurrence of disease was analyzed in terms of the subject's distance, measured in meters, from a point directly below the blast (both the Hiroshima and Nagasaki bombs were detonated above the city) and the dose of exposure. Some of the major findings that have emerged are shown in Figures 30a and 30b.

Figure 30a. Excess deaths from cancer in Hiroshima and Nagasaki, 1950-1972.

Causes of death	Observed	Expected	Excess
Leukemia	84	13.7	70.3
Other malignant cancers	1075	918.8	156.2
Breast	37	19.0	18.0
Respiratory organs	129	73.7	55.3
Digestive organs	678	652.4	25.6
Other organs	231	173.7	57.3
Benign and unspecified cancers	53	42.9	10.1
All cancer	1212	975.4	236.6

Source: Sztanyik, L.B., in Vol. I. Proceedings of a symposium: Late biologic effects of ionizing radiation, Vienna, Austria, March 1978, p. 66.

Question 29

Based upon the atomic bomb data and findings presented earlier associating x-ray and ionizing radiation and cancer, what concern do you have about annual screening examination by x-rays (mammography) to detect female breast cancer, given that:

(1) breast cancer is a common cancer in U.S. women;
(2) x-ray particles can cause changes in breast tissue;
(3) mammography would irradiate the local tissue with a dose of 500 milliroentgens compared to a 30-40 milliroentgen dose received in chest x-ray or the 30-44 milliroentgen dose received in dental x-rays?

Figure 30b.   Age-specific incidence of acute granulocytic leukemia in A-bomb survivors in relation to age at irradiation, as compared with that in nonirradiated populations.

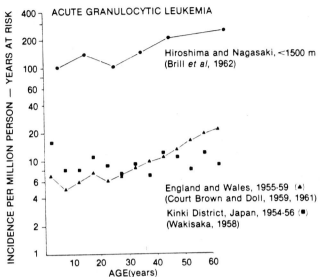

Source: Upton, A.C., Radiation injury: effects, principles and perspectives, Univ. Chicago Press, 1964, p. 64.

5.   Nutrition and Child Development

The health effects of obesity and diets with high cholesterol content concerns nutritionists and epidemiologists.   The results of their investigations may affect school lunch programs, agricultural practices, the food processing industry, and our eating habits in the future.

The subject of nutrition is one of the more difficult areas confronting researchers.   If, for example, one wanted to determine whether or not prenatal nutrition has an effect on the growth and development of a developing fetus and the mental or intellectual development of children, where would you obtain suitable populations for study?   Would mothers volunteer for an experiment that might jeopardize the health of their children?   Moreover, even if you could find volunteers, it is doubtful whether such studies would be performed due to the ethical, political, and legal problems that might result.

Before proceeding further, can you think of a population at risk or situation in which the relationship between prenatal nutrition and fetal growth and mental development might be studied?

Dr. Zena Stein and her co-workers recognized that birthweight and intellect, which are the factors to be measured in an investigation of the above questions, are subject to many other influences.   Because of the complexity of the subject and the ethical issues involved, an experimental study on humans would

Figure 31. Some factors that may affect birthweight and intellect.

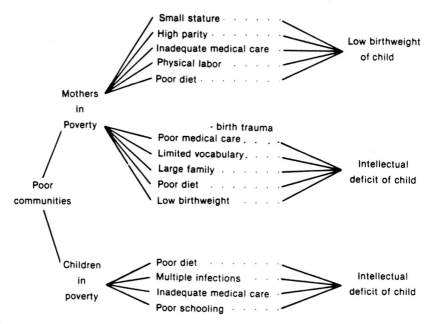

be impossible to perform.   Moreover, the results might not provide clear and unequivocal answers.

Stein et al. recognized that a "natural experiment" might provide useful in-sights in the absence of planned and controlled nutritional studies.   Such a natural experiment occurred in Europe during the last stages of World War II, when a famine took place in the western Netherlands.   Moreover, since that country also had good records of births and deaths, as well as documentation of the food rations, study of the famine in a rigorous scientific manner was feasible.   Thus, the question relating prenatal nutrition to fetal growth and development could be studied.

A second fact useful to the investigators was that all males were subject to military induction at age 18.   Therefore, Stein et al. were able to study 98% of all surviving males who were residing in Holland, in order to determine if the mental performance of military inductees was affected by exposure to the famine, during prenatal and infancy periods.

The main features of the study are reproduced from the book <u>Famine and Human Development</u> (Oxford Univ. Press, 1975), and article Nutrition and Mental Performance, Science 178:708, 1972 (copyright 1972, the American Association for the Advancement of Science), by Stein et al.

Figure 32. Average quarterly distribution of food rations in calories, protein, fats, and carbohydrates in the western Netherlands, 1941-1945.

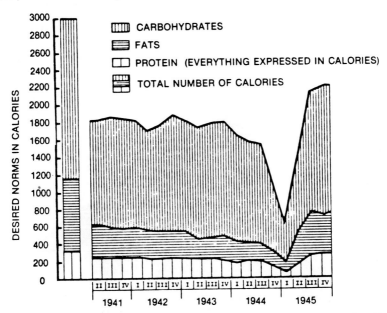

Source: Burger, G.C.E. et al., Malnutrition and Starvation in Western Netherlands, September 1944-July 1945. The Hague, Government Printing Office, 1948.

The design of the study consisted of measurements of birthweight and other indicators of fetal growth and development, and of mental performance at the time of military induction, in relation to the period of conception and birth for those males conceived and born between 1943 and 1946. Births occurring during a designated time period are referred to as a birth COHORT.

Several cohorts are shown below. Of particular interest are those whose prenatal or early postnatal life occurred during the famine. Since data were available for the entire country, it was possible to compare cohorts from famine and nonfamine areas. There are 36 cohorts grouped into 9 master cohorts (A_1-E_2) shown in Figure 33.

Figure 33.   Design of study, cohorts by month of conception and month of birth, in the Netherlands, 1943 to 1946, related to calories in the rations of famine cities. Solid vertical lines bracket the period of famine, and broken vertical lines bracket the period of births conceived during famine.

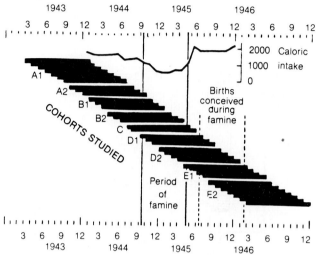

A few of the results of this study are given in Figures 34a-34d.

Figure 34a.   Birthweight by time and place (mean birthweight in grams for births in maternity hospitals) for seven birth cohorts in famine, northern and southern control areas, compared for the period August 1944 to March 1946.

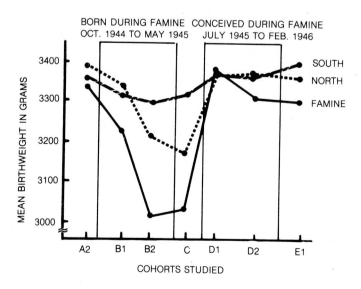

Figure 34b.   Infant length by time and place (mean infant length in centimeters for consecutive births in maternity hospitals) for seven birth cohorts in famine, northern and southern control areas, compared for the period August 1944 to March 1946.

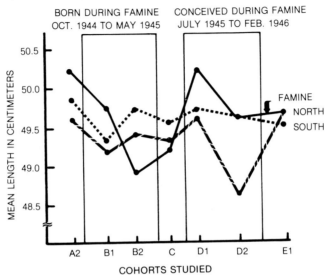

Figure 34c.   Head circumference of infants by time and place (mean head circumference of infants in centimeters for consecutive births in maternity hospitals) for seven birth cohorts in famine, northern and southern control areas, for the period August 1944 to March 1946.

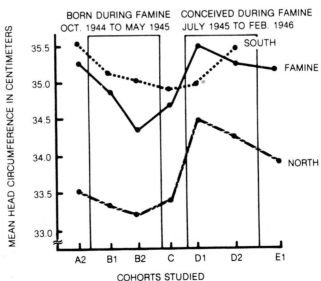

Figure 34d. Cohort deaths by cause and area (selected causes of death per 1000 total births compared in famine and combined control areas).

A. prematurity

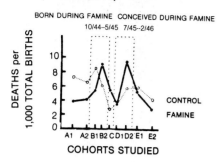

B. starvation and atrophy

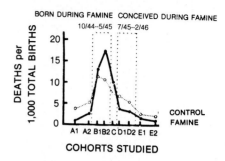

C. obstetric, all at ages under 90 days

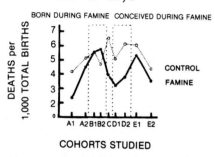

D. acute infections at ages over 90 days

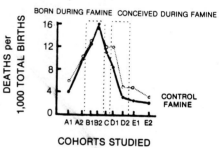

Mental performance of the 19-year-old, male military inductees was determined by their test scores (Raven progressive matrix). Note that in interpreting the Raven scores shown below, a higher score indicates a poorer performance. In each illustration, solid vertical lines bracket the period of famine, and broken vertical lines show the period of births conceived during the famine.

Figure 35a. Rates of mild mental retardation in 19-year-old military inductees by manual and nonmanual classes of father's occupation, and by cohort of birth in famine and control cities.

Figure 35b. Mean group scores on Raven progressive matrices test of 19-year-old military inductees by manual and nonmanual classes of father's occupation, and by cohort of birth in famine and control cities.

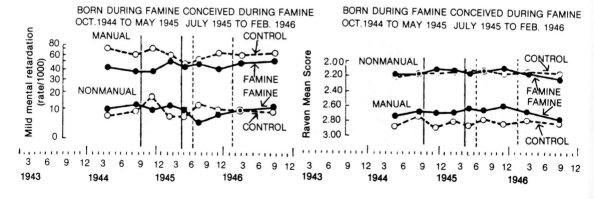

Figure 35c. Mean birth weight in maternity hospitals selected from famine and control cities (Rotterdam and Heerlen, respectively), by cohort of birth.

Figure 35d. Rates of severe mental retardation in 19-year-old military inductees, by cohort of birth in famine and control cities.

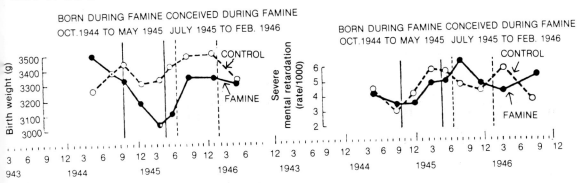

Question 30

You have seen how a natural experiment can provide a population at risk for study. What were the findings of the study with regard to fetal development and mental performance? Do you think these are valid findings?

IV. COHORT ANALYSIS

The term cohort was previously defined as a group of individuals born during a specified period of time. Although precisely defined, the term's usage has changed. Sartwell's essay, Cohorts: the debasement of a word (Am. J. of Epidemiol. 103:536, 1976) points out that:

> The present meaning seems to refer to any group of people, whatever their age or mode of selection, who are subjected to follow-up, of whatever duration.... Sometimes even the requirement of follow-up is omitted, and the term becomes just a synonym for any kind of a sample. It has even reached the point now that individuals who are associated [in any way] are referred to as cohorts.

> Whether or not we approve of the looser uses of the word cohort... certainly the term 'cohort analysis' if it is to have any meaning must adhere to the original Andvord-Frost usage at least to the extent that people of a given, restricted age group are followed forward in

time and their rates of disease or death are measured in successive
time intervals as they age.

Although Dr. Andvord's original paper on cohort analysis was not translated
into English, a treatise on this subject by Dr. Wade Hampton Frost, was published in the U.S. in 1939. Dr. Frost's paper is important in the development
of epidemiologic thought because it explains an unusual phenomenon observed
for tuberculosis mortality. In many infectious diseases recovery from infection
results in complete (or partial) immunity to later reinfection. Frost had observed that "age and prior exposure bring no such immunity against tuberculosis as they establish against many of the acute infections." Frost clearly
identifies the problem in paragraphs 2 and 3 of his paper and offers an in-
sightful analysis of the data. At the time it was written little was known of
the immunology of tuberculosis, its period of latency following initial infection,
and the possibility for reactivation of the disease. Frost's paper is reproduced below through the courtesy of the American Journal of Epidemiology.
The reader should review the unusual characteristics of the natural history of
tuberculosis (APHA handbook, Control of Communicable Diseases) before proceeding further.

The Age Selection of Mortality from Tuberculosis in Successive Decades*

As we pass along the age scale from infancy through childhood, to
early adult life, and on to old age, the curve of mortality from
tuberculosis shows a continuous movement either upward or downward. This is such a familiar fact that we are apt to take it for
granted; to dismiss it as characteristic of the disease, and to pass
on. But there is perhaps no single statistical record which is potentially of more significance. For every change in the rate of mortality as we pass from one age to another represents a shift in the
balance established between the destructive forces of the invading
tubercle bacillus and the sum total of host-resistance. If we could
accurately interpret this record, analyzing in detail each movement
upward or downward and assigning to each factor its due share in
the change, then we would be well on the way to knowing the epidemiology of tuberculosis.

But the record is peculiarly difficult to read with understanding,
because it is immediately apparent that the most striking changes in
mortality rate do not correspond to reasonably probable changes of
like extent in rate of exposure to infection. For instance, nothing
that we know of the habits of mankind and the distribution of the
tubercle bacillus would lead us to suppose that between the first and
the second five years of life there is, in general, a diminution in

*This article was first published, after Dr. Frost's death, in the American
Journal of Hygiene, 30:91, November 1939.

exposure to infection which corresponds to the decline in mortality rate. And there is little, if any, better reason to suppose that the extraordinary rise in mortality from age ten to age twenty, twenty-five, or thirty is paralleled by a corresponding increase in rate of exposure to specific infection.

We are forced, then, to recognize, as at least highly probable, that the predominant factor in the up-and-down movement of mortality along the age scale is change in human resistance. And this is a complex of which we have very little exact knowledge except the plain fact that age and prior exposure bring no such immunity against tuberculoses as they establish against many of the acute infections.

However, my purpose is not to attempt an interpretation of the age selection of tuberculosis; it is merely to call attention to the apparent change in age selection which has taken place gradually during the last thirty to sixty years, and to note that when looked at from a different point of view this change in age selection is found to be more apparent than real. The age-specific curve of mortality from tuberculosis for males in the United States Registration Area of 1900 is shown for the years 1900 and 1930 in Figure 1 and for Massachusetts males for the years 1880, 1910, and 1930 in Figure 2.

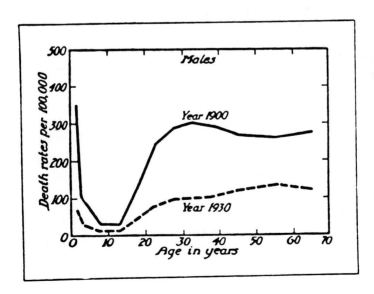

Figure 1. U.S. registration area of 1900 death rates from tuberculosis (all forms) by age, 1900 and 1930.

Figure 2. Massachusetts death rates from tuberculosis (all forms) by
age, 1880, 1910, 1930.

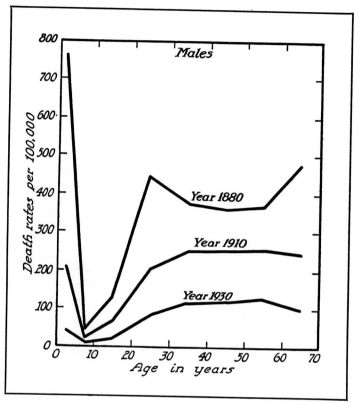

The tuberculosis mortality rates for Massachusetts used throughout
this paper are shown in Table 1. You will note that:

1. At every age mortality is lower in the later period.

2. In each period age selection is generally similar: mortality is
    high in infancy, declining in childhood, rising in adolescence to
    a higher level in adult life.

3. In the later period (1930) the highest rate of mortality comes at
    the age of fifty to sixty, whereas formerly it was at age twenty
    to forty.

Table 1.   Death rates* per 100,000 from tuberculosis, all forms for
Massachusetts, 1880 to 1930, by age and sex, with rates
for cohort of 1880 indicated.

Age	1880	1890	1900	1910	1920	1930
Males						
0— 4.....................	760	578	309	209	108	41
5— 9.....................	43	49	31	21	24	11
10—19.....................	126	115	90	63	49	21
20—29.....................	444	361	288	207	149	81
30—39.....................	378	368	296	253	164	115
40—49.....................	364	336	253	253	175	118
50—59.....................	366	325	267	252	171	127
60—69.....................	475	346	304	246	172	95
70+.....................	672	396	343	163	127	95
Females						
0— 4.....................	658	595	354	162	101	27
5— 9.....................	71	82	49	45	24	13
10—19.....................	265	213	145	92	78	37
20—29.....................	537	393	290	207	167	92
30—39.....................	422	372	260	189	135	73
40—49.....................	307	307	211	153	108	53
50—59.....................	334	234	173	130	83	47
60—69.....................	434	295	172	118	83	56
70+.....................	584	375	296	126	68	40

*They were obtained as follows: For the years 1910, 1920 and 1930—based on U. S. Mortality
Statistics—deaths from tuberculosis, all forms. For the years 1880, 1890 and 1900 the rates used are
calculated from data compiled by the late Dr. Edgar Sydenstricker from the state records. Because
of differences of classification in deaths, it has been necessary to base the rates on the deaths recorded as "tuberculosis of the lungs" to get comparable data for these years. The rate calculated
from the state records for "tuberculosis of the lungs" has been multiplied by a factor based on the
proportion such deaths bore to those from tuberculosis, all forms. This factor varied with the year
and age considered.

These characteristic changes from decade to decade can be demonstrated in the records for many different areas, both for males and
females.

Looking at the 1930 curve, the impression given is that nowadays an
individual encounters his greatest risk of death from tuberculosis between the ages of fifty and sixty.   But this is not really so; the
people making up the 1930 age group fifty to sixty have, in earlier
life, passed through greater mortality risks.

This is demonstrated in Figures 3 and 3a, which show for males and
females in Massachusetts the death rates at specific ages in the
years 1880 and 1930, and also those for each age of the cohort of
1880 or that group of people who were born in the years 1871 to
1880.   These graphs indicate that the group of people who were
children zero to nine years of age in 1880 and who are now aged
fifty to sixty years (if alive) have, in two earlier periods, passed
through greater risks.   They also indicate that the age selection in
the cohort of 1880 is quite different from that apparently indicated
by the age specific mortality rates for any single year.

Figure 3. Massachusetts death rates from tuberculosis (all forms) by age, in the years 1880 and 1930 and for the cohort of 1880.

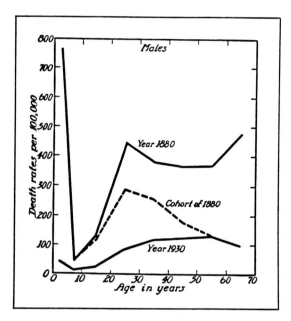

Figure 3a. Massachusetts death rates from tuberculosis (all forms) by age, in the years 1880 and 1930 and for the cohort of 1880.

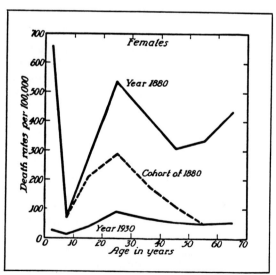

Figure 4 shows similarly for males the mortality at successive ages in cohorts of (1870), 1880, 1890, 1900, 1910. Note that "terminal" rates for these cohorts make the 1930 curve, and also that in successive cohorts the age selection has been uniform, with the mortality highest in the first five years and again from twenty to thirty years; thereafter it declines. This fact was previously noted by K.F. Andvord (1930). His interpretation was, in part, that this regularity of the age curve formed a basis for extending estimates of future mortality in the same cohort at higher ages. Such an interpretation is both tempting and encouraging but perhaps dangerous.

Figure 4.   Massachusetts death rates from tuberculosis (all forms) by age, in successive ten-year cohorts.

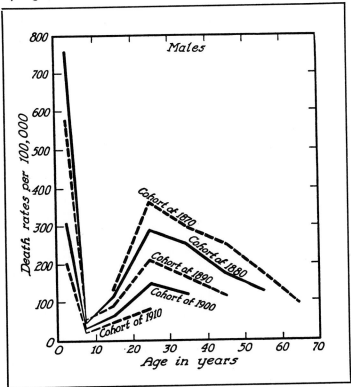

Without attempting to interpret the facts in detail, certain implications are noted.

1.   Constancy of age selection (<u>relative</u> mortality at successive ages) in successive cohorts suggests rather constant physiological changes in resistance (with age) as the controlling factor.

2.   If, as we may suppose, the frequency and extent of exposure to infection in early life have decreased progressively decade by decade, there is no indication that this has had the effect of exaggerating the risk of death in adult life due to lack of opportunity to acquire specific immunity in childhood.

3.   Present-day "peak" of mortality in <u>late</u> life does not represent postponement of maximum risk to a later period, but rather would seem to indicate that the present high rates in old age are the residuals of higher rates in earlier life.

References

1.   Andvord, K.F.,   What can we learn by studying tuberculosis by generations?   Norsk Magazin for Laegevidenskaben, 91:642-660, June 1930.

2.   Bureau of the Census.   Mortality Statistics, 1910, 1920, 1930.

Question 31

If you were to examine the age-specific rates of a disease for a given year, what might the curve look like if a cohort effect was present?

Question 32

Can you think of other diseases or health problems for which a cohort phenomenon occurs?

SUMMARY and REVIEW

You have completed a great deal of material in this exercise and you probably feel somewhat lost in the mass of details and facts.

Take a moment to review the goals of this exercise:

To understand the term population at risk and its relation to identifying patterns of disease and health problems in the community. To understand how particular populations can be utilized and the types of conclusions derived from their selection for epidemiologic study.

To achieve these goals we have demonstrated the following:

I.   AGE AND CAUSE-SPECIFIC RATES
II. DEFINITION OF THE TERM POPULATION AT RISK
III. POPULATIONS USEFUL IN IDENTIFYING EPIDEMIOLOGIC PROBLEMS.

    A.   Populations with exposure characteristics of interest

        1.   location
        2.   shared experience or event
        3.   vital events--birth or death
        4.   nonvital events--reporting of infectious disease
        5.   occupation
        6.   environment

    B.   Populations with biologic characteristics of interest

        1.   ethnic groups
        2.   families
        3.   twins

    C.   Populations involved in natural experiments

        1.   migrants
        2.   religious or social groups
        3.   the swine influenza immunization program
        4.   atomic bombing of Japan
        5.   famine in the Netherlands

IV. COHORT ANALYSIS

Having completed the first two exercises in this guide you should now understand WHAT epidemiologists do and WHY they do it. If you are still not sure, review the section in the Introduction that summarizes the purposes of epidemiology and the subjects with which epidemiology is concerned.

The remainder of the guide will help you to develop the skills concerned with HOW TO DO EPIDEMIOLOGY.

SUGGESTED RESPONSES
Exercise 2--Population At Risk

1a. The data show the magnitude of each of the causes of death. Heart disease is the leading cause of death for "all ages" in both 1968 and 1978. Cancer is second, cerebrovascular diseases are third, accidents fourth. These causes of death account for about 75% of all deaths in the U.S. There is variation in the leading causes of death in different age groups; among infants <1 year of age these four causes account for only 5-10% of all deaths. Until age 34, accidents and all other causes account for the majority of deaths. Heart disease, cancer, and cerebrovascular diseases become the major killers after age 45. Surprisingly, accidents are an important cause of death at all ages.

1b. For deaths from "all causes," there has been a decrease in the death rate in every age group. Notable improvement has occurred in every age group, particularly in infants. Heart disease has decreased in all ages except infants. Cancer has shown a slight decrease until age 54 but an increase after age 55.

Cerebrovascular diseases and accidents have decreased in all age groups. All other causes of death have decreased below age 14 and after age 35 but remained about the same for persons 15-34 in the 10-year period.

2a. You might compare lung cancer deaths to the size of the midyear population of the U.S. on July 1, or you might compare the deaths to the number of persons who are known to be smokers.

2b. You might compare the number of births to the midyear population of the U.S., a region, a state, a county, or a city, or you might compare the births to the number of women of child-bearing ages in each of the geographic areas mentioned.

2c. You might compare the total number of days during which a hospital bed was occupied compared to the midyear population of the U.S. or some other geographic area, or you might compare the total number of days during which the hospital bed was occupied to the number of persons admitted to a hospital.

NOTE: You also have the option of using age-specific rates for any population selected.

3a. Select females of child-bearing ages who are less than 19 years of age. From the operational viewpoint it is necessary to define the term "child-bearing ages." While documented cases of young girls (< 12 years) giving birth are rare, you might wish to include girls under the age of 14, especially since many of them have reached menarche and may have occasional or regular sexual contact. Menarche and sexual activity might be used as indicators of susceptibility and exposure.

3b. Census records, school rosters, special surveys, chamber of commerce records, etc., might be useful in identifying a denominator without regard to exposure considerations. If exposure were also of interest, you might contact social service agencies, family planning or birth control clinics, hospitals, and physicians in the county.

3c. Knowledge and use of birth control, frequency of sexual contacts, frequency of induced abortion, presence of sex education classes, availability of medical care for providing more effective contraception.

4. A population at risk comprised of the midyear population estimate of a nation or geographic region is usually easily determined. However, any population that includes all individuals might include certain individuals who are not susceptible or at risk of an event. For example, only females of child-bearing age are capable of having a baby. Any rate that compared births to the total population of the nation or area would include males and children who are not biologically "susceptible" to pregnancy. With regard to deaths, all persons will someday die, therefore, everyone in the population may be thought to be "susceptible" to death.

If a subgroup of the population is to be studied, an investigator must select a population on the basis of the type of disease and the degree of difficulty expected in locating or collecting usable data from the population of interest. A further consideration is whether susceptibility and degree of exposure can be determined.

5. Males have higher death rates than females in each country. Countries with high rates for males tend to have high rates for females as well. Countries with low rates tend to show low rates for both males and females. This raises the question of why. Do the excess death rates among males imply genetic factors or environmental differences in exposure? In general, environmental and behavioral factors are thought to play the more important role in both stomach (diet, and stress (?)) and skin (exposure to sunlight) cancers. Separating the genetic from the environmental and behavioral influences in searching for the cause of disease is one of the most difficult problems in epidemiology. Other questions that might be asked are whether the accuracy of the cause of death diagnosis and/or case finding is equally accurate among males and females and whether the completeness of reporting and accuracy of data are comparable in all countries.

6a. U.S. white males and females have higher death rates for each major cancer type except stomach. Male death rates exceed female rates for the particular site.

6b. Japanese diet is higher in salt, soy beans, tea, pickles, rice, and carbo-
     hydrates and lower in fats and protein compared to the U.S. In addition,
     Japanese males have a high rate of cigarette smoking and alcohol con-
     sumption. While the cause of stomach cancer is not known, much research
     is being done in this area. The role of stress and genetic factors also
     must be evaluated.

     Smoking is a known cause of lung cancer. Despite the high proportion of
     Japanese smokers, there are differences in the quality of smoking (inhal-
     ing, number of years smoked, use of filters, etc.), which may explain
     some of the higher death rates among Americans. There is also some evi-
     dence linking smoking and alcohol use to stomach cancer.

     Other gastrointestinal cancer including that of the colon, rectum, and
     pancreas may be linked to dietary factors such as dietary fiber or the
     quantity and type of fat in the diet.

     Bladder cancer has been linked to smoking, to occupational exposure to
     certain chemicals, and to infection. Differences in each of these factors
     exist between Japan and the U.S.

     Tumors of the reproductive system may be related to hormone production
     (breast and ovary), which in turn may have both dietary and genetic
     components. In addition, reproductive habits such as age at first deliv-
     ery and breast feeding of infants plays a role but it is not clear why.

7a. Before 1951 there was no immunity. All persons were susceptible because
     they all became infected when the measles virus was introduced into the
     population. After 1951 there was no disease. This implies that the infec-
     tion conferred complete immunity if the person recovered from the infec-
     tion, or that the virus disappeared.

     In the U.S., the cyclic pattern is due to an accumulation of new suscep-
     tibles due to births or immigration. The virus remains present in the
     population.

7b. While all individuals in the population are probably susceptible to measles
     and influenza viruses from infancy, the viruses affect the host in differ-
     ent ways. Clinical infection with measles virus results in complete immun-
     ity after recovery. Immunization against measles does not give complete
     immunity to all persons. Immunization protects some persons completely
     but gives only partial protection to others. A previous infection with
     influenza does not provide complete immunity although it seems to be more
     protective than immunization.

     Thus, we can see that the infectious processes of measles and influenza
     differ with regard to the immunity they confer. Some agents (measles)
     may confer complete immunity while others (influenza) confer only partial
     immunity to reinfection. The benefit of partial immunity is that illness
     resulting from reinfection is usually milder.

7c. The population at risk for measles should exclude persons with a known history of measles because that infection provides complete immunity. The population at risk for influenza would include all persons in the community because influenza gives only a partial immunity. Furthermore, the influenza virus is known to change periodically (types include A1, A2, B, and swine influenza) due to antigenic shift or drift.

7d. The answer depends upon the purpose of the study. The community population allows an epidemiologist to measure the "risk" in the city, state, etc. This might be useful in planning a health program when we need to know the amount of illness in the community. However, this would not tell us much about factors relating to the spread of the disease in the community. If we eliminate the "immunes" from the population at risk, we may be better able to study certain aspects of the way the disease spreads in those susceptible as well as to measure the effects of exposure to suspected causal factors of the disease with more precision. Choice of denominators also will be determined by the availability of data about the immune status of individuals.

8. A person's medical history, physical examination, health records, or special laboratory or diagnostic tests of blood, urine, X-rays, etc., can be used to determine susceptibility.

Frequently it will be impossible to determine the person's true immune status because of inadequate medical records, difficulties associated with remembering details of events occurring in the past, or lack of laboratory tests and diagnostic techniques specific for the disease or health problem to be studied. Knowledge of the person's medical history may be helpful, but absence of disease may mean full or partial immunity, no exposure to the infection, or that a mild infection was not diagnosed. You must also keep in mind that a doctor may have misdiagnosed an illness. Thus, absence of a particular disease does not guarantee that a patient did not have the disease, but rather it signifies that no one diagnosed it.

Evidence of susceptibility to infection or other illness may require special blood, urine, skin, or x-ray tests to rule out the possibility of previously undiagnosed illness. Unfortunately, not all diseases have specific diagnostic tests or physical findings. When positive, either can be useful to confirm a patient's medical history or to detect early stages of disease and/or mild disease for which a patient never saw a physician. Most infectious agents cause the host to produce antibody which can be detected in blood or other tissues. These antibody detection tests are usually quite specific and accurate, although some error will occur with any laboratory test.

Relying upon the patient or person responding to a health survey to provide reliable information is of limited value because memory may be incorrect. Laboratory tests or written medical records should be obtained to verify verbal accounts of prior illness.

Vaccination (immunization) history will also be useful. Diagnosis that depends upon written medical records from a doctor's office or a hospital may be helpful, but keep in mind that some records may be incomplete or not very useful, depending upon which disease or information is being investigated.

9a. Comparisons help to identify where health problems exist, to find where improvements in the medical care system can be made, and to evaluate the effectiveness of the medical care system. This study may reflect differences in the availability and access to follow-up treatment or other differences between wealthy and poor communities.

9b. One might prepare a list of all patients diagnosed as having (rather than being treated for) colon-rectal cancer at a large hospital in that community. You might then compare survival after diagnosis with some measure of economic status such as income or occupation.

10a. The distribution of positive tuberculosis skin test reactions by economic area and state residence among Navy recruits, 1958-64, is shown. Active recruiting in areas with poor economic conditions or with poor secondary schools might offer a choice to young people with poor employment or educational opportunities after high school. These areas might also be expected to have social crowding and perhaps inadequate health care, particularly an ineffective or inactive tuberculosis control program.

10b. A comparative study of residents of high- and low-income census areas. A comparative study of school age children by area of residence and ethnic groups.

Both of these alternative populations would get at the issue of TB distribution by studying groups that might be at high risk of infection.

11. Infection rates reflect the age of patients and the types of disease for which they are hospitalized; the composition, training, and experience of the professional staff; the amount of surgery performed; hospital policy regarding antibiotic use; hygiene practices by professional and nonprofessional staff and employees; use of catheters and intravenous medications, etc. Each of these factors would probably differ among different hospitals, thereby making appropriate comparisons difficult.

12. Age, immunity status, nutritional status, presence of other diseases (particularly certain debilitating chronic diseases or burns), necessity for surgical treatment, the use of catheters, or long-term intravenous medication, allergic sensitivity of patients.

13. One might determine the disease frequency in a population of persons having the same general characteristics of age, sex, and occupation as those who became ill. Several sources might be possible. You might

survey airline employees or airline travelers of similar age and sex as persons on the delayed flight. You would then compare the illness rates of those aboard the delayed flight to the surveyed group not aboard the delayed flight.

There is also a national study of disease that was carried out by the National Center for Health Statistics. This study uses a statistically selected sample of persons from the major geographical areas of the U.S. Health status is determined by an interview (the Health Interview Survey) or physical examination (the Health Examination Survey). Results are published and would be useful in determining the expected rate of disease among people of any given age and sex category for different parts of the U.S. The rate of expected disease could then be calculated and compared to the amount observed to help decide if an unusual rate of disease had occurred.

14. Useful features of birth and death certificates are that the events are readily observed and their occurrence is not subject to judgment. Second, in developed countries (U.S., Canada, Europe, Japan, etc.) birth and death registrations are virtually complete. Some care must be taken concerning the year the events occurred, e.g., vital registration in the United States was not truly national until 1933, when Texas became the last state to join the system. A third useful feature is the demographic information included.

Several limitations must be considered, however. The certificates are legal documents. Their use for health research is of secondary importance and information of interest to epidemiologists is not necessarily included. Because of the legal and confidential nature of this information it is not easy to obtain access to the records.

Second, some of the information may be of questionable accuracy, e.g., it is estimated that up to 30% of the cause of death diagnoses may be in error; and congenital defects are grossly underreported on birth certificates.

A third problem is that the use of a national standard registration system requires special training and procedures to assure that there is uniformity of procedures among different areas.

A serious problem is that in the U.S. births and deaths are separate registration systems, which are not linked together in all places. It is difficult to determine the survivorship of persons identified by birth certificates or details about the birth of individuals identified from death certificates. One reason is that there is not a unique number assigned to each individual at birth, which might be used to identify that person for all important events occurring throughout life. In many nations citizens have identity cards, which serve this purpose. In the U.S., perhaps the Social Security number could be used. A national record linkage system exists in many European nations. In 1982 the National Center for Health Statistics finally established a national death index that will permit some records to be linked after death.

A fifth problem is the fact that medical knowledge changes over time and the possibility that diagnostic categories of one era may not be similar to those of other eras. This is a particular problem in interpreting trends in causes of death determined from death certificates.

Also of concern is the completeness of reporting. In some developing countries all births or deaths may not be recorded, particularly if they occurred in rural areas. Even in the economically developed nations complete reporting might be a problem, particularly for events such as fetal deaths occurring in early pregnancy or in undiagnosed pregnancy. For this reason fetal deaths occurring before 20 or 28 weeks of pregnancy are largely undetected.

Finally, for use in epidemiologic study, population based rates must be calculated. These rates use the birth or death as the numerator (outcome to be measured) of the rate but require a denominator (the population at risk) based on a periodic national census, between census estimates of the population or special surveys to enumerate a particular population of interest.

15. Many studies are possible. The source of patients for study could be family planning clinics, Lamaze childbirth preparation courses, hospital maternity wards or outpatient prenatal care programs, or unwed mothers' homes. In addition, statistical analysis may be done from birth certificate data collected by the State Health Department Bureau of Vital Statistics or the National Center for Health Statistics.

Other sources of medical records or sources of access to patients might include large health clinics such as the prepaid Kaiser system in California and Oregon or large medical clinics such as the Kelsey-Seybold clinic in Houston or Mayo clinic in Minnesota.

16a. From Figure 14 it can be seen that farmers have almost 40% of all the leukemia deaths in Nebraska, but if farmers constituted 40% of the total population of the state, their percentage of leukemia deaths would not be disproportionate. If farmers comprised less than 40% of the population, then they would have a higher percentage of leukemia deaths than expected, assuming that the age and sex distributions of decedents of all other occupations is similar to that of farmers.

16b. From Figures 15a and 15b you can see that there is an excess of leukemia deaths in areas corresponding to the location of certain agriculture products, animals, and chemicals in the east, central, and northern portions of the state. However, in the wheat-producing areas of the west and southern counties, there is only a slight (6%) excess of leukemia deaths.

Further investigation would be necessary to determine if the cause of the excess deaths is related to specific activities of farming or to some non-farming exposure to leukemia carcinogens such as benzene or radiation, which might occur to a different degree in various regions of the state. Curiosity would almost certainly tempt an epidemiologist into taking a closer look at the problem of leukemia deaths in Nebraska.

17. Sources of data or access to patients include hospital or local physician records and out-patient medical departments, surveys of seafood restaurants or markets, drug abuse clinics, blood banks, health department clinics, hospital dental clinics, county medical or dental societies, hemodialysis centers, airline or travel agency records, and commercial tatoo or ear-piercing businesses licensed or identified by the city health department or by the telephone book. A survey of clinical laboratories to determine recent laboratory tests suggestive of hepatitis might be an additional source of study. Information would also be obtained from medical records or by interview or written questionnaire survey of infected persons or their family.

18. From Figure 17a the percentage of prostitutes with virus particles or with hepatitis antibody is seen to be much greater than for female blood donors and nuns. Obviously there are many differences between these three populations: age, sexual activity, socioeconomic status, number of children, marital status, etc., which might contribute to exposure or susceptibility. Other factors besides sexual activity might play a role and should be investigated. From other sources such as the APHA Handbook of Communicable Diseases, one becomes aware of the many ways in which hepatitis virus can be transmitted: person-to-person, food, blood, water, illicit drug use, etc. One wonders if the virus is transmitted by semen during intercourse, or orally such as through saliva during kissing.

From Figure 17b you can see the great excess of prostitutes with antibody compared to female blood donors of similar ages. The shape of the curve suggests that exposure increases with age more markedly for prostitutes than for other women. Other factors still need to be investigated; however, the possibility of sexual transmission is feasible but has not been conclusively proved.

19. A second occupational group exposed to the risk of hepatitis is hospital personnel. From Figure 18a the risk of hepatitis infection is seen to be greater for older persons, those employed more than 5 years, and those from the lowest socioeconomic level, all of which suggests exposure characteristics of interest. From the more detailed data it can be seen that there is a higher proportion of hepatitis among persons involved in food handling, contact with blood or blood products, and contact with patients. These data support the conclusion that hepatitis is an occupational health hazard and that the risk is related to the duration and type of exposure.

20a. The expected number of deaths can be derived from U.S. national age- and sex-specific mortality rates. These specific rates are multiplied by the number of persons in the group being observed. This will give an expected number of deaths in that population. The observed and expected numbers are then compared to determine if an excess number has occurred.

20b. Radiology technicians; children of pregnant mothers who were x-rayed during pregnancy; uranium mine workers; civilian residents of Utah and Nevada who resided near the Atomic bomb testing site in the 1950s; survivors of the atomic bombing of Hiroshima and Nagasaki, Japan; residents of the sunbelt states (U.S. southwest) exposed to ultraviolet radiation; women who had mammograms (x-ray screening tests) to detect breast cancer.

21. Pollution of the air can pose a definite health hazard under certain atmospheric conditions. Diseases of the respiratory system and cardiovascular system can be worsened to a sufficient degree to cause deaths. Following the large jump in the number of deaths, the curve shows a depression and then rises again. This suggests that the date of death of many people with severe disease may have been hastened as a result of exposure to the pollution. Relatively fewer persons for whom death was imminent were alive during the immediate postpollution period; thus a dip in the curve is noted. The dip (decrease) after a blip (elevation) of the curve is a characteristic of unusual events such as air pollution inversions, wars, and disasters, which affect one or several age-sex groups disproportionately. The number of deaths from motor vehicle accidents was unchanged. The fact that an important nonphysiologic cause of death was relatively unchanged strengthens the argument that the pollution exerts its effects primarily on the respiratory and circulatory systems.

22. The risk of developing diabetes increases with age, although some irregularity occurs in the percentages when small numbers of individuals are involved. There is an increased risk among persons with more Indian heritage; full-blooded Indians have 2.4 to 5.8 times as much disease as groups with mixed blood.

The ratio of excess disease for Pima Indians compared to whites is remarkable in both sexes, particularly in females. The cause of diabetes is not known, but data such as these raise the possibility of a genetic mechanism or some unusual factor in the Indian's environment, such as diet, having an important role. Also of interest is the fact that among the Pimas, females have higher rates than males, but in whites males show an excess. It is possible that the search for cases is more complete among Indian females than for whites.

23a. Studies of family members and populations with distinct genetic characteristics are approaches that epidemiologists use to determine the role of genetic inheritance (as opposed to environmental factors) in different diseases.

Thus, demonstration of excess risk among family members supports the possibility of genetic mechanisms. The evidence in Figures 24a and 24b supports the possibility of a genetic link in the mechanism of breast cancer, particularly in younger women (<39). However, there is also the possibility that environmental factors may act together with a genetic "predisposition" to the disease. One might also correctly argue that the data also support the hypothesis that environmental factors are involved, since family members would generally have similar dietary and social habits.

As you will discover in Exercise 9, the task of proving a cause-effect relation is not at all easy. Thus, determining the relative importance and unravelling the complex interplay of genetic and environmental factors is quite difficult. No single study is capable of solving the genetic/environmental puzzle. Rather, the epidemiologist looks for supporting evidence and gradually builds a web of evidence.

23b. If we assume that the finding has been duplicated in the general population, that it is a biological fact and not due to some unsuspected error in diagnosis or bias in the study design, then the health program should concentrate its case-finding efforts among female family members of known cases. Cases can be identified from death certificates, surveys of medical records, and admissions to hospitals or cancer centers. Local doctors should be contacted to alert them to the goals of the program and request their assistance. Such a health program would be expected to produce a higher yield of breast cancer identification for a given amount of expenditures; a more efficient program in terms of costs and benefits.

24. The spread of disease among contacts exposed to infection can often be studied in families. This is especially true for adults whose broad range of daily contacts (both the number and type) make quantitative risk assessment difficult. Among younger persons, school classmates (as well as family contacts) also are useful populations for studying the spread of disease.

Families, however, are quite efficient and convenient populations for study, and they are not subject to some of the logistical problems of attempting to study nonhousehold contacts.

The data from Figure 25 generally show higher attack rates and secondary attack rates as the size of the household increases. The table does not show a direct linear relationship, however.

Obviously, the spread of disease depends upon the exposed person receiving a sufficient dose of the infecting organism. Repeated exposure to contaminated air, food, water, or household articles affects the spread of different disease agents within the family.

25a. From Figure 26a it is seen that there is no statistically significant difference between the deaths from all causes in smokers and nonsmokers.
There is a hint of excess deaths among smoking male twins 45-59, but the
numbers are not large enough to form a definite conclusion. Among older
twins, there are no differences. One problem with these data is that
many causes of death are grouped together. There may not be enough
data to detect statistical differences for individual diseases. On the other
hand grouping different disease processes together may mask the effect of
smoking on specific disease processes that have distinct pathologic path-
ways, e.g., cancer and heart disease. Second, the quality of exposure
(inhalation and other smoking habits) and/or the quantity (dose) of
smoking may differ between the younger and older groups. Figure 26b
does not show a consistent pattern of excess deaths among moderate/
heavy smokers in different age groups.

25b. Monozygous twins are derived from a single fertilized ovum and therefore
should be genetically identical. Thus, if smoking is an important cause
of death, differences between the death rate of smoking and nonsmoking
twins ought to be attributable to differences in environmental exposures,
habits, diet, etc.

25c. One of the arguments used in an attempt to discredit the data showing
that smoking is a cause of lung cancer is that some persons may be
genetically predisposed to cancer. Smoking would cause cancer in only
those persons who were genetically predisposed.

Since these data do not show an excess number of deaths among smokers
or moderate/heavy smokers, one might conclude that the environmental
differences (i.e., smoking) do not produce an excess of deaths. This is
an unexpected finding! It supports the argument that genetic factors
might be more important than generally believed. In Exercises 10-12 you
will learn about study design. You may then wish to return to this
study of twins to examine the research methods used and whether or not
methodological problems may be a factor in producing the unanticipated
results.

26a. Migrants have similar genetic backgrounds as their nonmigrating country-
men. If disease patterns of the migrants or their descendants in the new
country differ from the patterns in the native country, it suggests that
environmental factors (such as diet, social customs, and lifestyle) may
play a role in the etiology of the disease. This is another approach by
which epidemiologists attempt to distinguish between genetic and environmental factors in the cause of disease. Japanese in Hawaii are thought to
have a lifestyle combining some elements of traditional Japanese and
modern Western life, whereas Japanese in the U.S. have the least traditional lifestyle. Thus, the higher mortality among more westernized
lifestyles for each age group suggests environmental factors may play a
major role in the disease. Identifying specific differences in the environmental factors might lead to control or prevention of a major cause of
illness and death.

26b. Diet in Japan is higher in fish, salt, and vegetables and lower in fat, beef, sugar, protein, and total carbohydrates than the U.S. Migrants would probably modify their diets in a new country. Another major difference is that traditional family life in Japan has emphasized living together in harmony and reduction of stress and competition. Migrants would encounter many stresses in acculturating to their new country. Thus, diet and stress might be factors contributing to the increased rates of migrating persons. The amount of increase would depend upon how much traditional lifestyles could be followed in the new country.

27. The data from Figure 28 are quite impressive in suggesting that age and lifestyle are important factors in the disease etiology. However, we do not have some important information such as whether Mormons and non-Mormons have lived in Utah for similar periods of time, or whether they are from similar genetic backgrounds. Data collected routinely from death certificates do not provide information about these or other factors such as smoking habits, which might play a role in the etiology of heart disease (special studies would be necessary to obtain these additional data). If we assume that Mormons and non-Mormons are similar with respect to some of these factors, then the data are useful because they show that differences in lifestyle are associated with acquired heart disease. If one is not willing to make the above assumptions, then the differences in death rates are not as meaningful. Despite these gaps in our knowledge, the data are quite impressive.

Even if other factors exert some influence on mortality, do you think that they would be sufficient to equal the 9-178% excess mortality observed for non-Mormons in the various age-sex-disease categories?

28. There appears to be a relationship between immunization and identification of G-B cases, although, we do not know if publicity in the news media contributed to finding new cases or whether all cases were correctly diagnosed. If the data do not result from unusual reporting practices (including differences in the case-finding methods for those vaccinated compared to the nonvaccinated) or diagnostic errors they suggest several possibilities:

1. G.B. syndrome might be caused by the swine influenza virus. The median incubation period would be 2-3 weeks after exposure.

2. The virus or the vaccine might alter the tissues of the host so that another organism (the real cause) can produce disease.

3. The virus or the vaccine might be needed to furnish some essential material required to produce the disease in a susceptible host.

29. Radiation is known to be capable of producing cancer in certain tissues or body organs (blood, thyroid, breast). Mass-screening for breast cancer

would be expected to cause cancer in some women who would otherwise not have developed the disease. The value of a large screening program would be judged by the number of lives saved (benefits) relative to the deaths caused by the test (risks).

30. Birthweight of those born and those conceived during the famine in famine areas is lower than the control areas. Infant length did not differ; nor was head circumference particularly affected by exposure to famine. Cohort deaths by cause suggest that premature infants in famine areas may have had higher death rates during the famine, but rates fell below those of control areas after the famine ended. Other causes of death were not appreciably changed by the famine.

Raven test scores do not suggest any remarkable differences between famine and control areas. However, those from families in which the father's occupation was nonmanual had better performance than offspring of workers with manual occupations.

There are many sources for error, such as the accuracy of measurements, the biological significance of some measures, the possibility of disproportionate out-migration by surviving offspring from the famine area, and the possibility that those males who survived the famine differ markedly from those who may have perished from malnutrition or intercurrent disease. The data seem to have been collected in a careful manner, however. The onus for discrediting the validity of these findings must fall upon readers who disbelieve the data.

31. A blip (an increased rate of death or disease) would occur in the affected age group, as reflected in Table 1 of Frost's paper; there is an elevation of mortality in different decades as the cohort of 1880 ages.

32. Lung cancer among smokers. Neonatal tetanus of newborns. Vaginal cancer among daughters of pregnant women exposed to diethyl stilbestrol.

PART II. MEASUREMENT

Part II of the guide includes Exercises 3-6, which are concerned with the techniques of measurement used by epidemiologists.

EXERCISE 3. ASSESSING RISK

Goals

Upon completion of this exercise you should be able (1) to quantify risk in several ways, and (2) understand the uses and limitations of common epidemiologic measures of risk.

Methods

In order to achieve these goals you will need to understand:

I.   CATEGORIES OF MEASUREMENT

    A.   Rates
    B.   Ratios
    C.   Proportions

II.   MISLEADING NUMBERS

    A.   Inappropriate Nomenclature
    B.   Imaginary numbers

III. MEASUREMENT OF MORBIDITY, MORTALITY, AND NATALITY

    A.   Morbidity

        1.   Prevalence
        2.   Incidence

    B.   Mortality rates

        1.   Crude
        2.   Case-fatality

    C.   Natality Rates

IV.   DENOMINATORS: USING MIDYEAR POPULATION VS. PERSON-TIME UNITS
V.   STANDARDIZATION--DIRECT AND INDIRECT ADJUSTMENT OF RATES
VI.   RELATIVE RISK AND ATTRIBUTABLE RISK
VII. DEFINITION OF FORMULAS

Terms

Ratios; indices; proportions; case-fatality rate; maternal mortality ratio; point and period prevalence; incidence; attack rate; infant mortality; crude birth rate; infection vs. disease; standardized mortality ratios (SMRs); attributable and relative risk; person-years.

Suggested Readings

Friedman, *Principles* of *Epidemiology*, 1980 (Statistics in Epidemiology, pp. 8-26; Adjustment, pp. 181-184)

Mausner and Bahn, *Epidemiology*: an *Introductory* Text (Measures of disease frequency, pp. 126-153; Relative and attributable risk, pp. 316-323)

Fox, Hall and Elvebach, *Epidemiology*, Man and Disease, pp. 127-150.

Lilienfeld and Lilienfeld, *Foundations* of *Epidemiology* (Morbidity statistics, pp. 133-144; Standardized mortality ratios, pp. 78-80)

MacMahon and Pugh, *Epidemiology* (Measures of disease frequency, pp. 57-72; Vital records, pp. 74-85; Relative and attributable risk, pp. 232-239)

Remington and Schork, *Statistics* with *Application* to *Biological* and *Health Sciences*, Chapter 13, pp. 326-340 (Age adjustment, pp. 330-338)

Descriptive statistics: rates, ratios, proportions, and indices, USDHEW, PHS, Center for Disease Control. Pub. No. 00-1834.

Physicians are concerned with the health of their individual patients. They describe that person's health with reference to body organs such as the heart, the lungs, and the liver. In order to assess the condition of each organ, physicians use a medical history and physical examination. The physical examination often requires specialized instruments to observe internal organs (stethoscopes, x-ray, CAT scanners) and laboratory tests of the blood, urine and feces to measure their function.

Epidemiologists are interested in assessing the health of a community and use surveys, vital statistics, health records, and health examinations of groups of people to determine the type and extent of health problems in the community.

The work of epidemiologists and physicians is often complementary. In some cases, an observation by an epidemiologist may be used to improve diagnosis or treatment of individuals, or to make possible new measures to prevent a disease or health problem, which can then be implemented by physicians. In other situations, clinical observation by a physician may stimulate epidemiologic interest in the problem, leading to increased knowledge of the extent to which the disease or health problem affects the community. Frequently, city, county, or state health departments and federal agencies will develop projects and health programs to control or prevent the disease or health problem.

While epidemiologists may sometimes be involved with assessing the health status of individual patients, that work is incidental to their primary concern, which is the community, or group experience. The status of the community requires epidemiologists to summarize their findings by grouping data for both ill and nonill persons. Summary data are presented in terms of rates, ratios, and percentages. A clear understanding of the definition, uses, limitations, and implications of these terms is important in interpreting epidemiologic data answering questions such as:

1. How much disease is present in the community?
2. Who has the disease?
3. What factors contribute to the frequency and distribution of a disease in a population?
4. Has a proposed solution been effective in controlling or preventing a health problem?

I.   CATEGORIES OF MEASUREMENT

A.   RATES

A rate measures the occurrence of some particular event during a given time period, in a population at risk. The form is

$$x/y \quad \cdot \quad k \text{ per unit of time}$$

In a rate, all the events counted as (x) are derived from the population at risk (y). Thus, the mortality rate indicates the total number of deaths (x) occurring in a given population or community (y) during a specified period of time, usually expressed as deaths per 1000 (or 10,000 or 100,000) population (k) per year.

Generally, the properties of rates may be summarized:

1. Rates are a statement of the risk of developing a condition.
2. Rates are not necessarily predictive for an individual in the group.
3. Rates may have predictive value for the group providing that no unusual changes in host, agent, or environment occurred that would affect the steady state of those components.

B.   RATIOS

A ratio expresses a relation between a numerator (x) and a denominator (y) in which the events or items counted as (x) are not necessarily derived from (y). The form is

$$\frac{x}{y}$$

where

x is the number of events or items counted and NOT NECESSARILY A PORTION of y,

y is the number of events or items counted and NOT NECESSARILY A POPULATION of persons exposed to the risk.

A base (as in the case of a rate), usually 1 to 100 when expressing ratios, and a period of time (either an interval or an instant in time) may be used if appropriate to the ratio.

When we are unable to formulate rates but still need a summary statistic to give us an impression of risk, other statistics including ratios may be substituted. Used in this way the statistic is termed an index.

C.   PROPORTIONS

A proportion is an expression in which the numerator is always included in the denominator. In a sense, a rate might be considered to be a proportion, insofar as the numerator is included in (and, therefore, derived from) the denominator. However, a rate must include the period of time over which the events occurred. Proportions other than rates do not require that time be included, although the period of time may be indicated if it is appropriate.

II.   MISLEADING NUMBERS

A.   INAPPROPRIATE NOMENCLATURE

Although we have gone to some lengths to stress the definition of the above terms and to suggest the clarity of thought and specificity of terms that epidemiologists employ, we shall now demonstrate inconsistencies with which you must contend.

1.   Maternal Mortality Rate

The maternal mortality rate is concerned with maternal deaths related to pregnancy and child-bearing. Without looking at any textbook, write an expression for the maternal mortality rate.

The definition of the maternal mortality rate is:

$$\frac{\text{Deaths from puerperal causes during pregnancy within 90 days of delivery or completion of pregnancy in a calendar year}}{1000 \text{ live births in that calendar year}}$$

The denominator obviously excludes all pregnancy events which do not result in a live birth (stillbirths, induced abortions, spontaneous abortions (miscarriages) and ectopic pregnancies). But maternal deaths occurring as a result of these excluded pregnancies WOULD be counted in the numerator. Thus, the denominator is not actually an expression of the population at risk of all pregnancy, but merely a convenient and readily available statistic to which maternal deaths can be related. The maternal mortality rate, therefore, is really a RATIO. However, due to the extent of common use of the term, it usually is called the maternal mortality rate, although the more appropriate term "ratio" should be used.

Question 1

a. Why are some categories of pregnancy excluded from the denominator?

b. What is the effect of using a denominator limited to live births?

2. Infant Mortality Rate

The infant mortality rate is concerned with infants (children < 1 year of age) who die from any cause. Without looking at any textbook, write an expression for the infant mortality rate.

The definition of the infant mortality rate is

$$\frac{\text{deaths under 1 year of age from any cause during a calendar year}}{1000 \text{ live births in that calendar year}}$$

This "rate" is not actually a true rate but is really a ratio. To understand why consider the hypothetical illustration of births and infant deaths in a 2-year period of time as shown in Figure 1.

Figure 1.   Conceptions, births and deaths in a hypothetical population, Feb. 1979-Jan. 1981.

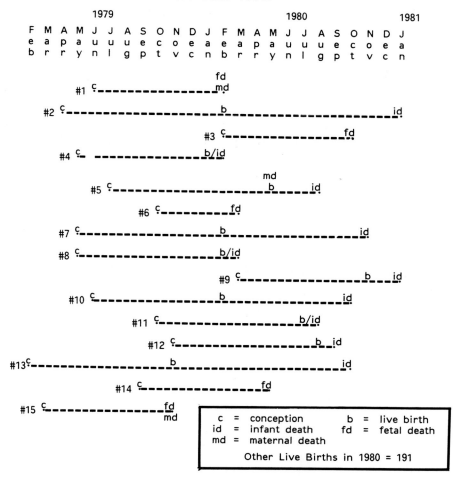

Question 2

Calculate the following:

a.   Total number of infant deaths for the period Feb. 1979-Jan. 1981.

b.   Total number of infant deaths occurring in 1980.

c.   Total number of children born in 1980 who also died in 1980.

d.   Infant mortality rate for 1980:

e.   The actual risk of death to an infant born in 1980 is not accurately measured by the infant mortality rate for that year. Why is this so?

f.   How could the infant mortality rate be computed so that it was a true rate rather than a ratio, i.e., the actual risk of death of an infant born in a certain year is obtained?

g.   What would be a difficulty with the new computation?

From these examples it is clear that there may be unexpected surprises in accepting the term "rate" at its face value. While the definition of rate and ratio will, in general, follow the expected format, you should CAREFULLY EVALUATE THE NUMERATOR AND DENOMINATOR OF EVERY FORMULA TO DETERMINE WHETHER THE DEFINITION ACCURATELY IDENTIFIES THAT STATISTIC AS A RATE OR RATIO. In time, you will become familiar with many of the commonly used formulas in epidemiology and the distinction between rates and ratios will become clear. However, when a new formula is encountered, it is important to determine whether it is a rate or ratio, so that you can draw the correct conclusion regarding the risk of the disease or health problem in the population being described. The manner in which a statistic is calculated is important to its correct interpretation.

From discussion of the maternal mortality and the infant mortality measures it should be clear that some health statistics may be used to describe a situation or health problem for which it is inappropriate or insensitive. Thus, the information conveyed by them may be difficult to interpret correctly. In instances where the most appropriate denominator cannot be easily obtained an epidemiologist may find it necessary to use the best available substitute denominator, and in some situations it might be necessary to <u>invent</u> a <u>new rate</u> or <u>ratio</u> when those in current use are not appropriate to the situation. When reading or reviewing health data, strive to develop your ability to distinguish whether the statistics used are appropriate to the health problem being presented.

Of special importance is the necessity for you to determine the source of the data being presented and the purpose for which they were collected, e.g., routine health or legal records, specific surveys or examinations performed to answer an "epidemiologic" question. If the data are specific to the intended use, there will usually be little problem in interpretation, but if the data were collected for other purposes, then they may sometimes be inappropriate to answer the question the investigator has raised.

B.   IMAGINARY NUMBERS

In epidemiology, rates, ratios, and numbers are used in describing groups of people. Therefore, it is as necessary to understand how to interpret rates and numbers as it is to know how to compute them.

The following article raises the issue of the inappropriate use of numbers as well as pointing out three important questions to be considered with regard to numbers, percentages, or rates of any kind:

(1) What is the denominator? Is it or isn't it the same population at risk from which the numerator came?

(2) How was the count taken? What are the reporting problems, such as the problem for the "rate of unemployment" mentioned in the article?

(3) What period of time is involved? How long is the period of observation or the duration of exposure of the population?

Of Imaginary Numbers

In the cloudland of higher mathematics, there is a whole area of study called "imaginary numbers." What is an imaginary number? It is a multiple of the square root of minus one. What is the good of knowing that? Imaginary numbers, according to mathematicians, are useful in figuring out such problems as the flow of air or water past a curved surface like an airplane wing.

In ordinary life, imaginary numbers of a somewhat different kind seem to have become even more useful. From solemn public officials and eager corporations, from newspapers, television (and even, some dare say, from newsmagazines) comes a googol of seemingly definitive and unarguable statistics. They tell us, with an exactitude that appears magical, the number of heroin addicts in New York and the population of the world. By simulating reality, they assure us that facts are facts, and that life can be understood, put in order, perhaps even mastered.

If this sounds fanciful, consider a few specimens from one issue of the New York <u>Times</u> last week:

BANGKOK: In 1965, only 17% of the people in northeastern Thailand were within a day's journey of a main road. Today the figure is 87%.

NEW YORK: The St. Patrick's Day parade cost the city $85,559.61, whereas Puerto Rico Day cost only $74,169.44.

ATLANTA: There are 1.4 million illiterates in the U.S.

KABUL: Caravans traveling between Afghanistan and Pakistan "commonly carry up to 1,200 pounds of opium at a time."

In assuredly reporting these statistics, the <u>Times</u>--like all other journalistic enterprises--is carrying on a tradition founded by Archimedes. He set himself the task of computing the number of grains of sand that could be encompassed within the area of the known universe. After a great deal of figuring, accompanied by many diagrams, he produced an answer that satisfied him. (It mattered not that his data on the universe were wrong.)

The tradition flourishes today at many levels. It has been computed, for example, that the offspring of 450 moths can eat the weight of a diesel locomotive in one year. And that the average housewife washes 2.5 million kitchen utensils during her lifetime, the equivalent of a stack of dishes 70 times as high as the Empire State Building. And that 9.2 billion strokes of a cat's back would generate enough electricity to light a 75-watt bulb for exactly one minute.

These statistics may well be true, and so may most of the <u>Times</u>'s figures--but obviously some are truer than others. A census of illiterates in an advanced, well-documented country carries considerably more conviction than a report from the remote corners of Thailand. Nobody is really sure exactly how many people there are in Thailand, after all, much less the distance that one of them can travel in a day, so the margin for error is presumably considerably larger than a precise figure like 17% implies. What makes such numbers imaginary is that most of them are basically collections of someone's estimates of the unknowable. We can assert with some confidence that there are, say, four birds on a branch. As the numbers get larger, we still believe in them, but with less reason.

In almost any area of life today, the best--certainly the most honest-- answer to a request for figures would be: Nobody knows. But that makes us feel that somebody has failed at his job; there must be a right answer, therefore a right answer is composed. Last week the Federal Government's Center for Disease Control announced that a certain drug company may have infected 5,000 hospital patients with contaminated intravenous solutions, contributing to the deaths of 500 people. When asked how this figure had been determined, a Government spokesman said that one estimate of 2,000 was "unrealistic" and another estimate of 8,000 was "unfair." So the authorities split the difference.

Imaginary numbers sound true--that is their function, after all--and so they may serve the cause of truth. But they can serve the purpose of falsehood just as well. At the highest levels of government, imaginary numbers can delude even the shrewdest of leaders with "quantifications" of reality. For years, the Pentagon demanded imaginary numbers from combat troops in Viet Nam: body counts, kill ratios, and even computations of the numbers of obscure villages that were free from Viet Cong control (to a certain percentage). With the figures produced, the computers could declare with statistical certainty that the war was being won. "Is it a coincidence," asks Arthur M. Ross, former U.S. Commissioner of Labor Statistics, "that the most elaborately measured war in American history is also the least successful?"

It is not that the figures are falsified, but that we create the figures we want to believe. If the numbers game involves fears and prejudices, imaginary numbers reinforce the prejudice, heighten the fear. Since many heroin addicts in New York commit crimes to buy drugs, to cite one example, it has often been stated that the addicts steal $2 billion to $5 billion worth of goods per year. Max Singer, president of the Hudson Institute, decided to inquire how the figure came to be computed. It turned out, as he reported in The Public Interest, that someone had multiplied an estimated 100,000 addicts by an estimated average habit of $30 per day to determine a collective need of $1.1 billion a year. And since a thief generally sells stolen property to a fence for about one-quarter of its value, four times $1.1 billion produces a theoretical total of $4.4 billion. Singer found, however, that the value of all the stolen goods in New York does not amount to nearly that much, and that the drug addicts probably take property worth about one-tenth of the popularly accepted figure. Conversely, then, there may not be 100,000 drug addicts in New York after all (Singer guesses 70,000 at most), but only in our nightmares.

If every statistic were regarded with similar skepticism, it might well be found that many of our most widely accepted figures are also, at least in part, imaginary numbers. The national rate of unemployment, for example, is now stated to be 5.6%, but that figure is based entirely on people who officially reported themselves out of work. Idle students, housewives who cannot find outside jobs, unsuccessful artisans--such people are not counted.

Statistics on crime are equally uncertain, since they mainly reflect police diligence in rounding up minor offenders and reporting all arrests. Then there are those "police estimates" that name a figure for the unknowable number of prostitutes in Los Angeles or the uncountable crowds outside the White House. If present figures are imprecise, beware of all projections that foretell the future, particularly those that talk of the increasing youthfulness of the "average American." Actually, because both birth and death rates have declined, the "average American" is getting older.

Is nothing, then, to be believed? Yes--the evidence of the senses and the observations of the mind, but not too many of the imaginary numbers that try to provide proof. How many is "not too many"? The computer is working on that.

Source: Otto Freidrich, 1964; reprinted by permission of Time magazine.

III. MEASUREMENT OF MORBIDITY, MORTALITY, AND NATALITY

A. MORBIDITY

Morbidity pertains to the sickness, disease, or disability within specific populations. The most commonly used measures include point prevalence, period prevalence, incidence, and attack rates. The distinctions between measures of prevalence and incidence are emphasized because these terms are among the principal measures encountered in epidemiologic and other public health reports. When expressed as rates time and place must always be specified.

1. Prevalence

Prevalence measures the frequency of all current cases of disease in a population at a specified time. Current cases include those previously diagnosed in other years and those diagnosed in the current year, or at the time of your survey or examination. Prevalence is of two types:

   a. POINT PREVALENCE: Point prevalence measures the frequency of all current cases of a disease at a given instant in time.

   b. PERIOD PREVALENCE: Period prevalence measures the frequency of all current cases of disease in a specified period of time.

2.   Incidence

Incidence measures the development of a disease or health problem in a population, i.e., the frequency of NEW cases in the population at risk during a
specified period of time.

   a.   ATTACK RATE: An attack rate is an incidence rate (usually expressed as a percent), used for exposed populations observed for limited
   periods of time, such as during an epidemic.

Question 3

A mathematical relationship exists between the incidence (I) and prevalence (P)
of a given disease.   Use the space below to explain that relationship.   Attempt
to write a mathematical expression for the relationship if you can.

Question 4

a.   Incidence rates and prevalence ratios tell different stories about the same
   health condition.   Which statistic provides the most useful information
   about the risk of illness?   Explain your opinion.

b.   Why would incidence data be helpful to a health agency administrator?

c.   Why would prevalence data be helpful?

Calculation of Incidence and Prevalence

Formulas for the most commonly used prevalence and incidence measures may
be found in Figure 13, at the conclusion of this exercise.

Question 5

A class has 100 students enrolled. During the month of October, some of the students became ill with sore throat. Calculate rates for sore throat in this class based on the following:

On 30 September, 5 of the students who attended class reported sore throat. All of them continued to be ill on 1 October but recovered within 3 days. On 14 October, 10 students had sore throat and 4 of them were absent due to illness. During October, 30 different students had sore throat and 8 of them were absent due to illness. None of these students was ill at the beginning of the month.

Calculate:

a.   A point prevalence rate:

b.   The period prevalence ratio:

c.   The incidence rate of sore throat for October:

Question 6

In a hypothetical survey of serum enzyme values in a group of 60 middle aged golfers, the results shown in Figure 2 were obtained.

a.   Calculate the frequency and cumulative frequency for each serum enzyme value and enter in columns (c) and (d).

Exercise 3-14

Figure 2. Distribution of serum enzyme values in golfers.

Serum enzyme values (a)	Number of golfers with this value (b)	Frequency percent (c)	Cumulative frequency percent (d)	Age in years	
				40-49 no.	>50 no.
30-34	2			2	0
35-39	3			2	1
40-44	6			4	2
45-49	9			4	5
50-54	12			7	5
55-59	10			4	6
60-64	9			5	4
65-69	7			3	4
70-74	2			2	0
Total	60			33	27

b.   Assuming 44 to be the upper limit of normal, calculate the age-specific prevalence ratios of elevated serum enzymes in golfers.

(1) 40-49 years

(2) >50 years

Using various measurement techniques, the status of tuberculosis in the United States in 1972 will be studied from data in Figure 3.

Definitions of Terms in Figure 3:

New Active case: active case of tuberculosis occurring for the first time this year and never before reported in any other year.

Reactivated case: active case of tuberculosis occurring this year, which in previous years had been active and then been diagnosed as inactive.

In the study of infectious diseases, a distinction is made between infection and disease.   Infection means that a person has been exposed to an infectious agent that has invaded the body of that person, however, the person does not exhibit any evidence of illness. Disease means that an infected person exhibits evidence of clinical illness.

Figure 3.   Selected information about tuberculosis, U.S., 1972.

Category	Numbers
U.S. Population	
July 1, 1972	208,232,000
Active TB cases on Register Jan. 1	44,000
Reactivated cases during 1972	3,500
New active cases reported during 1972	32,882
New active cases with contacts identified	18,768
TB deaths (provisional) among new active cases	4,550
Contacts of new active cases identified during year	145,890
Household contacts	54,522
Nonhousehold contacts	91,368
Contacts examined among those identified during year	132,061
Household contacts	49,401
Nonhousehold contacts	82,660
Contacts infected among those examined during year	28,280
Household contacts	14,383
Nonhousehold contacts	13,897
New active cases among contacts examined during year	1,150
Household contacts	819
Nonhousehold contacts	331

Source: Tuberculosis Programs, 1972, U.S. Dept. of HEW, Tuberculosis Program Reports, Nov., 1973.

Question 7

Calculate the following rates and ratios of tuberculosis (per 100,000 population) from Figure 3.

a.   Incidence in 1972

b.   Point prevalence of active cases on January 1, 1972

c.   Period prevalence of active cases for 1972

d.   New active case rate in 1972

e.   Tuberculosis death rate in 1972

f.   Provisional TB case fatality rate in 1972

Question 8

a.   Why is there a difference between the incidence rate of TB and the new active rate?

b.   Why do TB reports exclude reactivated cases and those active on Jan. 1 from the denominator when calculating the new active case rate?

c.   Why is the case-fatality rate difficult to interpret?

d.   What do the measurements you have calculated suggest about the control or prevention of tuberculosis?

e.   What other information would you need to better understand the epidemiology of tuberculosis?

Question 9

a.   Complete Figure 4 for household (HH) contacts and nonhousehold (NH) contacts using data from Figure 3.

b.   Summarize the findings you calculated in Figure 4.

Exercise 3-17

Figure 4. Household and nonhousehold contacts of TB cases, U.S., 1972.

	Percent type of contact of total identified (a)		Number of contacts identified per new active case (b)		Percent examined of contacts identified (c)		Percent infected of contacts examined (d)	
	HH	NH	HH	NH	HH	NH	HH	NH
Numerator								
Denominator								
Rate per 100 or percent								

Question 10

a. Calculate the secondary attack rate for household and nonhousehold contacts. (This rate is defined in Figure 13.)

HH rate =

NH rate =

b. What is the implication of these rates for a tuberculosis control program?

c. Difficulty is encountered in defining the denominator for the secondary attack rate. Although it should include all exposed persons, not all exposed persons were examined. If one were to use a denominator of all exposed persons regardless of whether they were examined or not, what assumptions would have to be made?

d. What subgroup of the total population is excluded from the denominator in the calculation of the secondary attack rate?

e. Why did fewer NH contacts develop TB when more of them were at risk?

f.   What does the disparity between the percent infected among NH and HH contacts examined suggest about the disease?

g.   Calculate the ratio of infecteds to secondary cases for:

   Households:
   Nonhouseholds:
   What does this ratio suggest about control effectiveness?

B.   MORTALITY RATES

Mortality rates measure the frequency of deaths within specific populations for a specified time interval and place.

Question 11

a.   In 1970, there were 1,920,312 deaths in the U.S. and a midyear population estimated at 203,210,158. The death rate for 1970 was 9.44 per 1000. This is referred to as the CRUDE MORTALITY RATE. Why?

b.   In 1974, there were 165,812 deaths in Colombia, South America, and a midyear population estimated at 21,595,000. The crude mortality rate for Colombia was 7.67 per 1000. Does this correctly imply that Colombians have a lower risk of death than residents of the U.S.?

c.   How might the death rates of the U.S. and Colombia be compared to give a better idea about which country has the higher risk of death?

Case-Fatality Rate

The case-fatality rate is concerned with persons (cases) who die from a particular disease. Without looking at any textbook, write an expression for the case-fatality rate.

The Definition of the case-fatality rate is:

$$\frac{\text{deaths assigned to a particular disease}}{\text{number of cases of the disease}} \text{ per specified time period} \times 100$$

Question 12

a. What information is conveyed by this rate?

b. How is the interpretation of the rate affected when considering acute short illness such as infectious diseases compared to chronic diseases of long duration?

c. Calculate the deaths-to-cases ratio for Figure 5.

Figure 5. Estimated new cases and deaths for major cancer sites, U.S., 1981.

Site	No. of cases	Deaths	Deaths-to-cases ratio
Lung	122,000	105,000	
Colon-Rectum	120,000	54,900	
Breast	110,900	37,100	
Uterus	54,000	10,300	
Prostate	70,000	22,700	
Oral	26,600	9,150	
Skin (melanoma)	14,300	6,700	
Leukemia	23,400	15,900	
All sites	815,000	420,000	

Source: Cancer facts and figures, American Cancer Society, 1981.

d. What information does the deaths-to-cases ratio provide? Why is it an inappropriate statistic for studying the lethality of cancer? What would be a better measure?

C.   NATALITY RATES

Natality rates measure the frequency and the probability of births within specific populations and are calculated for a given time interval and place. A variety of measures relating to fertility and population growth have also been proposed. Most fertility rates are more commonly used by demographers than by epidemiologists. However, they may be useful in epidemiology when estimates of the population size are needed for intercensal years.

<u>Question 13</u>

The crude birth rate is defined as

$$\frac{\text{number of live births per calendar year}}{\text{midyear population}} \quad \text{per 1000}$$

a.   Why is this called the crude birth rate?

b.   Suggest a modification of the denominator of the crude birth rate that would be appropriate for epidemiologic uses.

c.   Is the birth rate an adequate statistic to determine the overall change in population size in a given period of time?   Explain.

IV.   DENOMINATORS: USING MIDYEAR POPULATION VS. PERSON-TIME UNITS

Many rates use the midyear population as the denominator. The midyear population is estimated as the arithmetic average of those alive and present on January 1 and December 31 of the year being observed. Thus, on average, all persons in the midyear population will have been present for one year. The denominator of a rate in which the midyear population at risk is estimated at 2 million persons could also be expressed as 2 million person-years of risk. By convention the midyear population is rarely expressed as person-years of risk even though it is implied.

Underlying the use of the midyear population are two assumptions: first, that all persons estimated to be in the midyear population are present for the same amount of time (i.e., one full year); second, that the change in population (either increase or decrease) occurred uniformly throughout the year. In many situations, neither of the assumptions is correct. Persons in the population may be present and/or exposed for varying lengths of time during a calendar year, and therefore they may not actually be at risk for certain types of events for the entire period (this is true particularly for occupational exposures in the workplace). Thus, to calculate the most accurate rates, the actual period of time that each person in the population was present and at risk should be determined and incorporated into the denominator.

Another problem with rates that use the midyear population is that they may not reflect the duration of the exposure or the incubation period of the disease. In diseases that require cumulative exposure of long duration or that have long and uncertain incubation periods (15-25 years for leprosy and some cancers), or diseases with very slow development between the initial and the end stage of the disease (tuberculosis), the usual incidence measures do not actually reflect the rate at which disease develops. Incidence rates that use the midyear population as the denominator express the proportion of the population with newly developed disease in any given year, but they do not relate the disease to the period of time during which the disease develops. Several modifications of the denominator are possible to remedy this problem: the denominator could be defined as the estimate of the midinterval population; or it could be defined as the number of persons present at the time of exposure. A useful modification of the denominator could also reflect the period over which new cases of disease develop. One could compute the number of persons and their years of exposure of all members who were present for all or any portion of the specified interval. Frequently, this is an impossible task and the midyear population is used as the denominator because it is more convenient and easier to determine, even when studying the risk of diseases with long exposure time or incubation periods.

Computation of the time at risk is done by calculating and adding the days, weeks, months, or years each individual in the study population was at risk. The denominator of the rate is expressed in terms of person-time units. Rates using person-time units are usually expressed per 100 or 1000 person-time units. Person is a nonspecific term that can refer to men, women, children, etc. Time units may be expressed as hours, days, weeks, months, or years. For example, in a study population composed of 1000 persons observed for varying lengths of time, during which 30 cases of disease occurred:

200 persons observed for 1 month	=	200 person-months of observation
500 persons observed for 6 months	=	3000 person-months of observation
300 persons observed for 11 months	=	3300 person-months of observation
TOTAL: 1000 persons observed	=	6500 person-months of observation

To calculate the disease rate for this example, the numerator (x) is the number of cases (30) that occurred among the 1000 individuals while they were under observation. The denominator (y) is 6500 person-months or 6500/12 = 541.67 person-years of exposure.

To convert this example to a rate, it must correspond to the form

$$x/y \cdot k, \quad \text{or} \quad (30/541.67)\,1000 = 55.4 \text{ per 1000 person-years.}$$

Rates calculated in person-time units are also very useful in situations in which patients die or are unable to be followed until the completion of the desired period of observation or follow-up, or if they have periods of illness and illness-free intervals during the calendar year or specified time.

Question 14

a.   What problem is there in interpreting the following person-year measures?

     30 persons followed for 20 years = 600 person-years of risk
    600 persons followed for 1 year   = 600 person-years of risk

b.   What problem is presented in interpreting the risk of tuberculosis for a person who contributed 30 years of exposure compared to someone contributing 5 years?

c.   A total of 10 meetings were scheduled for a club with 100 members for December.   A total of 15 persons missed one meeting each.   Due to faulty lighting in the room many persons had headaches at different times.   A total of 30 people reported 65 instances of headaches during the meetings for the entire month.

    Calculate headache attack rates for December using a denominator of person-time units of exposure and another rate using the number of club members as the exposed population.

d.   When might illness rates calculated in person-time units be advantageous?

The following data from a tuberculosis study give the experience in White and Black families during the observation period according to the sputum status of the index case in each family.

Question 15

a. Calculate the family-years of observation for Figure 6a and enter it in the space for sputum-positive Whites in Figure 6b.

Figure 6a. Family-years of observation.

Number of families in the study at each observation period	Years of observation	Family-years observed
305	1	305
150	2	300
100	3	
100	4	
98	5	
95	6	
TOTAL FAMILY-YEARS OBSERVED		

Figure 6b. New cases of TB, deaths from TB, and deaths from all causes among White and Black household contacts.

Event	Character of index case							
	Sputum positive				Sputum negative			
	White		Black		White		Black	
	No.	Rate	No.	Rate	No.	Rate	No.	Rate
Family-years observed			1316		7122		751	
New cases	18		27		17		5	
TB deaths	5		22		5		2	
Deaths, all causes	29		44		60		11	

Source: Puffer, R.R., et al. Tuberculosis in household associates. Am. Rev. Tuberculosis 52:89, 1945. Reproduced with permission of the American Review of Respiratory Disease.

b. Calculate the rates in Figure 6b based on the denominator of family-years observed for each column.

c.   What are your conclusions about the relationship between the positivity of
      the sputum of the index case, and the TB attack rates and death rates?

d.   Why would Black/White differences in family size be important to consider?

V.   STANDARDIZATION--DIRECT AND INDIRECT ADJUSTMENT OF RATES

In a previous problem, comparison of the crude death rates for Colombia and
the U.S. yielded an unexpected conclusion. In this section you will learn how
and when to adjust or standardize rates so that more useful comparisons of
data from differing populations can be performed.

Question 16

Complete the calculation for Figure 7.

Figure 7. Population distribution and deaths for Arizona and Alaska, 1970.

Age in years	Arizona				Alaska			
	Deaths	Population		Death rate per 1000	Deaths	Population		Death rate per 1000
		Number	Percent of population			Number	Percent of population	
<15	1,028	538,480			236	103,004		
15-44	1,629	728,363			388	149,964		
45-64	3,839	341,956			436	40,699		
≥65	8,358	162,094			368	6,715		
Total	14,854	1,770,893			1,428	300,382		

Source: 1970 Census of the Population. U.S. Volume I--Characteristics
          of the Population; Part 4--Arizona; Part 3--Alaska. Vital
          Statistics of the United States--1970. Volume II, Mortality,
          Part B, Table 7-3.

Question 17

a.   What interpretation would you give to these data?

b. Why does a difference in the age structure of these two states make it preferable to standardize the rates before making further comparisons?

c. Epidemiologists commonly will age-adjust or standardize crude rates. In general, what condition must prevail so that it is necessary to adjust or standardize for age or other factors?

The two most common types of adjustment are termed the direct method and the indirect method.

The Direct Method

To age-adjust using this method, a commonly available standard population of known age distribution should be selected, for example, the U.S. population for 1970.

Complete Figure 8 by calculating the expected deaths for Arizona (columns a x b) and Alaska (columns a x d) based upon the standard population distribution of the U.S. in 1970. The age-specific death rates can be obtained from your calculations in Figure 7.

Figure 8.   Expected number of deaths in Arizona and Alaska based upon the U.S., 1970 standard population.

Age in years	Standard population (USA-1970) (a)	Arizona		Alaska	
		Age-specific death rate per 1000 (b)	Expected deaths (c)	Age-specific death rate per 1000 (d)	Expected deaths (e)
<15	58,017,845				
15-44	83,270,951				
45-64	41,820,193				
≥65	20,101,169				
Total	203,210,158				

Source: 1970 Census of Population, U.S. PC(1)-D1. Table 189.

Question 18

a. To calculate the age-adjusted rates, add the expected deaths for each state [columns (c) and (e)]. Divide the expected total deaths in each state by the total standard population of the U.S. The age-adjusted death rate per 1000 of

        Arizona = ____   Alaska = ____

b.   What information does the age-adjusted rate convey?

c.   Are adjusted rates real or artificial numbers, i.e., should they be considered real estimates of actual risk?

d.   What steps are performed when calculating an age-adjusted rate by the direct method?

The Indirect Method

It is not possible to use the direct method where adjustment may be necessary but deaths by age group in the population are not known; in such cases the indirect method is used. The following problem illustrates how to perform the indirect method of adjustment. Calculate the crude death rates and compare the proportional age distributions to establish that age-adjustment is necessary. Then calculate the U.S. age-specific death rates per 1000 in Figure 9; then complete Figure 10 to get the expected number of deaths in Colombia.

Figure 9. Population distributions and mortality by age for Colombia, South America, 1974, and the U.S., 1970.

Age in years	Colombia			United States			
	Population			Population			
	number	percent of total	deaths	number	percent of total	deaths	Age-specific death rate per 1000
<5	3,780,000	17.5	n.a.	17,115,336	8.4	86,215	
5-14	5,932,000	27.5	n.a.	40,902,509	20.2	16,847	
15-44	9,714,000	44.9	n.a.	83,270,951	40.9	157,071	
45+	2,169,000	10.1	n.a.	61,921,362	30.5	1,660,179	
Total	21,595,000	100.0	165,812	203,210,158	100.0	1,920,312	

                Crude death rate =   Crude death rate =
                      per 1000   per 1000

n.a. = not available.

Figure 10. Calculation of expected deaths in Colombia if U.S. rates are applied.

Age in years	Colombian population	Age-specific death rate per 1000 in the U.S.	Expected deaths in Colombia
<5			
5-14			
15-44			
45+		_____	
Total		_____	

Source:
1. U.S.A. 1970 Census of the Population, Table 189, PC(1)-D1.
2. Vital Statistics of the United States--1970, Vol. II, Mortality, Part B, Table 7-3.
3. 1974 Colombian Health Sector Analysis. US AID/Colombia, pp. 10, 15, 16.

Question 19

a.   Calculate the age-adjusted rate by dividing the total expected deaths in Colombia by the total population of Colombia. The age-adjusted death rate is _____.

Age-adjustment using the indirect method also enables us to calculate the STANDARDIZED MORTALITY RATIO (SMR). To calculate the SMR simply divide the observed deaths for Colombia by the expected deaths in that country. SMRs are expressed as if the expected number of deaths was equal to 100. Thus to calculate the SMR for Colombia, simply multiply the ratio of observed to expected deaths by 100.

b. $\dfrac{\text{observed deaths in Colombia}}{\text{expected deaths in Colombia}}$ × 100   =

c.   What does an SMR greater than 100 mean?

d.   What does an SMR less than 100 mean?

e.   In what circumstances would it be necessary to use the indirect rather than the direct method to adjust rates?

f.   What are the steps necessary to calculate an age-adjusted rate using the indirect method?

g.   In Exercise 2 the examples of leukemia in Nebraska farmers, breast cancer in female relatives of nurses, and Guillain-Barre Syndrome, included an expected number of cases or an expected rate of disease for each situation. How can an expected number of cases or the expected rate of disease be computed?

VI.   RELATIVE RISK AND ATTRIBUTABLE RISK

One of the important tasks of epidemiologists is to make a statement about the degree of risk in a population. Until now we have used incidence, prevalence, crude and specific rates, and ratios to express the actual or estimated risk in a population.

The rates and ratios whose denominators are a population at risk are measures of ABSOLUTE RISK that do not distinguish illness among those exposed from illness due to exposure. For example, some smokers may develop lung cancer from cigarettes or from other causes as well. Thus, measures of absolute risk do not provide a direct answer to one of epidemiology's basic questions, which is, how much excess disease a factor such as smoking might produce in the population or how much of the disease might be prevented. To make these determinations epidemiologists calculate ATTRIBUTABLE AND RELATIVE RISK and the ATTRIBUTABLE RISK PERCENT for a factor related to or believed to be a cause of the disease. Calculations may be from either mortality or morbidity rates of the disease. For the purpose of this exercise relative and attributable risk for the disease lung cancer and the factor smoking will be illustrated using mortality rates. You should be aware that some authors use the term "risk ratio" to refer to relative risk, and "risk difference" to refer to attributable risk.

RELATIVE RISK is defined as:

$$\frac{\text{death rate from lung cancer among persons EXPOSED (smokers)}}{\text{death rate from lung cancer among persons NOT EXPOSED (nonsmokers)}}$$

ATTRIBUTABLE RISK is defined as:

death rate from lung cancer among persons EXPOSED (smokers) MINUS the death rate from lung cancer among persons NOT EXPOSED (nonsmokers).

The ATTRIBUTABLE RISK PERCENT is the attributable risk divided by the rate among exposed persons, expressed in percent:

$$\frac{\text{death rate among exposed MINUS death rate among nonexposed}}{\text{death rate among exposed}} \quad X \quad 100$$

Relative risk, attributable risk, and the attributable risk percent may be computed from the hypothetical data for a 1-year period, for alcoholism and tuberculosis, presented below in the form of a 2 X 2 table (sometimes referred to as

Exercise 3-29

a fourfold table). The numbers in each of the four cells refer to the number of individuals who may be classified according to the designated categories.

	persons with TB	persons without TB	Total
alcoholics	40	10	50
teetotalers (nondrinkers)	10	90	100

Incidence rate of tuberculosis for alcoholics = 40/50 × 100 = 80 per 100/year

Incidence rate of tuberculosis for teetotalers = 10/100 × 100 = 10 per 100/year

A. Relative risk = 80 per 100 / 10 per 100 = 8.0

B. Attributable risk = 80 per 100 minus 10 per 100 = 70 per 100 per year

C. Attributable risk percent =

$$\frac{80 \text{ per } 100 \text{ minus } 10 \text{ per } 100}{80 \text{ per } 100} \times 100 = \frac{70}{80} \times 100 = 87.5\%$$

Thus,

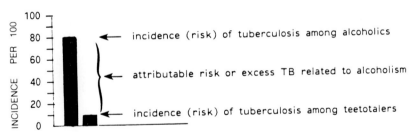

Question 20

What is the essential difference between attributable risk and relative risk and of what value are these statistics in disease prevention?

Question 21

Is the statement of relative risk a rate or a ratio?

Doll and Hill sent questionnaires on smoking habits to all of the 59,600 physicians in the United Kingdom in October 1951. Usable replies were received from 40,701 physicians, 34,494 men and 6,207 women. The respondents were followed for 4 years and 5 months by obtaining notifications of physicians' deaths from the Registrars General, the General Medical Council and the British Medical Association. For every death certified as due to lung cancer, confirmation was obtained by writing to the physician certifying the death and also, when necessary, to the hospital or consultant to whom the patient had been referred. Some of the results are shown in Figure 11.

Figure 11.   Standardized death rates per year per 1000 physicians aged 35 years or more, in relation to the most recent amount smoked.

Cause of death	No. of deaths	Death rate among men					
		All men	Non-smokers	All smokers	By daily average of cigarettes smoked		
					1-14	15-24	25 or more
Lung cancer	84	0.81	0.07	0.90	0.47	0.86	1.66
Other cancer	220	2.02	2.04	2.02	2.01	1.56	2.63
Other respiratory diseases	126	1.10	0.81	1.13	1.00	1.11	1.41
Coronary thrombosis	508	4.78	4.22	4.87	4.64	4.60	5.99
Other causes	779	6.79	6.11	6.89	6.82	6.38	7.19
All causes	1,714	15.48	13.25	15.78	14.92	14.49	18.84

Source: Doll, R., and Hill, A.B. Brit. Med. J. 2:1071, 1956.

Question 22

Complete Figure 12 by calculating the relative risk, attributable risk, and attributable risk percent of smoking, for deaths from lung cancer, coronary thrombosis, all causes, and for lung cancer by smoking dose from the data in Figure 11. What do your calculations indicate about the importance of smoking to the various causes of death given in the table?

Exercise 3-31

Figure 12. Risk assessment, smokers vs. nonsmokers, for selected causes of death, British physicians, 1951.

Cause of Death	Relative Risk	Attributable Risk per 1000	Attributable Risk Percent
Lung Cancer Death Rate per 1000			
Smoker Nonsmoker			
0.90 0.07			
Coronary Thrombosis Death Rate per 1000			
Smoker Nonsmoker			
4.87 4.22			
All Causes Death Rate per 1000			
Smoker Nonsmoker			
15.78 13.25			
Lung Cancer Death Rate per 1000			
1-14 cig Nonsmoker			
0.47 0.07			
Lung Cancer Death Rate per 1000			
15-24 cig Nonsmoker			
0.86 0.07			
Lung Cancer Death Rate per 1000			
25+ cig Nonsmoker			
1.66 0.07			

Question 23

How do you assess the importance of the following situations:

a. Relative risk greatly in excess of 1.0; low absolute risk (low incidence rate)--a rare disease.

b. Relative risk slightly in excess of 1.0; a common disease having a high
    incidence rate.

c. Relative risk slightly in excess of 1.0; attributable risk is low to medium.

d. Relative risk greatly in excess of 1.0; attributable risk percent greater
    than 60.

e. Relative risks below 1.0.

VII. DEFINITION OF FORMULAS

Figure 13. Frequently used rates, ratios, proportions, and indices for describing natality, morbidity, and mortality.

Name of rate or ratio	Variations of presentation	Numerator (x)	Denominator (y)	Expressed per number at risk (k)

Death rate	1. Crude rate
	2. Specific rates by:
	  cause
	  age
	  race
	  sex
	  occupation
	  other
		Total number of deaths reported during a specified time interval.	Estimated mid-interval population	As desirable
				per 1,000
				per 10,000
				per 100,000

Birth rate	1. Crude rate
	2. Specific rates for:
	  maternal age
	  sex of child
	  race
	  marital status
	  other
		Number of live births reported during a specified time interval.	Estimated mid-interval population.	1000

Fertility rate		**Theoretical**		
		Number of live births reported during a specified time interval from mothers aged 15-44 years.	Estimated number of women in age group 15-44 years at midinterval.	1000
		In general use		

	1. Crude rate
	2. Specific rates for:
	  maternal age
	  race
	  socioeconomic
	    status
	  other
		Number of live births reported during a specified time interval.	Estimated number of women in age group 15-44 at midinterval.	1000

Low birth weight ratio	1. Crude rate
	2. Specific rates for:
	  maternal age
	  race
	  socioeconomic
	    status or
	    area
	  other
		Number of live births under 2,500 grams (or 5½ lbs) during a specified time interval.	Number of live births reported during the same time interval.	100

Figure 13 (continued)

Name of rate or ratio	Variations of presentation	Numerator (x)	Denominator (y)	Expressed per number at risk (k)

Incidence rate	1. Crude rate by cause
	2. Specific rates by:
	  age
	  race
	  sex
	  socioeconomic status
	  stage of disease
	  other
		Number of new cases of a specified disease reported during a specified time interval.	Estimated mid-interval population at risk.	As desirable:
				per 100
				per 1,000
				per 10,000
				per 100,000
				per 1,000,000

Attack rate	1. Crude rate by cause
	2. Specific rates by:
	  age
	  race
	  sex
	  socioeconomic or residence area
	  other
		Number of new cases of a specified disease reported during a specified time interval.	Susceptible population at risk during the same time interval.	As desirable:
				per 100
				per 1,000
				per 10,000
				per 100,000
				per 1,000,000

Secondary attack rate	1. Crude rate by cause
	2. Specific rates by:
	  age
	  race
	  sex
	  households
	  families
	  other
		Number of new cases of a specified disease occurring within the incubation period of that disease reported following identification of an index case in a household, family or other appropriate epidemiological unit.	Susceptible number of persons exposed to the index case during the same time interval.	per 100
				(usually)

Point prevalence ratio	1. Crude rate by cause
	2. Specific rates by:
	  age
	  race
	  sex
	  socioeconomic status
	  stage of disease
	  other
		Number of current cases of a specified disease existing at a specified point in time.	Estimated population at risk at the same point in time.	As desirable:
				per 100
				per 1,000
				per 10,000
				per 100,000
				per 1,000,000

Figure 13 (continued)

Name of rate or ratio	Variations of presentation	Numerator (x)	Denominator (y)	Expressed per number at risk (k)
Period prevalence ratio, also called case-load ratio	1. Crude rate by cause 2. Specific rates by: age race sex socioeconomic or residence area stage of disease other	Number of current cases of a specified disease existing during a specified time interval.	Estimated mid-interval population at risk.	As desirable: per 100 per 1,000 per 10,000 per 100,000 per 1,000,000
Proportionate mortality ratio	1. Crude ratio 2. Specific ratios by: age race sex socioeconomic status occupation other	Number of deaths assigned to a specified cause.	Total number of deaths from all causes reported during the same interval.	100 or 1000
Case-fatality rate, also called death-to-case ratio	1. Crude rate 2. Specific rates by: age sex race other	Number of deaths assigned to a specified disease.	Number of cases of that disease during the same time interval.	100
Infant mortality rate	1. Crude rate 2. Specific rates by: age of infant race socioeconomic status prenatal care marital status cause of death other	Number of deaths under 1 yr of age reported during a specified time interval, usually a calendar year.	Number of live births reported during the same time interval.	1000
Maternal mortality rate	1. Crude rate 2. Specific rates by: age race cause of death other	Number of deaths within 90 days of delivery, assigned to causes related to pregnancy during a specified time interval.	Number of live births reported during the same time interval.	1000

Figure 13 (continued)

Name of rate or ratio	Variations of presentation	Numerator (x)	Denominator (y)	Expressed per number at risk (k)
		In general use		

Fetal death rate	1. Crude rate
	2. Specific rates by:
	    maternal age
	    race
	    marital status
	    socioeconomic status
	    cause of death
	    other
		Number of fetal deaths of 28 weeks or more gestation reported during a specified time interval usually a calendar year.	Number of fetal deaths of 28 weeks or more gestation reported during the same time interval plus the number of live births occurring during the same time interval.	1000

		(May be used if reporting of early fetal deaths is good)		
		Number of fetal deaths of 20 weeks or more gestation reported during a specified time interval, usually a calendar year.	Number of fetal deaths of 20 weeks or more gestation reported during the same time interval plus the number of live births occurring during the same time interval.	1000
		In general use		

Fetal death ratio (this is sometimes mistakenly termed the fetal death rate)	1. Crude rate
	2. Specific rates by:
	    maternal age
	    race
	    prenatal care
	    socioeconomic status
	    cause of death
	    other
		Number of fetal deaths of 28 weeks or more gestation reported during a specified time interval.	Number of live births reported during the same time interval.	1000

		(May be used if reporting of early fetal deaths is good)		
		Number of fetal deaths of 20 weeks or more gestation reported during a specified time interval.	Number of live births reported during the same time interval.	1000

Neonatal mortality rate	1. Crude rate
	2. Specific rates by:
	    maternal age at birth
	    race
	    socioeconomic status
	    birth weight
	    cause of death
	    other
		Number of deaths under 28 days of age reported during a specified time interval, usually a calendar year.	Number of live births reported during the same time interval.	1000

Figure 13 (continued)

Name of rate or ratio	Variations of presentation	Numerator (x)	Denominator (y)	Expressed per number at risk (k)

Perinatal mortality rate	1. Crude rate
	2. Specific rates by:
	  maternal age
	  race
	  prenatal care
	  socioeconomic status
	  cause of death
	  other
		In general use
		Number of reported fetal deaths of 28 weeks or more gestation plus the reported number of infant deaths within 7 days of life during a specified time interval.
			Number of reported fetal deaths of 28 weeks or more gestation plus the number of live births reported during the same time interval.	1000

		(May be used if reporting of early fetal deaths is good) Number of reported fetal deaths of 20 weeks or more gestation plus the reported number of infant deaths within 7 days of life during a specified time interval.	Number of reported fetal deaths of 20 weeks or more gestation plus the number of live births reported during the same time interval.	1000
Postneonatal mortality rate		**Theoretical** Number of deaths from 28 days of age, up to but not including, 1 year of age, reported during a specified time interval, usually a calendar year.	Number of live births reported during the same time interval less the number of deaths under 28 days of age.	1000

	1. Crude rate
	2. Specific rates by:
	  maternal age at birth
	  race
	  socioeconomic status
	  cause of death
		In general use
		Number of deaths from 28 days of age, up to but not including, 1 year of age, reported during a specified time interval, usually a calendar year.
			Number of live births reported during the same time interval.	1000

SUGGESTED RESPONSES
Exercise 3--Assessing Risk

1a. There is great difficulty in enumerating certain pregnancy outcomes. The number of stillbirths can be determined from fetal death certificates but it would require a search of those records, and possibly (nonfetal) death certificates, to discover fetal deaths that may have been misclassified.

Induced abortions are not included since there is not mandatory reporting in all states. Some states have mandatory reporting, but others have voluntary and others such as Texas have no official mechanism for reporting. Before 1973, abortions were illegal in the U.S. and no reliable information is available.prior to that year.

Spontaneous abortions below 20 or 28 weeks of gestation do not require a fetal death certificate. Also, many early pregnancies (below 8-10 weeks) may not be diagnosed and therefore are not detected. Others may not be suspected if the woman has had a history of irregular menstrual periods. Thus, the extent of reporting practices for both induced and spontaneous abortions affects estimates of these pregnancy outcomes.

By agreement, live births are used because they are reliable, easy to obtain, and readily verified.

1b. The denominator is smaller than it would be if all pregnancies were included. Thus, the ratio of maternal deaths to live births is likely to be larger than it would be if outcomes other than live births were also included in the risk estimate.

2a. Infants must be born alive and die within one year of birth to qualify. Deaths in which the baby was not born alive are fetal deaths. There are 10 infant deaths (#2, 4, 5, 7, 8, 9, 10, 11, 12, 13).

2b. There are 8 infant deaths during 1980 (#4, 5, 7, 8, 10, 11, 12, 13).

2c. There are 9 live births during 1980 (#2, 4, 5, 7, 8, 9, 10, 11, 12) who died within their infancy. However, two of these (#2 and #9) died in 1981, leaving a total of 7 births from calendar year 1980 who also died in the calendar year of birth.

2d. The infant mortality rate for 1980 is

$$8/(191+9) \ = \ 8/200 \ = \ 40 \text{ per 1000 live births}$$

2e. One infant who died (#13) in 1980 was not born in that calendar year. Thus, the numerator and denominator of the infant mortality rate do not represent the same birth cohorts.

2f. Infant deaths should be assigned to their appropriate denominators, i.e., the year of birth, even if the baby died in the following calendar year.

2g. Deaths are registered by year of death and not birth (refer to the sample death certificate in Exercise 2). While the death certificate does contain space for the year of birth, that item may not be completed, or may not be accurately recorded. In any event, the new computation would require that birth and death records use 2 calendar years of data in order to correctly assign infant deaths to the year of birth. This would complicate the task of record keeping since data would need to be maintained for 2 years so that deaths in 1980 would be properly assigned to either the 1979 or 1980 birth cohorts, while 1981 deaths could be properly assigned to the 1980 or 1981 birth cohorts. Thus, the expense and difficulty in linking two separate types of vital statistics would complicate the task of collecting and maintaining births and death certificates. Finally, you must recognize that vital registration of births and deaths is not primarily for the purpose of compiling health or epidemiologic data but to provide LEGAL RECORDS. Use of these legal documents (either from the originals or from computerized tapes prepared to protect the confidentiality of individuals) by epidemiologists or health agencies is a secondary purpose. For this reason certain information that might be of great use to epidemiologists and health agencies is not collected.

3. Incidence refers only to new cases of a disease. Prevalence includes both newly discovered and previously diagnosed cases. The number of prevalent cases depends upon the rate of cure or recovery, i.e., how many cases survive the initial episode with complete recovery (cures) or partial recovery. Partial recovery may be manifested by the continuous, chronic persistence of disease or by intermittent episodes of the illness. In years following the initial (incident year) onset, persons with chronic or intermittent disease are considered to be known (old or previously diagnosed) cases, and some will die of their disease. In epidemiologic terms, the prevalence of a disease (P) reflects the Incidence (I) and the duration of that disease (D). Mathematically, $P \cong I \times D$.

4a. INCIDENCE implies that people were free of disease at the start of the observation period but developed disease during the period. Incidence is a more useful measure of risk because it measures the development of disease and thus is a true rate (x disease derived from y persons at risk). PREVALENCE describes the amount of disease in the population at a point in time or during an interval. Prevalence does not measure the rate of development of disease and is more properly termed a ratio. "Usefulness" is a relative term because either statistic can be informative in a variety of situations depending upon your need and the availability of data.

4b. Increasing incidence rates might provide clues to the etiology of a disease if we were able to determine what exposures occurred prior to the disease onset. Decreasing incidence rates might be due to the benefits of disease control or prevention programs. Increasing rates might indicate failure or ineffectiveness of the current programs, or changes in host or agent characteristics.

Rising incidence rates might suggest the need for a new disease control or prevention program or that reporting practices had improved or diagnostic procedures were more sensitive to the presence of the disease (better case-finding).

4c. Prevalence measures would help to estimate the magnitude of health problems and identify potential high risk target populations.

5a. In all calculations be sure to remember the k term and EXPRESS IT.

On October 1:   5 per 100   On October 14:   10 per 100

5b. For the period October 1-10, 15 per 100 (5 old cases present on 1 October, 10 new cases were present on 10 October). For the month of October the period prevalence ratio is 35 per 100.

5c. The incidence rate is 30 ÷ 95 (5 were ill in September) or 31.6 per 100.

6a. The table for question 6 should look like this.

Figure 2. Distribution of serum enzyme values in golfers.

Serum enzyme values (a)	Number of golfers with this value (b)	Frequency percent (c)	Cumulative frequency percent (d)	Age in years	
				40-49 no.	>50 no.
30-34	2	3	3	2	0
35-39	3	5	8	2	1
40-44	6	10	18	4	2
45-49	9	15	33	4	5
50-54	12	20	53	7	5
55-59	10	17	70	4	6
60-64	9	15	85	5	4
65-69	7	12	97	3	4
70-74	2	3	100	2	0
Total	60			33	27

6b. 1. The prevalence ratio for 40-49 is 25/33 × 100 = 75.8 per 100.
     2. The prevalence ratio for >50 is 24/27 × 100 = 88.9 per 100.

7a. <u>incidence</u>

$$\frac{\text{New active} + \text{reactivated cases in 1972}}{1972 \text{ population} - \text{those with TB}} = \frac{32,882 + 3,500}{208,232,000 - 44,000} \times 100,000 = 17.5 \text{ per } 100,000$$

7b. <u>point prevalence</u>

$$\frac{\text{Existing cases on Jan. 1, 1972}}{\text{total population, on survey date (if known) or midyear population}} = \frac{44,000}{208,232,000} \times 100,000 = 21.1 \text{ per } 100,000$$

7c. <u>period prevalence</u>

$$\frac{\text{Old} + \text{reactivated} + \text{new cases}}{\text{person-years of observation (or the mid-year population) during the period}} = \frac{44,000 + 3,500 + 32,882}{208,232,000} \times 100,000 = 38.6 \text{ per } 100,000$$

7d. <u>new active case rate</u>

$$\frac{\text{New active cases}}{\text{total population} - \text{those with TB} - \text{reactivated cases}}$$

$$\frac{32,882}{208,232,000 - 44,000 - 3,500} \times 100,000 = 15.83 \text{ per } 100,000$$

In the event that the above denominator cannot be calculated, the total mid-year population can be used and the rate would be the usual form seen in the TB reports:

$$\frac{32,882}{208,232,000} \times 100,000 = 15.79 \text{ per } 100,000$$

7e. <u>tuberculosis death rate</u>

$$\frac{\text{deaths}}{\text{person-years of observation or midyear population during the calendar year}} = \frac{4,550}{208,232,000} \times 100,000 = 2.2 \text{ per } 100,000$$

7f.   <u>provisional case-fatality rate</u>

The ideal rate:

$$\frac{\text{TB deaths}}{\text{New active} + \text{reactivated}} = \frac{4,550}{32,882 + 3,500} \times 100 = 12.5 \text{ per } 100$$
$$\text{cases} \qquad \text{cases}$$

The usual calculation of the rate:

$$\frac{\text{TB deaths}}{\text{new active cases}} = \frac{4,550}{32,882} \times 100 = 13.8 \text{ per } 100$$

8a.   Reactivated cases are included in incidence rate but not the new active case rate.

8b.   It is done for ease in calculation. The number of reactivated cases is actually an estimate. It is a small number compared to the denominator, and does not affect the rate much one way or another. Also, it is hard to clear Registry files of all nonactive cases. It takes a lot of time and money to do that accurately.

8c.   The numerator only takes deaths from new cases into account and ignores the possible effect of the duration of the disease. One may be at highest risk of dying from TB the longer one has it. The case-fatality rate should reflect prevalent cases (old and new) not just the incidence (new) cases. This example is unusual because the provisional deaths are limited to new active cases, whereas deaths from cases occurring in prior years are usually included in calculating this rate.

8d.   New cases of disease still occur, but the number of deaths (2.2/ 100,000) appears low. This suggests a chronic disease of long duration. The point prevalence ratio and new active case rates of 21.1 and 15.8/100,000, respectively, indicates that old cases contribute more to period prevalence than new ones. However, both types of cases make a sizable contribution, which means that TB control programs must be concerned with finding new cases and with surveillance of old ones over a long period of time.

8e.   Trend data, rates by age, sex, race, geographic region, mode of transmission, secondary attack rates, and other data to describe the disease in terms of person-place-time or characteristics of host-agent-environment or factors related to host susceptibility and exposure would be useful.

9a.

Figure 4.   Household and nonhousehold contacts of tuberculosis cases, U.S., 1972.

	Percent type of contact of total identified (a)		Number of contacts identified per new active case (b)		Percent examined of contacts identified (c)		Percent infected of contacts examined (d)	
	HH	NH	HH	NH	HH	NH	HH	NH
Numerator	54,522	91,368	54,522	91,368	49,401	82,660	14,383	13,897
Denominator	145,890	145,890	18,768	18,768	54,522	91,368	49,401	82,660
Rate per 100 or percent	37.4	62.6	2.9	4.87	90.6	90.5	29.1	16.8

9b.   It is more difficult to find cases among nonhousehold contacts. From a cost-effectiveness viewpoint, case finding is easier and more productive if efforts are concentrated among household contacts.

10a.

$$SAR = \frac{\text{\# contacts developing the disease within the incubation period}}{\text{Total \# susceptible and exposed persons (contacts) examined}} \times 1000$$

$$HH = \frac{819}{49,401} = 16.6 \text{ per } 1000 \qquad NH = \frac{331}{82,660} = 4.0 \text{ per } 1000$$

10b. The data suggest that case finding is more efficient if efforts are concentrated on household contacts.

10c. It would be assumed that those not examined developed the disease at the same rate as those who were examined.

10d. Index cases, those who introduce the disease into the household, are excluded.

10e. The quality of contact with the index case was probably different for NH members. NH contacts with the primary case probably involve less time in closed rooms or in close proximity, than contacts of family members with the primary case.

10f. Infection is more likely to occur among HH members. Exposure probably occurs more often and perhaps HH members receive a larger dose than NH contacts. However, both HH and NH percentages show that most contacts with cases do not develop infection. Various factors of the environment or the host resistance play a role in determining whether or not a person becomes infected.

10g. HH = 14,383/819 = 18 to 1   NH = 13,897/331 = 42 to 1
      NH are at less risk of developing disease.

      Infection with TB does not necessarily produce disease (illness). If
      infection is treated properly (prophylaxis) it usually can prevent the
      infection from progressing to a clinical case. Nonhousehold contacts have
      a higher infected-to-case ratio than household contacts, i.e., it takes 42
      NH compared to 18 HH infecteds to produce one active case of disease.
      If priorities must be established household contacts should be treated
      first.

11a. The crude rate is a summary statistic for an entire population. The rate
      is called a crude rate because we have no idea of the types of people who
      died, the types and distribution of causes of death, or the composition of
      that population: the proportions of young and old or males and females.

11b. The crude death rate of Colombia is lower than the U.S. This is sur-
      prising given the economic status of Colombia. The populations of Colom-
      bia and the U.S. differ in the percentage of young and old, males and
      females, and other demographic characteristics. In the U.S., most deaths
      are due to chronic illness, which occurs in older persons, while in less
      developed nations, a large percentage of deaths is caused by infectious
      diseases among infants and young children. The crude death rate does
      not accurately reflect the risk of death when populations have large
      differences demographically.

11c. We should compare age-specific death rates for each country. By con-
      vention, we group ages into 5 or 10 year age groups: 0-4, 5-9, 10-14,
      etc., or 0-9, 10-19, 20-29, etc. Infants are frequently separated from
      the youngest age group due to the unusual risk associated with birth and
      early life; thus a special category of < 1 year is often used.

      A second set of techniques is termed adjustment or standardization of
      rates. These techniques allow you to eliminate the differences in rates
      that occur because the two populations have different proportions of
      persons with a characteristic known to influence the risk of disease.
      Age, sex, social class, and occupation are attributes for which data are
      sometimes standardized.

12a. The case-fatality rate indicates the lethality or deadliness of the disease.
      Some diseases such as lung cancer and pancreatic cancer are very lethal
      while others such as hepatitis and measles are not.

12b. When the deaths are limited to those occurring among new (incident)
      cases of disease in a short period of time, as might occur in acute infec-
      tious diseases of short duration, the calculation of deaths-to-cases would
      represent a true rate if death occurred in the same year the disease
      began.

However, in diseases that do not cause death within a short period of time, for example, chronic diseases, the onset of disease might be in a different year than that in which the death occurred. With regard to case-fatality, someone diagnosed in 1975 would be assigned to the denominator (cases) for 1975. If that person died in 1982 death would be assigned to the numerator in 1982. Thus, numerators and denominators in different years do not necessarily reflect the same cases of illness; therefore, the measure of deaths-to-cases is sometimes a ratio.

12c.

Figure 5. Estimated new cases and deaths for major sites of cancer in the U.S., 1981.

Site	No. of Cases	Deaths	Deaths-to-cases ratio
Lung	122,000	105,000	86.1
Colon-rectum	120,000	54,900	45.8
Breast	110,900	37,100	33.5
Uterus	54,000	10,300	19.1
Prostate	70,000	22,700	32.4
Oral	26,600	9,150	34.4
Skin (melanoma)	14,300	6,700	46.9
Leukemia	23,400	15,900	67.9
All sites	815,000	420,000	51.5

Source: Cancer facts and figures, American Cancer Society, 1981.

12d. The ratio tells us the relative severity of these cancers by site. Lung cancer is the most and uterine cancer the least fatal of those shown. The ratio is inappropriate because the denominator consists of new (incident) cases but the numerator includes deaths from disease which may have been discovered prior to the specified year, 1981. Because cancer patients might not die in the year during which their illness is diagnosed, the numerator contains deaths from "incidence" and "prevalence" categories. The death-to-cases ratio is not a useful statistic for evaluating the survival of persons with cancer. Suppose that a disease kills 50% of new cases within the year of diagnosis and 30% over the next 3 years. Over the period 80% of new cases would have died but it would be impossible to determine this from the ratio because of the way data are tabulated. The ratio underestimates lethality unless the patient dies in the year of diagnosis. Other statistics such as 5-year survival rates are more useful measures. Cause-specific mortality rates by age are also useful when it is not possible to determine the total number of prevalent cases.

13a. The birth rate is not strictly a measure of the probability of birth among the susceptible population at risk, i.e., females of child-bearing ages. In its present form the birth rate underestimates the probability of birth because the denominator includes many who are not at risk and who do not contribute to the numerator; it include males, old persons, and children, who are not "susceptible to" or at risk of giving birth.

13b. Birth rates limited to age-specific categories of women ages 15-45 would be appropriate to define the population at risk. There are also a variety of demographic measures of fertility that have special use in estimating population growth. These measures are covered in any standard text on demography.

13c. The birth rate provides information about part of the reasons for change in population size. A truer measure of population growth should reflect additions minus losses. Thus

$$\frac{(\text{births} + \text{in migration}) \text{ minus } (\text{deaths} + \text{outmigration})}{\text{midyear population}}$$

14a. The total period of observation is the same for both groups but we do not know if persons at risk for a longer time are more likely to get the disease than persons at risk for a short period. The period of exposure necessary to develop a disease differs for many diseases. It is short for most infectious diseases and long for most chronic diseases. Study of chronic illnesses including cancer requires several years of observation to correctly assess risk due to exposure to the suspected agent.

14b. One might assume that the risk of developing disease is constant throughout the observation period. A study in which different birth cohorts entered the observation period (remember the Frost article about the cohort effect) for different periods of time would certainly not have equal risk. A second possibility is if the disease agent became less pathogenic over a period of years or if the population immunity changed over time. Persons observed for the longer period of time would probably have a different disease risk than those with shorter exposure period.

14c. Using person-time units the risk of headaches is

$$65 \ / \ (10 \ \text{X} \ 100) - 15 \ = \ 65/985 \ = \ 66.0 \text{ per 1000 person-classes}$$

Using club members, the risk of headache is

$$65/100 \ = \ 65 \text{ per 100}$$

The rates could also be calculated for the number of persons who became ill. Denominators would be the same but the numerator would be the number of of persons ill (30).

Thus, the rates would be 30/985 = 30.5 per 1000 person-classes or

$$\frac{\text{no. ill}}{\text{exposed population}} \ = \ \frac{30}{100} \ = \ 30 \text{ per 100}$$

14d. Rates expressed in person-time units are useful for conditions in which a person might be ill and not ill one or more times during the same period of observation, or not be present for part of the observation period.

15a.

Figure 6a. Family-years of observation.

Number of families in the study at each observation period	Years of observation	Family-years observed
305	1	305
150	2	300
100	3	300
100	4	400
98	5	490
95	6	570
TOTAL FAMILY-YEARS OBSERVED		2365

15b.

Figure 6b. New cases of TB, deaths from TB, and deaths from all causes among White and Black household contacts.

Event	Character of index case							
	Sputum positive				Sputum negative			
	White		Black		White		Black	
	No.	Rate	No.	Rate	No.	Rate	No.	Rate
Family-years observed	2365		1316		7122		751	
New cases	18	7.6	27	20.5	17	2.4	5	6.7
TB deaths	5	2.1	22	16.7	5	0.7	2	2.7
Deaths, all causes	29	12.3	44	33.4	60	8.4	11	14.6

15c. Sputum-positive cases are more likely to transmit infection and death rates are higher than for sputum-negative cases. Regardless of race, the phenomenon is the same whether one uses attack rates or death rates to compare them.

15d. More people are exposed in large families. Blacks tend to have larger families and lower incomes than Whites. Closeness of contact and factors associated with low socioeconomic status are important in the spread of tuberculosis.

16.

Figure 7.   Population distribution and deaths for Arizona and Alaska, 1970.

Age in years	Arizona				Alaska			
	Deaths	Population		Death rate per 1000	Deaths	Population		Death rate per 1000
		Number	Percent of popu- lation			Number	Percent of popu- lation	
<15	1,028	538,480	30.4	1.91	236	103,004	34.3	2.29
15-44	1,629	728,363	41.1	2.24	388	149,964	49.9	2.59
45-64	3,839	341,956	19.3	11.23	436	40,699	13.5	10.71
≥65	8,358	162,094	9.2	51.56	368	6,715	2.3	54.80
Total	14,854	1,770,893	100.0		1,428	300,382	100.0	

17a. The total (crude) death rate is higher in Arizona than Alaska. Because the age distribution is different for these states (there is a higher pro- portion of older persons in Arizona) the crude rates are not suitable for comparison.   The age-specific rates can be compared but they do not indicate whether the two states have similar proportions of males and females in each age group.

Alaska has higher age-specific death rates for those below age 45 and above age 65.   The crude death rates give an erroneous impression concerning the risk of death in the two states because of differences in the age structure of the population in these states.

17b. Because mortality is correlated with age, the crude death rates in states (or countries) with a high proportion of older persons will disproportion- ately emphasize the older age groups when comparisons are made with states (or countries) having a lower percentage of old persons.   The problem may also be present if comparisons are to be made for two popu- lations selected from hospitals, medical records, or other sources in which the age distributions differ.

17c. Age is not the only factor that might need to be adjusted.   Adjustment would also be necessary IF THE TWO POPULATIONS DIFFER in their proportions of males/females, smokers/nonsmokers, urban/rural residence, severe/nonsevere illness, etc., IF THE CHARACTERISTIC IS KNOWN TO BE ASSOCIATED WITH THE HEALTH OUTCOME being studied.

In other words, when comparisons are made between populations, those populations should be as similar as possible with regard to factors related to the disease, i.e., compare apples to apples rather than apples to oranges.   Unfortunately, epidemiologists cannot control the age, sex, place of residence, etc., of human populations.   Adjustment techniques permit epidemiologists to mathematically eliminate the major differences in the disease-related characteristics (<u>confounding</u> <u>variables</u>) of the two populations.

18a.

Figure 8. Expected number of deaths in Arizona and Alaska based upon the U.S., 1970 standard population.

Age in years	Standard population (U.S.-1970) (a)	Arizona		Alaska	
		Age-specific death rate per 1000 (b)	Expected deaths (c)	Age-specific death rate per 1000 (d)	Expected deaths (e)
<15	58,017,845	1.91	110,814	2.29	132,861
15-44	83,270,951	2.24	186,527	2.59	215,672
45-64	41,820,193	11.23	469,641	10.71	447,894
≥65	20,101,169	51.56	1,036,416	54.80	1,101,544
Total	203,210,158		1,803,398		1,897,971

The age-adjusted rates are Arizona = 1,803,398/203,210,158 × 1000 = 8.87 per 1000; Alaska = 1,897,971/203,210,158 × 1000 = 9.34 per 1000.

18b. It represents the expected number of deaths divided by the total U.S. population, per 1000. The adjusted rate eliminates the age differences between the two populations and shows us what would happen to the death rate in these populations if both groups had the same age structure as the standard population.

18c. Adjusted rates are artificial numbers that do not represent the actual rates of death (or other health outcome) for these populations. Adjustment is performed to eliminate the effect of differences in age (or other important characteristics) between populations that we wish to compare.

18d. 1.   Select a standard population of known age distribution.

2.   Calculate age-specific death rates for two populations to be compared.

3.   Calculate the expected number of deaths in each of the two populations by multiplying the age-specific rates by the number of persons in that age group for the standard population.

4.   Add the expected number of deaths calculated for each of the two populations and divide by the population of the standard population.

Figure 9. Population distributions and mortality by age for Colombia, South America, 1974, and the U.S., 1970.

Age in years	Colombia			United States			
	Population			Population			Age-specific death rate per 1000
	number	percent of total	deaths	number	percent of total	deaths	
<5	3,780,000	17.5	n.a.	17,115,336	8.4	86,215	5.04
5-14	5,932,000	27.5	n.a.	40,902,509	20.2	16,847	0.41
15-44	9,714,000	44.9	n.a.	83,270,951	40.9	157,071	1.89
45+	2,169,000	10.1	n.a.	61,921,362	30.5	1,660,179	26.81
Total	21,595,000	100.0	165,812	203,210,158	100.0	1,920,312	

n.a. = not available.

Crude death rates per 1000 are:

Colombia = 165,812/21,595,000   = 7.68 per 1000

U.S.   = 1,920,312/203,210,158 = 9.45 per 1000

Figure 10. Calculation of expected deaths in Colombia if U.S. rates are applied.

Age in years	Colombian population	Age-specific death rate per 1000 in the U.S.	Expected deaths in Colombia
<5	3,780,000	5.04	19,051
5-14	5,932,000	0.41	2,432
15-44	9,714,000	1.89	18,359
45+	2,169,000	26.81	58,151
Total	21,595,000		97,993

19a. The age-adjusted death rate for Colombia is 97,993/21,595,000 × 1000 = 4.5 per 1000. This is the death rate Colombia would be expected to have if the age distribution of Colombia was similar to the U.S.

19b. SMR = observed/expected deaths × 100 = 165,812/97,993 × 100 =169.2

19c. An SMR greater than 100 means that the standardized ratio has an excess of mortality compared to the amount expected. In the above example, Colombia had a 69.2% excess mortality (169.2/100) compared to the U.S.

19d. An SMR below 100 means that the observed mortality is below that expected. In Exercise 2, comparison of observed and expected mortality among Mormons and non-Mormons was expressed in relation to unity (1.0). The observed/expected death rates could have been modified in order to present them as SMRs. Mormons would have an SMR below 100.

19e. The indirect method of adjustment is useful in two situations: first, when the age-specific death rates are known for only one of the populations to be compared; second, when the number of persons in an age group is very small, so that the death rates might show large fluctuations due to the inclusion or exclusion of a few deaths. Thus, the indirect method might also be useful in mortality studies where a limited number of observations or cases is available for study.

19f. 1. Apply the age-specific death rates for a standard population to the number of persons in each age group of another population to determine the expected number of deaths for each age group.

2. Add the expected number of deaths to obtain the total.

3. Divide the total expected deaths by the total population to obtain the adjusted death rate.

4. To convert to an SMR divide the observed by the expected number of deaths and multiply by 100.

19g. The expected number for any age is merely the age-specific rate multiplied by the number of individuals in the age group of interest.

20. Attributable risk is the difference between the rates of disease in exposed and unexposed populations. The relative risk is the ratio of the rates in exposed and unexposed populations.

Attributable risk describes the excess rate of disease above the "baseline" of disease that would be present if the population had not been exposed to the factor of interest. The relative risk is an index of the strength of association. Thus, a relative risk of 2:1 would indicate that the exposed population had double the rate of disease found among nonexposed persons. When the relative risks are 2:1, 3:1, 4:1 an epidemiologist would speak of 2-fold, 3-fold, 4-fold, etc. differences.

21. The form is the ratio of the rates.

22.

Figure 12. Risk assessment, smokers vs. nonsmokers, for selected
causes of death, British physicians, 1951.

Cause of death	Relative risk	Attributable risk per 1000	Attributable risk percent
Lung Cancer Death Rate per 1000			
Smoker Nonsmoker			
0.90 0.07	12.86	0.83	92.2
Coronary Thrombosis Death Rate per 1000			
Smoker Nonsmoker			
4.87 4.22	1.15	0.65	13.4
All Causes Death Rate per 1000			
Smoker Nonsmoker			
15.78 13.25	1.19	2.53	16.0
Lung Cancer Death Rate per 1000			
1-14 cig Nonsmoker			
0.47 0.07	6.7	0.40	85.1
Lung Cancer Death Rate per 1000			
15-24 cig Nonsmoker			
0.86 0.07	12.3	0.79	91.9
Lung Cancer Death Rate per 1000			
25+ cig Nonsmoker			
1.66 0.07	23.7	1.59	95.8

22a. Among smokers there is an excess of deaths from lung cancer, coronary
thrombosis, and deaths from all causes. The relative risk is greatest for
lung cancer (a 12-fold difference). The relative risk shows an increase
with more smoking. As the dose increases, the risk of death increases.
This is termed dose-response. The relation between lung cancer and
smoking is one of the most impressive demonstrations of a dose-response
relationship that can be found in epidemiology.

The relative risk in all smokers is 12.86. Among smokers, the relative
risk rises from 6.7 to 23.7 in light and heavy smokers, respectively.

Such high relative risks are rarely seen in epidemiologic studies. Statistics such as these are strong evidence in establishing proof that smoking is a cause of lung cancer. Proving causation will be discussed in more detail in Exercise 9.

The attributable risk shows the death rate occurring due to the presence of the suspected cause. The attributable risk of lung cancer due to smoking shows the rise with increased exposure dose. The data also show that lung cancer and coronary thrombosis death rates comprise over half the death rate attributable to smoking. The attributable risk percent suggests the amount of disease that might be eliminated if the factor under study could be controlled or eliminated. Thus, smoking is calculated to play a role in 92% of lung cancer, 13% of coronary thrombosis, and 16% of all causes of death in the population studied. The attributable risk percent rises from 85 to 92 to 96% as smoking dose increases.

23a. High relative risk suggests a strong association between a disease and a suspected cause; however, if the disease is rare, few people are likely to be affected. An example is thrombophlebitis associated with oral contraceptives.

23b. The relation between smoking and coronary thrombosis is an example of this situation. Although the relative risk is low, it is greater than unity (1.0). Since the disease is very common, there is much potential for benefiting the general level of health in the population.

23c. Both the strength of association and the attributable risk are not very high. The attributable risk percent would also be relatively low, suggesting that not much of the disease could be prevented. The effect on the public's health would depend upon whether the disease was common or rare, or if the disease trend was changing, particularly if increasing.

23d. This is an epidemiologist's dream. The factor is likely to be a cause of the disease. Smoking as a cause of lung cancer is a good example of this situation. Rarely can we show such a clear relationship between a suspected cause and its effect on health. The benefit of eliminating the cause may have either large or small effects on the general level of health in a population depending on whether the disease is common or rare and whether the trend is changing. Fortunately, lung cancer is a relatively uncommon disease despite the large number of smokers, however, it is an important health problem due to its increasing incidence in males and females and the clear demonstration of the etiologic disease agent.

23e. Relative risks below 1.0 suggest that there is no excess of disease due to exposure to the factor being considered, and that disease is not strongly associated with that factor to which the groups were exposed.

EXERCISE 4. PRESENTATION OF DATA

This exercise presents alternative ways to describe the patterns of diseases in populations at risk.

Goals

Upon completion of this exercise you should (1) be familiar with the methods and format of presenting epidemiologic data, (2) be able to distinguish charts, graphs and tables that display data clearly from those that do not, and (3) be able to interpret measurements and graphical displays of epidemiological data.

Methods

In order to achieve these goals you will need to understand:

I. METHODS FOR PRESENTING AND INTERPRETING HEALTH-RELATED DATA*
    A. Tables
    B. Graphs
    C. Charts
    D. Suggestions for the design and use of tables, graphs, and charts.
II. IMPROPERLY PREPARED GRAPHS
III. DIVIDING DATA INTO CATEGORIES
IV. DEPENDENT AND INDEPENDENT VARIABLES

Terms:

Coordinates, axes, independent and dependent variables, histogram, frequency polygon, scatter diagram, bar chart, pictogram, pie chart, flow chart, organization chart, mutually exclusive, qualitative and quantitative variables, discrete and continuous variables, dependent and independent variables.

Suggested Readings

Campbell, S.K. <u>Flaws</u> <u>and</u> <u>Fallacies</u> <u>in</u> <u>Statistical</u> <u>Thinking</u>, Prentice-Hall, Inc., 1974.
Huff, D. <u>How</u> <u>to</u> <u>Lie</u> <u>with</u> <u>Statistics</u>, Norton Publishing Co., New York, 1954.
Bancroft, H. <u>Introduction</u> <u>to</u> <u>Biostatistics</u>. Hoeber and Harper, Inc. New York, N.Y., 1962.
Swaroop, S. <u>Introduction</u> <u>to</u> <u>Health</u> <u>Statistics</u>. E. & S. Livingstone, Ltd., Edinburgh and London, 1960.
Schor, S.S. <u>Fundamentals</u> <u>of</u> <u>Biostatistics</u>. G.P. Putnam's Sons, New York, N.Y., 1968.

---

*Adapted from the monograph, Descriptive Statistics: Tables, Graphs, and Charts, U.S. Department of Health, Education, and Welfare, Public Health Service, Center for Disease Control.

I. METHODS FOR PRESENTING AND INTERPRETING HEALTH-RELATED DATA

Tables, Graphs, and Charts

A. TABLES

Although there are no absolute rules governing table construction, certain general principles have become accepted as more or less standard.

1. Tables should be as simple as possible. Two or three small tables are preferred to a single large table containing many details or variables. Generally, three variables are a maximum number that can be read with ease.

2. Tables should be understandable without reference to text.

   a. Codes, abbreviations, or symbols should be explained in detail in a footnote.
   b. Each row and each column should be labeled concisely and clearly.
   c. The specific units of measure for the data should be given.
   d. The title should be clear, concise and to the point, and should answer the questions: what? when? where?
   e. Totals should be shown.

3. The title is commonly separated from the body of the table by lines or spaces. In small tables, vertical lines separating the columns may not be necessary.

4. If the data are not original, their source should be given in a footnote or in the title.

5. Specific examples.

   a. The simplest table is a two-column frequency table. The first column lists the classes into which the data are grouped. The second column lists the frequencies for each classification. An example is shown in Table 1.

Table 1. Classification of live births by education of father, Anystate, 1968.

Education of father	Number of live births
High school graduate	50,684
Less than 12 years of school	31,774
TOTAL	82,458

Source: "Vital statistics of the United States," 1968, volume 1, p. 81.

Exercise 4-3

Table 1 may be enlarged to include subclassifications, such as place of delivery and attendant at birth, as shown in Table 2.

Table 2. Classification of live births by education of father, place of delivery, and attendant at birth, Anystate, 1968.

| Education of father | Number attended by | | | | Total |
| | Physician | | Midwife | Other and not specified | |
	In hospital	Not In hospital			
High school graduate	46,606	3,014	910	154	50,684
Less than 12 years of school	14,334	3,094	13,930	416	31,774
TOTAL	60,940	6,108	14,840	570	82,458

Source: "Vital statistics of the United States," 1968, volume 1, p. 81.

All tables presenting the same basic data (as do Tables 1 and 2 above) should be checked compulsively to assure that the grand total and the marginal totals agree from one table to another. If they do not agree, the discrepancies should be explained in a footnote.

Table 3. Admissions to any hospital in 1968, classified by age, residence, and sex.

| Age in years | Urban | | | Rural | | | Total | | |
	Male	Female	Total	Male	Female	Total	Male	Female	Total
<1									
1-4									
5-9									
10-14	C								
.									
.									
.									
Total	A			B					

b. Summarization of data will be expedited and simplified by initially preparing a master table. In this table, all available data should be completely classified.

From the general format of a master table as shown in Table 3, we can determine several facts including how many URBAN PERSONS (A), how many MALES (B), and how many URBAN MALES IN A SPECIFIED AGE GROUP (C), were admitted to the hospital.

B. GRAPHS

Definition: A graph is a pictorial display of quantitative data using a coordinate system where x is the horizontal axis and y is the vertical axis.

Although several different types of graphs exist, we will limit ourselves to rectangular coordinate graphs.

1. General Concept

Rectangular coordinate graphs consist of two sets of lines at right angles to each other, each line containing a scale of measurement. Figure 1 presents the general structure of the rectangular coordinate graphs. Generally, the variable assigned to the x-axis (the horizontal axis), is considered the IN-DEPENDENT VARIABLE (method of classification), and the variable assigned to the y-axis (the vertical axis) is the DEPENDENT VARIABLE (frequency or rate of occurrence of some event or other indicator of the risk of disease). In drawing a graph, we plot a change in "y" with respect to "x".

2. General Principles

When graphs have been drawn correctly, they allow the reader to rapidly obtain an overall grasp of the data. Some of the most important principles of graphing are:

a. The simplest graphs are the most effective. No more lines or symbols should be used in a single graph than the eye can easily follow.
b. Every graph should be self-explanatory.
c. The title may be placed either at the top or bottom of the graph.
d. When more than one variable or relation is shown on a graph, each should be differentiated clearly by means of legends or keys.
e. No more coordinate lines should be shown than are necessary.
f. Frequency is usually presented on the vertical scale (y axis) and method of classification on the horizontal scale (x axis).
g. On an arithmetic scale, equal increments on the scale must represent equal numerical units.
h. Scale divisions and the units into which the scale is divided should be indicated clearly.

Figure 1.   General Graph.

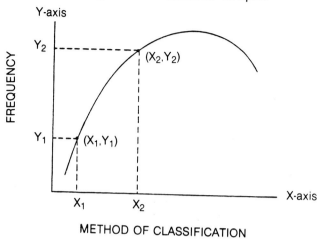

METHOD OF CLASSIFICATION

3.   Specific Examples

a.   Arithmetic Scale Line Graph

An arithmetic scale line graph is one where an equal distance represents an equal quantity anywhere on an axis, although the scales on the two axes may differ.   Care must be exercised in the choice of whether we use equal intervals on both axes, wide intervals on the x axis in relation to the y axis, or vice versa.   The scales should be defined in such a way that the final graph is pleasing to the eye.   A scale break may be used in either axis of a scale line graph, but if used, care must be taken to avoid misinterpretation.   Figure 2 is an example of a line graph.

Figure 2.   Reported rubella case rates by 13 four-week periods, U.S., 1968.

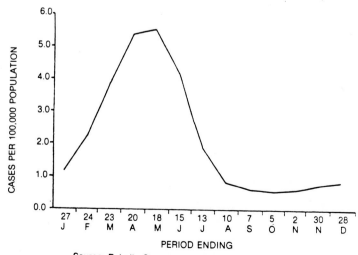

Source: Rubella Surveillance Unit, Center for Disease Control

b.   Semilogarithmic scale-line graph

The semilogarithmic scale-line graph is one where one coordinate or axis, usually the y axis, is measured in logarithms of units, whereas the other axis is measured in arithmetic units.   This is useful when we are inter- ested in the relative (or rate of) change rather than the absolute (actual amount of) change in a series of data over a period of time.   The advan- tages of semilog graphing are:

(1)   a straight line indicates a constant rate of change,
(2)   the slope of the line indicates the rate of increase or decrease,
(3)   two or more lines following parallel paths show identical rates of increase or decrease.

An illustration of this type of graph is shown in Figure 3.

c.   Histogram

A histogram is a graph used only for presenting a frequency distribution of quantitative data.   There is no space between the cells (often referred to as tic-marks) on a histogram.   This graph is not to be confused with a bar chart, which has space between the cells.   A scale break should not

Figure 3. Reported annual incidence rates, death rates, and death-to-case ratios for diphtheria, U.S., 1920-1968.

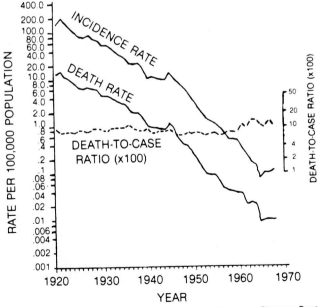

Source: Diphtheria Surveillance Unit, Center for Disease Control

Figure 4. Cases of rash illness, elementary school, sample city, Feb. 22-Mar. 23, 1970.

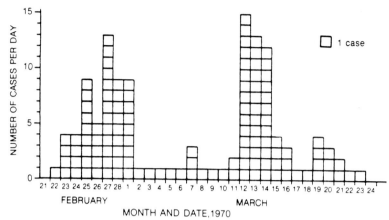

be used in the histogram because the <u>histogram</u> <u>depicts</u> <u>the</u> <u>total</u> <u>area</u> <u>under</u> <u>the</u> <u>curve</u>. Because of this characteristic the easiest type of histogram to construct will be one with equal class intervals as shown in Figure 4.

For illustration, Figure 4 shows the area under the curve partitioned into each case of illness. Ordinarily, only the line representing the height of each column would be drawn and partitioning of cases is not shown.

In order to construct the histogram, we let the y axis (height) represent the number of cases per unit of measurement (number of cases per day) and the x axis (width) be the method of classification (interval of time in days). Therefore, the height times the width will equal the number of cases within a day, just as height times width is equal to the area of a rectangle.

Figure 5. Reported cases of tetanus by five year age groups, U.S., 1968.

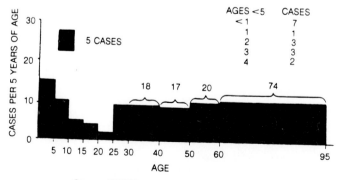

Source: MMWR Annual Supplement, 1968

A histogram with unequal intervals requires more thought in its construction because of the total area concept. Figure 5 has been selected to illustrate this situation. Ages 35, 45, 55, 65, 70, 75, 80, 85, and 90 are omitted because we do not want to imply that the cases per 5 year age group occur uniformly for the omitted ages. Rather, we show the data as a <u>summary</u> or average for 2 or more categories grouped together.

In general, only one set of data should be shown on a histogram; however, it is quite common in public health to present data showing cases-deaths, males-females, etc., by a histogram.

d.   Frequency Polygon

When presenting more than one set of data in terms of a frequency distribution, the data should be presented as a frequency polygon. A frequency polygon is constructed from a histogram by a series of straight lines connecting the <u>midpoints of the class intervals</u>. This is illustrated in Figure 6.

Figure 6. Number of cases of influenza-like illness by week, sample city, 1970.

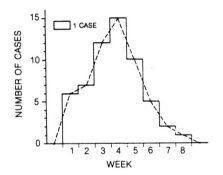

Since a frequency polygon is constructed from a histogram, the rules pertaining to area under the curve will hold. The frequency polygon should be constructed in order to maintain the correct area. This is done by connecting the first and last points with the base of the graph.

Figure 7. Correct method of closing frequency polygon.

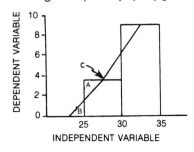

Figure 8. Incorrect method of closing frequency polygon.

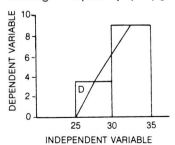

The area in the frequency polygon must be approximately equal to that which would have been in the histogram. Figure 7 shows the correct method of constructing the frequency polygon, while Figure 8 shows the incorrect method.

In Figure 7 the area designated by A would be part of the histogram if data were plotted by histogram. In order to compensate for this area, which is excluded when a frequency polygon is drawn, the point C is connected to the x-axis so that the area designated by B will be approximately equal to area A.

Figure 8 illustrates the incorrect method of closing a frequency polygon because the entire area designated by D is omitted and there is no provision for compensation.

In Figure 9 a frequency polygon having equal class intervals is shown. Additionally, Figure 10 illustrates a frequency polygon with unequal class intervals.

Figure 9. Number of cases of influenza like illness by week, sample city, 1970.

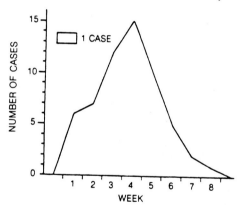

Figure 10. Reported cases of tetanus by 5-year age intervals, U.S., 1968.

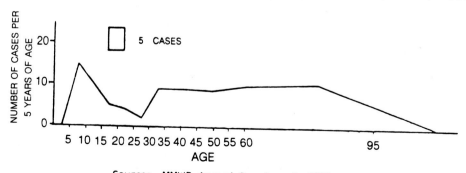

Source: MMWR Annual Supplement, 1968

A frequency polygon illustrating three sets of data is shown in Figure 11.

Figure 11. Reported cases of encephalitis by month and etiology, U.S. 1965.

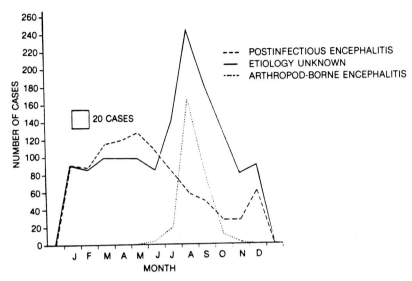

e.   Scatter Diagram

In a scatter diagram a pair of measurements is plotted as a single point
on the graph.   The value of one variable of each pair is plotted on the x
axis, and the value of the other variable is plotted on the y axis.   The
pattern formed by the points represents different pairs and is a function
of the magnitude and nature of the association between the two variables.
The pattern made by the plotted points is indicative of a relation that
might be linear (if they tend to follow a straight line), or curvilinear (if
the pattern does not follow a straight line).   If the pattern is a random
scatter of points, then probably little or no relation exists.   The graph
may depict two measurements made for one individual at different times or
compare measurements made by 2 separate observers.   Figures 12a and b
show scatter diagrams.

Figure 12a.   Relations depicted by scatter diagrams.

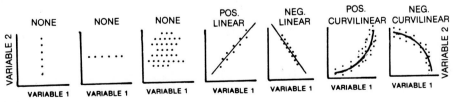

Figure 12b. Histoplasmin skin tests: comparison of two readers, South Carolina, 1963.

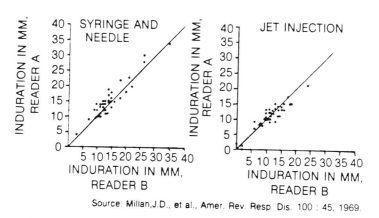

Source: Millan, J.D., et al., Amer. Rev. Resp. Dis. 100 : 45, 1969.

C. CHARTS

Definition: Charts are methods of presenting statistical information pictorially.

Charts can convey many different types of information including length, proportion, geographical distributions, and special relationships.

1. Charts Based on Length

Two of the most important charts are <u>pictograms</u> and <u>bar</u> <u>charts</u> (bar graphs).

a. Pictogram

The pictogram uses a series of small identifying symbols to present the data. The figures are usually arranged horizontally, but may be arranged vertically. Each symbol will represent a fixed number of persons, items, or units. The number of items per symbol is determined by the length of the x axis. Figure 13 illustrates a pictogram with two persons being represented by a symbol.

b. Bar Chart

This kind of chart uses bars all of the same width (unlike the histogram). There are also spaces between the columns (also unlike the histogram). This type of chart is ideally suited for presenting comparative data for discontinuous or discrete variables. The bars may be arranged horizontally or vertically (as illustrated in Figures 14 and 15). It is best to arrange the bars in either ascending or descending order for ease of reading. A scale break should be avoided if at all possible because

breaks may lead to misinterpretation. Bars may be shaded, hatched or
colored, to emphasize differences between them. The bars should not be
labeled within the field of the chart itself, as this may detract from the
visual impact of the chart. When comparisons are made, the space between bars in the same group is optional, but space between groups is
mandatory.

Figure 13. Vaccination status of smallpox cases and deaths, United Kingdom,
1962, and Sweden, 1963.

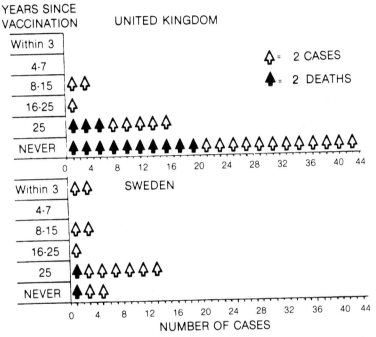

Source: Smallpox Eradification Program, Center for Disease Control, 1963

Figure 14. Death rate per 100,000 from cancer by site, U.S. males, 1974-75.

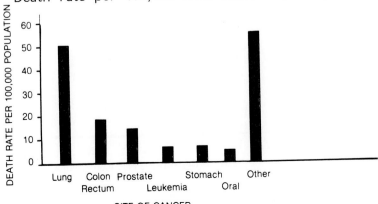

Source: World Health Statistics Annual, 1977-1978.

Continuous variables such as age should not be illustrated by bar graphs. Instead, frequency polygons or histograms should be used because they convey information about the <u>area</u> included within the curve. Also, the categories selected for illustration on the horizontal axis may not be of equal size or importance. Bar graphs should be used only when discontinuous categories of data are presented.

Figure 15.   Annual rate of selected operations in short-stay hospitals, by age and sex per 1000 population, U.S., 1978.

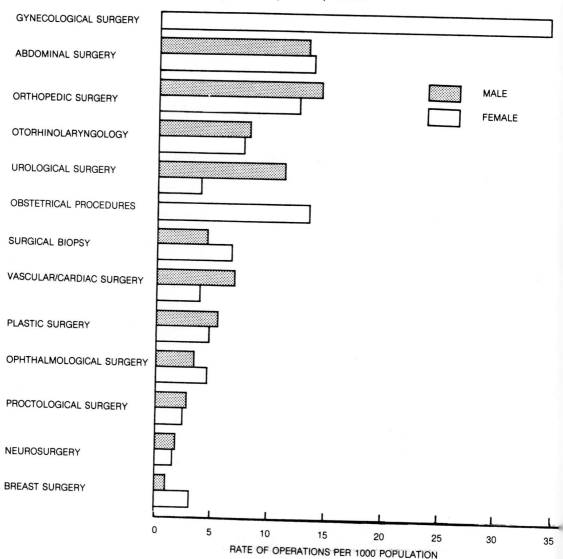

Source: National Center for Health Statistics, <u>Data from the National Health Survey</u>, Series 13, No. 61.   USDHHS, 1982.

2.   <u>Charts Based on Proportion</u>

Two of the most important charts in this category are <u>component bar charts</u> and <u>pie charts</u>.

a.   Component Bar Chart

A component bar chart uses bars that are either colored or shaded to show the relative contribution of each of its components. An example of a component bar chart is given in Figure 16.

Figure 16. Poliomyelitis immunization status for central cities (pop. ≧ 250,000) by age and financial status, U.S., 1969.

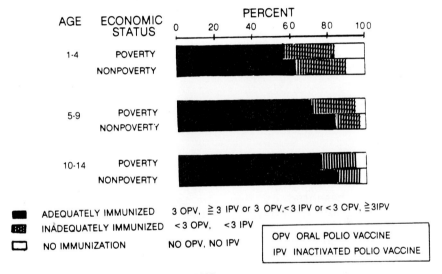

Source: U.S. Immunization Survey, 1969.

b.   Pie Chart

Pie charts use wedge-shaped portions of a circle to illustrate the division of the whole into segments. The convention is to start at the 12 o'clock position and arrange segments in the order of their magnitude, largest first, and proceed clockwise around the chart. To convert from percentage to degrees, multiply the percentage by 3.6°, since 360°/100% = 3.6%. Figure 17 is an example of a pie chart.

Figure 17.   Poliomyelitis immunization status of children age 1-4 in central cities (pop. ≧ 250,000) by financial status, U.S., 1969.

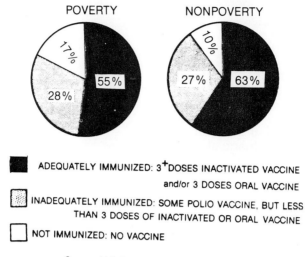

Source: U.S. Immunization Survey, 1969.

3.   Flow Charts

The sequence of a series of events is often illustrated by a flow chart. Materials flowing through a sewage treatment or a water treatment plant can be readily presented by flow charts.   A simple example of food flow through a restaurant is shown in Figure 18.

Figure 18.   Food flow in a restaurant, sample city, 1970.

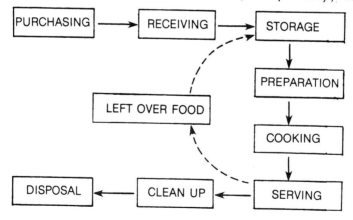

4. <u>Geographic Coordinate Charts</u>

Geographic coordinate charts are those which show the geographic distribution of diseases using maps. Also, percentages showing immunity levels, etc., can be shown in this fashion by distributing the dots in the correct proportions. Figure 19 is an illustration of a geographical coordinate chart.

Figure 19. Counties reporting one or more cases of animal rabies, U.S., 1968.

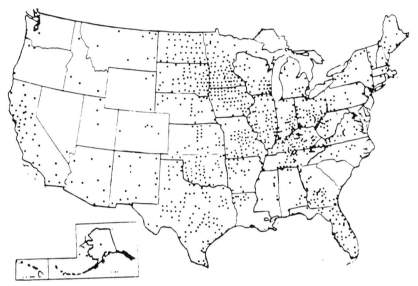

Source: MMWR Annual Supplement, 1968.

D. <u>SUGGESTIONS FOR THE DESIGN AND USE OF TABLES, GRAPHS, AND CHARTS</u>

In conclusion, it would be good to review and reinforce what has been discussed up to this point.

1. <u>Choose the method most effective for data and purpose</u>

Some methods of presentation call for more complete data than others; a few require special configuration of data. Within such limitations, decide upon the precise idea that you wish to communicate, then choose the method: continuous line graphs are suitable for a comparison of trends; bar charts clearly compare separate quantities of limited number; pie charts have advantages in comparing parts to their whole; scatter diagrams are excellent for showing tendency.

2.   <u>Point out one idea at a time</u>

Confine the presentation to one purpose or idea; limit the amount of data
and include only one kind of data in each presentation. Different viewpoints on the information (unless they are being compared) call for separate presentations. So do large quantities of information or various kinds
of information.

3.   <u>Use black and white for exhibits that are to be reproduced</u>

Few copying machines can reproduce color--and all color reproduction is
expensive. Color can be adequately replaced: for areas, by cross-
hatching or dotted fields; for lines, by continuous marks, dots, dashes
(of different length in different lines), or combinations of the foregoing.

4.   <u>Use adequate, properly located titles and labels</u>

Titles should include the "what, where, and when" that completely identifies the data they introduce. All other labels should be clear, complete,
and easy to understand--and, like the title, they should be outside the
frame of the data. Only keys or legends (and these in a neat "box" that
sets them apart from the data) should appear within the field of a graph
or chart.

5.   <u>Give your sources</u>

Where or how (or both) the data were obtained is vital. Verification or
further analysis by readers is difficult if not impossible without full disclosure of sources. Also, access to the original information can prove as
useful to the audience as either the excerpts that you present or the
conclusions that you propose from them.

6.   <u>Use care in proposing conclusions</u>

In particular, draw conclusions that reflect the full body of information
from which excerpted data were taken; propose only such conclusions as
the data that you present can support. But keep in mind that tables,
graphs, and charts emphasize generalities--at the expense of detail.
Compensate for this distortion by careful design of your presentation and
by noting (an asterisk or footnote) in a prominent way any important
detail that has been obscured. Avoid conclusions that do not take such
distortion into account.

<u>Question 1</u>

How might methods of putting information into graphs, charts, and tables influence the interpretation of them?

II.   IMPROPERLY PREPARED GRAPHS

As well as being able to construct a proper graph, one must be able to recognize a bad example when one sees it.   Read the following example:

Daly Jogger of Ozone, Texas, says his times to run a 6-kilometer race were diminishing the more he ran in Ozone compared to his times when he ran in Clear Air, Utah.   He produced a graph to prove it:

Figure 20.

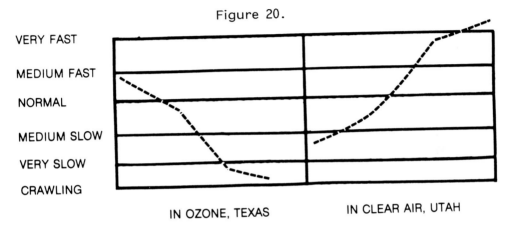

Question 2

What missing items should be included so that the observer is not misled? What other features of this graph might be misleading?

The following figures represent the incidence for diseases A, B, and C in the U.S. from 1960 to 1975.   For each of the figures comment on the pattern of illness.

Question 3

a.   Comment on Figure 21a.

Figure 21a.   Incidence of Disease A in U.S., 1960-1975.

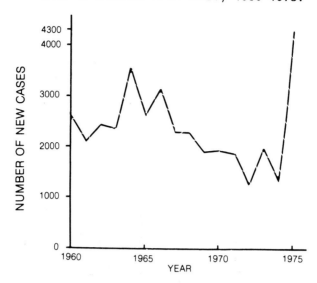

Figure 21b.   Incidence of Disease B in U.S., 1960-1975.

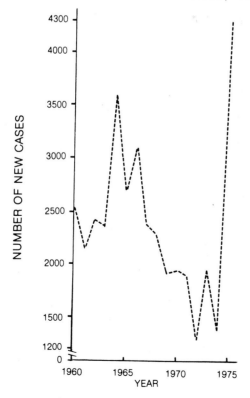

Exercise 4-20

Question 3 (continued)

b.   Comment on Figure 21b.

Figure 21c.   Incidence of Disease C in U.S., 1960-1975.

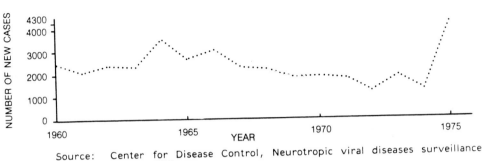

Source: Center for Disease Control, Neurotropic viral diseases surveillance report, 1976.

c.   Comment on Figure 21c.

d.   Diseases A, B, and C depict the same condition, viral encephalitis, except that Figures 21a, -b, and -c show the information in different forms.   How do the axes and the units of measurement of Figures 21b and -c differ from Figure 21a?

e.   Assume that you have been running the viral encephalitis control program for several years.   In your progress report for 1976 you want to include a pictorial representation that emphasizes the success of your adminis- tration.   Which figure would you use and why?

f.   Which of the three figures is correct?   Explain.

Question 4

Here is a graph that presents data on cancer survival.

Figure 22.   Five-year cancer survival rates for selected sites.

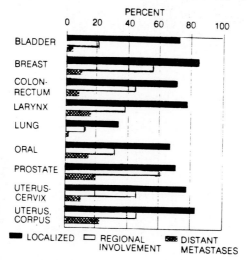

Source: Cancer Facts and Figures, 1981.   American Cancer Society, 1981.

a.   Is this graph complete?   What more (if anything) should it contain?

b.   What does this graph suggest to you?

c.   If you had money for a cancer program, what would you recommend, based on the information presented in this chart?

Exercise 4-22

Question 5

The following graphs show data presented in different ways for different reasons.

Figure 23a. Frequency distribution of visit rates for husbands and wives.

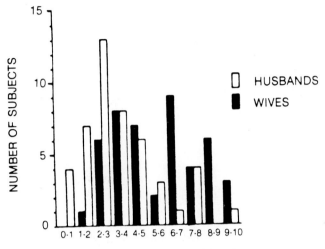

a.   What kind of graph is Figure 23a?

b.   Are the classes on the x axis clearly defined and easily distinguishable?

c.   What kind of graph is Figure 23b?

d.   Make a frequency polygon out of Figure 23b.

e.   When is the frequency polygon preferable to the histogram?

Now examine the data for husbands shown below.

Figure 23b.   Frequency distribution of visit rates for husbands.

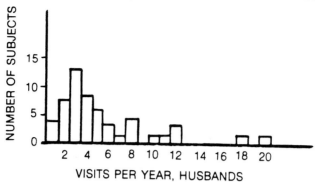

Source: Chien, A., and Schneiderman, L.J.,   A comparison of health care
          utilization by husbands and wives, J. Comm. Health 1: 118, 1975.

III.   DIVIDING DATA INTO CATEGORIES*

When a mass of data is to be presented, there is always a problem of how to
divide the data into categories.   The datum that the population of Texas in
1980 numbered 14,000,000 scarcely deserves a table, but if the population is to
be presented according to age, sex, and race, then the problem of categori-
zation exists.   Take the variable "age," for example.   We have to decide
whether to show our data for every year of age, for every five-year age
group, or for some other divisions.   The particular intervals that we choose
will depend on the purpose of the table, but the example below illustrates that
we must observe some general rules in establishing categories.   In this example, age is divided into several intervals, as follows:

Age in years

20 - 34
27 - 40
30 - 40
30 - 48
35 - 54
40 - 54

Suppose we were to use this set of intervals for showing the population of a
community by age, and were going through the census records, assigning each
person to an age interval.

---

*Adapted from Yurushalmy, J., and Chin-Long-Chiang, University of Cali-
fornia, School of Public Health, Department of Biostatistics.

Question 6

a.   How would you categorize a person of 33 years of age, and what effect might this have on your ability to present the age distribution in a clear and unambiguous manner?

b.   How would you categorize a person of age 62?

c.   What two essential requirements of any set of categories are illustrated by questions 6a and b?

It will be useful to look a little more closely at the possible kinds of measurements that may be taken from the point of view of dividing them into categories.   The most obvious division of measurements is into <u>quantitative</u> groups, which can be described numerically, and <u>qualitative</u> groups, which cannot.   Typical quantitative measures are height, weight, number of children, and antibody titer.   Typical qualitative measures are marital status, race, sex, and place of residence.

Quantitative variables

Quantitative measures may be subdivided into discrete and continuous variables.   Discrete variables (or measures) are the result of counting, while continuous variables are the result of other processes giving numerical results, including weighing on a scale and measuring with a ruler.

<u>Discrete variables</u> are easily divided into categories, e.g., number of prenatal visits, which might be made by a group of patients in a maternity ward.   Some possible groupings of this measurement are:

Number of prenatal visits	or	Number of prenatal visits
0 and 1		3 or less
2 and 3		4 - 7
4 and 5		8 - 11
6 or more		over 11
Unknown		Unknown
Total		Total

Strictly speaking, the category "total" does not belong in the sets, but tabular presentations of sets of categories usually add on a "total" category for the convenience of the reader. Notice that as long as the same number of visits does not appear in two categories, there is no possibility of overlapping. Also, with discrete categories partial scores are not possible, since a patient cannot make half a visit to a physician. All observations are easily and unequivocably assignable to some category.

The situation with <u>continuous</u> <u>variables</u> is a little more complicated. For one thing, a continuous variable, such as height, can never be measured with complete precision because of the coarseness of our measuring devices. The measure is made with reference to divisions on a scale, and there is a practical, though not a theoretical limit to how fine we can make the divisions. We might measure height to the nearest inch or nearest tenth of an inch. But, no matter how sensitive the measurement, two persons for whom we record the same height will almost certainly differ by an amount too small to be measured.

Consequently, a recorded value for a continuous variable really indicates an interval within which the true value lies. The size of the interval depends upon the sensitivity of our measurement instrument. For example, if we say John Smith is 70 inches tall, to the nearest half inch, we mean that his "true" height is closer to 70 inches than it is to either 69.5 inches or 70.5 inches. If we say that his height to the last completed half inch is 70 inches, we mean that he is taller than 70 inches, but shorter than 70.5 inches. If we measure his height as 70 inches by taking it to the next complete half inch, we mean that he is taller than 69.5 inches but not taller than 70 inches, .

Here is a diagrammatic illustration of the three kinds of statements:

Nearest half-inch:

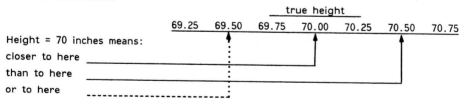

Therefore, the true height lies in the interval between 69.75 and 70.25.

Last half-inch

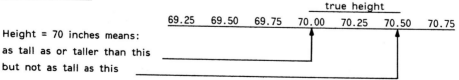

Therefore, the true height lies in the interval between 70.00 and 70.50.

Next complete half-inch

	true height					
69.25	69.50	69.75	70.00	70.25	70.50	70.75

Height = 70 inches means:

taller than this _____

but no taller than this _____

Therefore, the true height lies in the interval between 69.50 and 70.00.

The interval defined in measurement of a continuous variable depends on whether we use the nearest unit (the most common practice), the last complete unit (usually done when measuring age), or the next complete unit. If we select an interval such as "10-14," the boundaries of this interval will depend on which of the three types of categories was used. The following table illustrates how the boundaries for ages 10-14 can vary. By convention the age at last birthday is used. However, a subtle change such as illustrated below would produce different midpoints (average age) for the classes.

Reported interval	Date of reference	Lower boundary	Upper boundary	Mid-point
10-14	Age in years at last birthday	10 yrs	15 yrs	12.5
15-19		15 yrs	20 yrs	17.5
10-14	Age in years at nearest birthday	9½ yrs	14½ yrs	12
15-19		14½ yrs	19½ yrs	17
10-14	Age in years at next birthday	9 yrs	14 yrs	11.5
15-19		14 yrs	19 yrs	16.5

In the example of "height" the measured units were half-inches, while in the table for age they are years. The boundaries of the intervals in the age table can be deduced by using the same sort of reasoning that was used for height.

Notice that in the upper row, age at last birthday, the boundaries are exactly 10 and 15. This means that anyone who is included in the reported interval "10-14" must be at least 10 and less than 15 years old. If he is 15 he belongs to the next interval, 15-19. In the lower row, age at next birthday, the same reasoning holds. The interval 10-14 (boundaries 9-14) includes persons who currently are not less than 9 years old or those who are 14 or older.

Now we may define exclusive intervals for any continuous variable. For example, if we write the following set of intervals:

Age in years at last birthday	Weight to the nearest pound
Under 1	50 and under
1-4	51-100
5-14	101-150
15-34	151-200
35-44	201-250
45 and over	251 and over
unknown	unknown

We can see that each one is an <u>exclusive</u> and <u>inclusive</u> set of intervals. There is no doubt about which interval the "space" between 14 and 15 years belongs to, for example. The fact that the measurement is "age in years at last birthday" means that the boundaries of the interval 5-14 are 5-15, so that the "space" belongs to that interval. Similarly, the fact that the weights are to the nearest pound tells us that the boundaries of the intervals 50-100 and 101-200 are, respectively, 50.5-100.49 and 100.5-200.49. Therefore, the "space" between 100 and 101 is evenly divided between the two intervals.

The problem of dividing <u>qualitative</u> measurements into exclusive categories is primarily one of precise definition. In some cases the definition of a category may be an objective one. Often, however, it is at least partly subjective. If subjective, two observers may disagree on how to categorize an observation. Moreover, observers may even change their minds from one day to the next.

For example, suppose a public health nurse is reporting on a home visit. She is asked to classify the living quarters as "adequate" or "inadequate." The criteria she is told to use may be objective, as follows: "living quarters will be considered inadequate if there are more than 3 persons per room, or if there is no interior plumbing, or if there is no interior running water." This definition is objective, and there is not much chance of two nurses disagreeing on whether or not a given home is inadequate. Suppose, however, that the criteria were subjective, as follows: "living quarters will be considered inadequate if conditions exist which are detrimental to the health of the inhabitants." It is clear that two nurses might very well disagree on whether or not a given home was inadequate, and that the same nurse, on two different visits, might come to opposite conclusions.

This inconsistency, which seems to be inherent in subjective definitions, does not necessarily mean that they are bad. In the above example any purely objective criteria would probably be incomplete, and we might well prefer the nurse's subjective judgment in spite of its variability. The point of the example is that <u>qualitative</u> <u>categories</u> <u>usually</u> <u>have</u> <u>an</u> <u>unavoidable</u> <u>subjective</u> <u>element</u> <u>in</u> <u>their</u> <u>definition</u>, and that this element gives rise to inconsistencies when the judgments of different individuals are compared.

In summary, there may always be criticism about how you select your categories. This can be minimized by using those in common use when possible. If you do not use the common categories you should explain your reasons and alert the reader that the choice of categories may make it difficult to compare the study's observations to those in the literature.

IV. DEPENDENT AND INDEPENDENT VARIABLES

The purpose of tabulating data is to show the values of one variable according to different values of a second variable. One variable is called the independent variable, while the second is called the dependent variable. Designation of which variable is independent and which is dependent is a function of how the research question is phrased. An independent variable is a factor, characteristic, or condition that we are interested to study. The dependent variable is the health status observed or measured for different categories of the independent variable. The independent variable is sometimes termed the method of classification and if shown in a graph, it would be illustrated on the x-axis. The dependent variable is sometimes termed the outcome variable or outcome measure, and if shown in a graph, it would be illustrated on the y-axis.

In a table, the independent variable is usually shown in a column on the left side and the frequency, percentage, or rate of the dependent variable presented in rows to the right of each category of the independent variable.

Question 7

For each of the following problems identify which is the independent and which is the dependent variable; identify if the measurement unit is discrete or continuous, and suggest an appropriate set of intervals for the category of measurement.

a.   You wish to study the effect of suspended particulates (some of the stuff that pollutes air) on the function of the lungs.

b.   You wish to study if the use of medication is effective in the control of mild hypertension (elevation of blood pressure > 140/90 mm Hg).

c.   You wish to study the effectiveness of the health services provided in your clinic on the health status of clients from the community.

d.   You wish to determine whether middle-aged men who have premature heartbeats are at greater risk of developing a myocardial infarction (heart attack).

e.   You wish to study whether or not the infant mortality rate in an area is influenced by socioeconomic status.

SUGGESTED RESPONSES
Exercise 4--Presentation of Data

1. In the words of a noted poet, "Let me count the ways." The methods and types of presentations vary greatly and errors or distortions might intentionally or unintentionally occur. How to Lie with Statistics, and Flaws and Fallacies in Statistical Thinking are useful books to read.

2. The vertical and horizontal scales of measurement, title, source of graph information, and time scale should be indicated. The y axis looks like it may consist of unequal units. The speeds are subjective and it is difficult to know what they mean. The curve exceeds the margins of the graph.

3a. The x and y axes are in proportion. The curve shows 3 years with high frequency of disease, 1964, 1966, and 1975.

3b. The y axis is elongated and the x axis is comparatively short. This tends to exaggerate peaks and dips in the curve. The scale break reduces the length of the y axis. There appears to be much fluctuation from year to year.

3c. There is elongation of the x axis and shortening of the y axis. Large units of measurement on the y axis tend to flatten the curve. The incidence seems more stable from year to year than disease incidence in curves 21a and 21b.

3d. Figure 21b: y axis is exaggerated and x axis is diminished in length, thus overemphasizing the y axis. Units of measurement have different lengths. A small increment in disease incidence relative to one year of time may not be realistic. Figure 21c: The opposite distortion is presented. Here the x axis is very long and therefore changes in disease incidence do not seem very striking except in 1975.

3e. Figure 21c shows the least amount of fluctuation, suggesting that everything is under control. Especially, it decreases the impact of the increased incidence in 1964, 1966, and 1975.

3f. All are correct. Only the manner of presentation has been changed. No major "charting" rules have been violated. One must be alert that the manner of presentation can influence the impression that we get from the picture. The impression may not be accurate even though the graph is technically correct.

4a. The graph appears complete, but the denominator is ambiguous. It needs better x and y axis identification. The percentages for each disease do not total 100%, for example, breast cancer totals = 151%. Obviously some cases have been counted more than once. Other questions arise: Are new and old cases included in the rate? What years are covered? At what stage of illness were cases diagnosed? Were cases treated? It would be useful to have the time period of ascertainment indicated and other factors such as age at diagnosis, stage of disease at diagnosis, and treatment type.

4b. It suggests that localized cancer has a lower 5 year mortality rate (better survival) associated with it than cancer with regional or distant spread. But we don't know whether the data refer to survival after diagnosis or after being treated when cancer was localized or regional. The lack of information makes it difficult to understand exactly what the graph is attempting to say.

4c. Screening patients to diagnose cancer while it is still localized seems like a good idea.

5a. It is a bar graph.

5b. No, the categories are not mutually exclusive. There appears to be overlap in the categories. A person with 2 visits could belong to 2 groups. Categories should be defined so that there is no question about where the person is included.

5c. It is a histogram.

5d. Connect the midpoints of the intervals of Figure 23b. The left side of the graph does not have enough room to extend the curve to the x axis and so the categories comprising the x axis should be shifted to the right.

5e. It is preferred when more than one set of data will be presented on the graph.

6a. There are several categories from which to choose: 20-34, 27-40, 30-40, 30-48. Classification of the person's age might be different if two investigators were making the assignments. Two or more overlapping categories make presentation of the data confusing. While few classifications are so blatant as those presented here, some might be more subtle, 0-1, 1-2, etc. Into which category would a child be included if the observation is made on the first birthday? The visit rates from Question 5 were concerned with this sort of problem.

6b. There is no category available. You would need a miscellaneous category such as "other," to permit inclusion of all observations. For some data sets a category for "not stated" or "unknown" might be needed.

6c. Avoid overlapping categories by having clear and unambiguous groups. Provide a category for all persons who participated in your study.

7a. The independent variable is exposure to polluted air (qualitative) or the concentration of pollutants known to be in the air (quantitative). Pollutants are usually measured in parts per million. The U.S. government regulations of permissible concentration would vary for different chemicals (ozone, solid particulates, sulfur oxides, etc.). Intervals should include concentrations below and above the permitted concentrations. The dependent variable is lung function as measured by vital capacity or the expiratory flow rate.

Tests of respiratory function will have different normal values depending upon the age, physique, and sex of the person. Normal values can be obtained from standard texts of clinical medicine or the Merck Manual.

7b. The independent variable is the use or nonuse of medication (qualitative) or the dose of prescribed medication (quantitative). The dependent variable is the measurement of systolic and/or diastolic blood pressure in mm Hg.

Use or nonuse of medication could be categorized as "yes-no" or "everyday, occasionally, or never." Categories for quantity of medication ingested would depend upon the medication used. Because each medication has a different dosage, you would have to quantify the dose in terms of the outcome; for example, reducing the blood pressure by 10 mm Hg requires 100 mg of elixir y but only 10 mg of pill x.

Blood pressure reduction might be categorized in absolute terms--stepwise decreases of 5 (0-4, 5-9, 10-14) mm Hg or 10 mm Hg (0-9, 10-19, 20-29). Another way might be to determine the percentage reduction. One would also need to specify whether the top number alone (140, the systolic blood pressure), the bottom number alone (90, the diastolic blood pressure), or both numbers together were to be considered.

7c. The independent variable is the use or availability of the health service e.g., immunization. The dependent variable is some health status index, outcome of treatment, stage of illness or death, etc., in your clinic population. The outcome might be measured by the attack rate or the serum antibody levels among vaccinees. Evaluation of effectiveness implies comparison to some standard value to learn if the service is better than, equal to, or worse than other health (or no health) services. You might need to have a "control" or comparison group, which received other services or no services.

As with the other questions, your evaluation variables could have qualitative or quantitative categories.

7d. The independent variable is premature heartbeats. Categories for premature heartbeats could be discrete, (yes-no; occasional-frequent-never;) or continuous (0-1, 2-5, 6-10, 10+ per minute, hour, or day). Determination would be best made by having an ECG (electrocardiogram). A second way might be to ask how many times per minute (day, week, etc.) the patient felt "palpitations" in the chest. The second way is more difficult to evaluate objectively.

The dependent variable is myocardial infarction, which can be measured by presence or absence (qualitative) of ECG changes compared to a previous ECG examination. Other useful units of measurement could be presence or absence of chest pain; blood pressure and pulse measurements, evaluation of body temperature. Finally, serum enzymes are known to change during and/or following a heart attack. These enzymes (SGOT, SGPT, LDH, etc.) have normal values published in clinical texts and the Merck manual.

7e. The independent variable is socioeconomic status and the dependent variable is infant mortality. Socioeconomic status can be categorized by continuous variables such as income (in dollars) or education (in years); or discrete variables such as occupation (doctor, athlete, truck-driver, homemaker, teacher, construction worker, etc.), or other useful indicators related to housing, diet, or lifestyle.

Infant mortality can be categorized as all-or-none, i.e., the infant survived or died prior to the first birthday, or as a continuous variable--months of survival. One might also wish to look at specific causes of death.

EXERCISE 5.   CLASSIFICATION SYSTEMS

Goals

Upon completion of this exercise you should understand (1) the principles and major types of classification systems useful in epidemiology and (2) how the classification of data affects their interpretation.

Methods

In order to achieve these goals you will need to understand

I.   DEFINITION AND PURPOSE OF CLASSIFICATION
II.   CLINICAL AND EPIDEMIOLOGIC CLASSIFICATION OF DISEASES
III.   THE INTERNATIONAL CLASSIFICATION OF DISEASES
IV.   EFFECT OF GROUPING ON INTERPRETATION OF DATA
V.   DEFINING THE NUMERATOR: WHAT IS A CASE?

Terms

Observer error, nomenclature, signs, symptoms

Suggested Readings

ICD-9-CM, International Classification of Diseases, 9th revision, Clinical Modification, Vols. 1, 2, and 3, Commission on Professional and Hospital Activities, Published by Edwards Brothers, Inc., Ann Arbor, Michigan, 1978.

   Vol. 1, Foreword: pp. iii-v; Introduction: pp. xxi-xxix; Appendix A: pp. 1055-1076; Appendix B: pp. 1077-1126.
   Vol. 2, Introduction: pp. iii-xii; Section 2: pp. 763-861; Section 3: pp. 865-910.

Hospital Adaptation of ICDA, H-ICDA, 2nd Edition, Vols. 1 and 2, Commission on Professional and Hospital Activities, Ann Arbor, Michigan, 1973.

Sokal, R.R., Classification: Purposes, principles, progress, prospects. Science 185:1115, 1974.

Fox, Hall and Elveback, Epidemiology: Man and Disease, 1970, pp. 31-46.

MacMahon and Pugh, Epidemiology: Principles and Methods, 1970, pp. 47-56.

Humphreys, N.A. (Ed.), Vital Statistics: A Memorial Volume of Selections from the Reports and Writings of William Farr (1885). Reprinted, Metuchen: Scarecrow Press, 1975.

I.   DEFINITION AND PURPOSE OF CLASSIFICATION

Classification may be defined as the arrangement into groups of objects, concepts or information based on their relationships or properties. The term implies both a process, that is, how we arrange the groups, and also an end result, that is, what the arrangement looks like at the completion of the process.

The purposes of classification are <u>to</u> <u>summarize</u> <u>the</u> <u>information</u>, <u>to</u> <u>facilitate</u> <u>retrieval</u> <u>of</u> <u>information</u>, and most importantly, to describe the structure and relation of the items to similar items in order <u>to</u> <u>simplify</u> <u>relationships</u> <u>so</u> <u>that</u> <u>general</u> <u>statements</u> <u>can</u> <u>be</u> <u>made</u> <u>about</u> <u>the</u> <u>group</u>.

As a result of classification, it might be possible in some cases to formulate hypotheses relating to the underlying mechanisms governing the group. In other cases, the grouping may be so broad that the justification for it is merely one of convenience in summarizing disparate items.

There are two major ways of categorizing information. The first includes groups that have <u>one</u> <u>characteristic</u> <u>in</u> <u>common</u>. The second type includes groups in which the items have <u>several</u> <u>or</u> <u>many</u> common <u>properties</u> <u>but</u> <u>do</u> <u>not</u> <u>necessarily</u> <u>agree</u> <u>in</u> <u>any</u> <u>one</u> <u>characteristic</u>. In this second group, no single property is required for the definition of a group, and no combination of characteristics will necessarily define it. Classifications based on many properties are not likely to be specific and, therefore, may have use in a variety of situations, while those categorized on few properties would be less suited for general use (Sokal, 1974).

Three general problems are inherent to classification. The first may be likened to a "keyhole effect." Imagine the object to be classified to be a room and the classification system to be the keyhole. While one can place the keyhole in different positions and even increase the size or alter the shape of the hole slightly, we are still limited to what can be seen of the room by looking through the keyhole.

The second problem concerns how new information may be included in the classification system. If one had a system in which items are grouped as A or B, then all information, old and new, must be included in one or the other group. If the classification system were in error and another category C existed but was not recognized, information rightly belonging to C must, by definition, be placed in A or B. Any conclusions based upon data in groups A and B will be in error depending upon the number of C that are incorrectly located. In addition to introducing error, a rigid system of classification forces all items or observations to be placed in some category and may prevent the observer from modifying the original notion of A and B to include a new category C.

The final problem concerns another type of error that may be introduced in classification. Suppose we have a suitable system of 3 groups (A,B,C) but the observer mistakenly places items belonging in one group into another group, for example, A's items are placed in B or C. The error may be due to carelessness, incomplete or inaccurate determination of A's correct properties by the observer, or lack of equipment that can properly and accurately measure A's properties. In other words A will be misclassified due to <u>observer</u> <u>errors</u> of omission or commission.

II.   CLINICAL AND EPIDEMIOLOGIC CLASSIFICATION OF DISEASES.

Classification schemes differ with regard to the discipline being served and the purpose of the classification system. Epidemiologists are involved in a great variety of clinical, administrative, and research activities involving the public and private sectors of the health industry, so that a comprehensive listing of all classification systems is not possible in this manual. Several systems are widely employed and are mentioned below.

Question 1

For each of the following list the categories that might be included when diseases are classified by:

a.   Nature of the etiologic agent

b.   Nature of the disease process (pathology)

c.   Body organ systems affected

d.   Method of treatment

e.   Method of transmission of the disease agent

f.   Method of entry to and exit from the body

g.   Factors influencing exposure and/or susceptibility of the host.

h.   Degree of incapacity resulting from the disease

III. THE INTERNATIONAL CLASSIFICATION OF DISEASES*

Classification is fundamental to the quantitative study of any phenomenon. It is necessary for all scientific generalization and is therefore an essential element in [epidemiologic] methods. Since uniform definitions and systems of classification are prerequisites in the advancement of scientific knowledge about illness and death, therefore, a standard classification of disease and injury is essential.

There are many approaches to the classification of disease. The anatomist may desire a classification based on the part of the body affected, while the pathologist is primarily interested in the nature of the disease process. The clinician must consider disease from these two angles, but needs further knowledge of etiology. In other words, there are many axes of classification and the particular axis selected will be determined by the interests of the investigator. A statistical classification of disease and injury will depend upon the use to be made of the statistics to be compiled.

The purpose of [epidemiologic] classification is often confused with that of a <u>nomenclature</u>. Basically a medical nomenclature is a list or catalog of approved terms for describing and recording clinical and pathological observations. To serve its full function, it should be extensive, so that any pathological condition can be accurately recorded. As medical science advances, a nomenclature must expand to include new terms necessary to record new observations. Any morbid condition that can be specifically described will need a specific designation in a nomenclature.

The complete specificity of a nomenclature prevents it from serving satisfactorily as an [epidemiologic] classification. When one speaks of statistics, it is at once inferred that the interest is in a group of cases and not in individual

---

*Source: W.H.O., <u>International Classification of Diseases Adapted, Seventh Revision</u>, 1957, pp. vii-x. For use in this guide, the more appropriate term ["epidemiologic"] has been substituted for the word "statistical," which appears in the original W.H.O. text.

occurrences. The purpose of an [epidemiologic] compilation of disease data is primarily to furnish quantitative
data that will answer questions about groups of cases.

This distinction between an [epidemiological] classification
and a nomenclature has [long] been clear to [epidemiolo-
gists]. The aims of [epidemiologic] classification of disease cannot be better summarized than in the following
paragraphs written by William Farr, a century ago:

The causes of death were tabulated in the early Bills of
Mortality (Tables Mortuaries) alphabetically; and this
course has the advantage of not raising any of those nice
questions in which it is vain to expect physicians and
statisticians to agree unanimously. But statistics is emi-
nently a science of classification; and it is evident, on
glancing at the subject cursorily, that any classification
that brings together in groups, diseases that have considerable affinity, or that are liable to be confounded with
each other, is likely to facilitate the deduction of general
principles.

Classification is a method of generalization. Several classifications may, therefore, be used with advantage; and the
physician, the pathologist, or the jurist, each from his
own point of view, may legitimately classify the diseases
and the causes of death in the way that he thinks best
adapted to facilitate his inquiries, and to yield general
results.

The medical practitioner may found his main divisions of
diseases on their treatment as medical or surgical; the
pathologist, on the nature of the morbid action or product;
the anatomist or the physiologist on the tissues and organs
involved; the medical jurist, on the suddenness or the
slowness of the death; and all these points well deserve
attention in a statistical classification.

In the eyes of national statists the most important elements
are, however, brought into account in the ancient subdivision of diseases into plagues, or epidemics and en-
demics, into diseases of common occurrence (sporadic
diseases), which may be conveniently divided into three
classes, and into injuries the immediate results of violence
or of external causes.

An [epidemiologic] classification of disease must be confined to a limited number of categories which will encom-
pass the entire range of morbid conditions. The categories

should be chosen so that they will facilitate the statistical study of disease phenomena. A specific disease entity should have a separate title in the classification only when its occurrence, or its importance as a morbid condition, justifies its isolation as a separate category. On the other hand, many titles in the classification will refer to groups of separate but usually related morbid conditions. Every disease or morbid condition, however, must have a definite and appropriate place and be included in one of the categories of the classification.

Before a statistical classification can be put into use it is necessary to [specify] the inclusions for each category. If medical nomenclature were uniform and standard, such a task would be simple and quite direct. Actually, the doctors who practise and who will be making entries in medical records or writing medical certificates of death were educated at different medical schools and over a period of more than fifty years. As a result, the sickness records, hospital records and death certificates are certain to be of mixed terminology which cannot be modernized or standardized by the wave of any magician's wand. All these terms, good and bad, must be provided for as inclusions in an [epidemiologic] classification.

The construction of a practical scheme of classification of disease and injury for general statistical use involves various compromises. Efforts to provide a statistical classification upon a strictly logical arrangement of morbid conditions have failed in the past. The various titles represent compromises between classifications based on etiology, anatomical site, age, and circumstance of onset, as well as the quality of information available on medical reports. Adjustments must also be made to meet the varied requirements of vital statistics offices, hospitals of different types, medical services of the armed forces, social insurance organizations, sickness surveys, and numerous other agencies. While no single classification will fit the specialized needs for all these purposes, it should provide a common basis of classification for general statistical use.

The statistical study of disease began for all practical purposes with the work of John Graunt on the London Bills of Mortality in the 1600's. The kind of classification which this pioneer had at his disposal is exemplified by his attempt to estimate the proportion of liveborn children who died before reaching the age of six years, no records of age at death being then available. He took all deaths classed as thrush, convulsions, rickets, teeth and worms, abortives, chrysomes, infants, liver-grown, and overlaid, and added to them half the deaths classed as smallpox, swine pox, measles, and worms without convulsions. Despite the crudity of this classification, his estimate of a 36 percent mortality before the age of six years appears from later evidence to have been a good one. While three centuries have contributed something to the scientific accuracy of disease classification, there are many who doubt the usefulness of attempts to compile statistics of disease, or even causes of death, because of the difficulties of classification. To these one can quote Greenwood: "The scientific purist, who will wait for medical statistics until they are nosologically exact, is no wiser than Horace's rustic waiting for the river to flow away.

Fortunately for the progress of preventive medicine, the General Register Office of England and Wales, at its inception in 1837, found in William Farr (1807-1883)--its first medical statistician--a man who not only made the best possible use of the imperfect classifications of disease available at the time, but labored to secure better classification and international uniformity in their use.

The International Classification of Diseases Adapted (ICDA), now in its Ninth Revision, is a standardized coding system for causes of death and morbidity published by the W.H.O. The system is used for coding of death certificates and for hospital and outpatient medical records of fatal and nonfatal diseases. It is revised periodically to reflect new knowledge and better understanding of the disease process. The Ninth Revision Clinical Modification was printed in 1978 and the major categories in this revision are given below. Code numbers designating the diseases in each category are in parentheses.

1. Infective and Parasitic Diseases (001-139)
2. Neoplasms (140-239)
3. Endocrine, Nutritional, and Metabolic Diseases, and Immunity Disorders (240-279)
4. Diseases of the Blood and Blood-forming Organs (280-289)
5. Mental Disorders (290-319)
6. Diseases of the Nervous System and Sense Organs (320-389)
7. Diseases of the Circulatory System (390-459)
8. Diseases of the Respiratory System (460-519)
9. Diseases of the Digestive System (520-579)
10. Diseases of the Genitourinary System (580-629)
11. Complications of Pregnancy, Childbirth, and the Puerperium (630-676)
12. Diseases of the Skin and Subcutaneous Tissue (680-709)
13. Diseases of the Musculoskeletal System and Connective Tissue (710-739)
14. Congenital Anomalies (740-759)
15. Certain Conditions Originating in the Perinatal Period (760-779)

16.   Symptoms, Signs, and Ill-Defined Conditions (780-799)
17.   Injury and Poisoning (800-999)
V Code.   Supplementary Classification of Factors Influencing Health Status and Contact with Health Service (V01-V82)
E Code.   Supplementary Classification of External Causes of Injury and Poisonings (E800-E998).

Another useful reference is the Symptom Classification found in Series 2, number 63 of the National Center for Health Statistics "Rainbow Series" in the library. This classification is especially useful for surveys in which people are asked about their health status.

Question 2

a.   What are the similarities between the clinical and epidemiologic classification systems considered in question 1 and the system used in the International Classification of Diseases?

b.   What are the differences?

c.   What are the advantages of each system?

d.   What are the disadvantages?

Question 3

a. List some reasons why the International Classification of Diseases Adapted (ICDA) may be of value to an epidemiologist.

b. What considerations are important if the ICDA is to be a useful tool in epidemiologic research?

c. The ICDA periodically revises the definition of various diseases. Of what importance is this to an epidemiologist?

d. What problem does the passage of time pose for use of the ICDA system?

e. What scheme would be most appropriate for epidemiologic classification of diseases?

IV   EFFECT OF GROUPING ON INTERPRETATION OF DATA

To illustrate the effect of varying the classification system on the interpretation of data, consider the following example of the hypothetical disease, Sasquatch fever. For ease of illustration epidemiologic characteristics are not used.   However, the idea presented could easily be applied to a clinical disease by changing the characteristics of shape, size, angles, or position used in the example, to age, sex, race, mode of transmission, or other epidemiologic characteristic.

The Problem of Sasquatch Fever

Suppose a community consisted of 120 individuals of varying size and shape (characteristics of person) and position (characteristic of place).   During the calendar year 1981, several members were discovered to have a disease called Sasquatch fever, which is indicated in black, as shown in Figure 1.

Figure 1. Sasquatch Fever in a
          community, 1981.

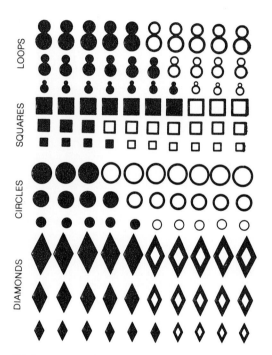

This space for calculation.

Figure 2. Specific rates for Sasquatch
          fever by selected character-
          istics per 100 persons, 1981.

Characteristic	Incidence per 100 persons
Shape	
Diamonds	
Circles	
Squares	
Loops	
Size	
Small	
Medium	
Large	
Angles	
None (circles, loops)	
Four (diamonds, squares)	
Position	
Upper 6 rows	
Lower 6 rows	
Total	

As an epidemiologist you are interested in describing the disease as it occurs in the community. Observation suggests that four characteristics may be important in uncovering clues to the disease etiology. Classification by diseased and nondiseased individuals in terms of their characteristics of person (shape, size, number of angles) and place (position on the upper 6 rows versus those on the lower 6 rows) permits calculation of incidence rates. There were no deaths associated with illness. Complete Figure 2, using data from Figure 1.

Inspection of the characteristic-specific rates calculated for Figure 2 suggests that the incidence of disease grouped by angles or by position does not depart appreciably from the total community incidence of 50.0 per 100 (the expected rate) to warrant further investigation. However, the characteristics of shape and size reveal wider range of incidence, i.e., that some individuals are at greater risk than others. Perhaps the disease etiology has something to do with either or both of these characteristics. Determine the contribution of each characteristic to the disease etiology by calculating the rates for the combined characteristics by completing Figure 3.

Figure 3. Sasquatch fever by size and shape per 100 persons, 1981.

Size and Shape	Incidence per 100 persons
Small diamonds	
Medium diamonds	
Large diamonds	
Small squares	
Medium squares	
Large squares	
Small circles	
Medium circles	
Large circles	
Small loops	
Medium loops	
Large loops	
Total	

The next step in understanding the factors contributing to the distribution of disease in this community might be to RANK ORDER all the characteristics in decreasing order of incidence as given below in Figure 4.

Figure 4. Rank order of incidence rates of Sasquatch fever per 100 persons, 1981.

Group	Incidence per 100 persons	Group	Incidence per 100 persons
Large squares Small loops Small diamonds Medium loops All loops Small size		Large size 4 angles No angles Lower rows All squares Medium size	
All diamonds Upper rows Medium diamonds Large diamonds Small circles Large loops		Medium circles Small squares All circles Large circles Medium squares Total	

From these data the following observations can be made.

1. All groups in which the incidence rate is greater than 50.0 per 100 are at increased risk while all groups whose incidence rate is less than 50.0 per 100 are at decreased risk of contracting the disease when compared to the overall population incidence rate, which is 50.0 per 100 persons.

2. From Figure 2, shape is best able to separate diseased and nondiseased persons (range of incidence 40.0-59.9 per 100); size is next best (range of incidence 45.0-55.0. per 100); position is next best (range of 46.7-53.3 per 100); angles, whose incidence is 50.0 per 100, shows no difference from the general population incidence and does not appear to offer any clues to the etiology.

3. From Figures 3 and 4 we would derive clues that shape and size were somehow related to the appearance of Sasquatch fever. However, there appears to be a more complex relation between characteristics thought to be involved in the etiology. For example, large squares and small loops have 70.0 per 100 incidence rate, well above the population incidence of 50.0 per 100, while large circles and medium squares have an incidence rate of 30.0 per 100, which is below the population incidence. Thus, neither size nor shape alone is sufficient to produce the disease or to afford protection from it. Further study would be necessary to uncover the way(s) in which the characteristic(s) act to produce the disease.

From the preceding discussion some general ideas concerning the effects of classification become evident:

1. The <u>choice</u> <u>of</u> <u>grouping</u> <u>and</u> <u>classification</u> influences <u>the</u> <u>presentation</u> <u>of</u> <u>observations</u> <u>and</u> <u>therefore</u> <u>the</u> <u>conclusions</u> <u>that</u> <u>are</u> <u>drawn</u>. Selecting an

unimportant characteristic such as position or angles might lead to the incorrect conclusion that there are no subgroups at increased risk of disease in this community and that further investigations are not warranted.

2. The more one can define the inherent or acquired host characteristics in precise and specific terms the better is the likelihood of identifying groups at increased risk of disease, and understanding the factors or determinants of the observed distribution. For example, a specific grouping might include white males age 40-59 while a more general grouping would refer to all residents of a city, which includes males and females of all ages.

3. The more general the classification, the easier it is to extrapolate the observations to the general population or community. There is a trade-off that must sometimes be made, however, the more diverse or heterogeneous the population at risk, the more difficult it is to determine the way(s) in which the characteristic under study exerts its effects in the population of interest.

It follows, therefore, that the choice of classification system must be carefully made in accordance with the researcher's intended purpose, and that knowledge of the pattern of disease and characteristics of susceptible persons (derived from the published literature or one's prior experience) will be very useful when defining, selecting, or classifying the categories to be studied.

Having discovered, through a suitable method of grouping data, some population subgroups in which the risk of disease is aggregated, you might now proceed to apply some statistical tests to the data to determine if the differences of the observed incidence rates are significantly different (in a statistical sense) from the population incidence.

Statistical theory tells us there is an expected probability that even rare events will eventually occur by chance, for example, a coin will occasionally fall face up (heads) on 10 consecutive tosses rather than the expected number of 5 face up (heads) and 5 face down (tails). In studying disease occurrence in human populations, epidemiologists assume that the observed incidence rates are due in part to biologic and physical factors such as exposure, susceptibility, age, sex, and occupation. However, there could be fluctuation in the incidence rates observed for different populations because of random variation in the composition of those populations, for example, the relative proportions of young/old, males/females, and smokers/nonsmokers. Statistical tests of significance are used to assist the epidemiologist in assessing the importance of observed differences in disease occurrence in population samples, where the differences may be due to the biologic influence of some factor related to the disease etiology, or the differences result from chance or random variation of the sampling process.

Observations thus derived from the above data may suggest clues to the relation between one or more characteristics of the host or its environment and the occurrence or nonoccurrence of disease. For example, study of persons in groups with a high incidence rate may suggest that a certain characteristic (factor) is somehow involved in the mechanism producing disease. The disease may be caused by that factor or by another factor, which may or may not have been identified. Study of Sasquatch fever suggests that size and shape are involved but other factors also might play a role. Further study might reveal size and shape to have a common mediating characteristic such as proximity in time or space making certain groups susceptible to Sasquatch fever. In realistic terms, a mediating or promoting characteristic might be vitamin intake, genetic inheritance, or perhaps the competence of the immune system.

The epidemiologist continues to search for and examine evidence that can be used to support or discredit existing hypotheses or that might lead to new explanations of disease occurrence. Through trial and error, a body of observable facts and conclusions emerges, the purpose of which is to develop preventive or control measures for diseases that affect the community. An essential element of this process is the means of classifying and categorizing data.

V. DEFINING THE NUMERATOR: WHAT IS A CASE?

Much attention has been devoted to the issue of defining denominators and identifying populations at risk. Of equal importance are the issues of defining the numerator, i.e., the criteria used to determine "what is a case," and identifying the manner in which cases are ascertained.

Included in the numerator are health conditions or events, cases of disease or changes in health status which are observed and counted. Some are easy to define, for example, births or deaths, and there is little doubt that the event occurred. The source from which the events are counted is also quite easy to determine: official registration of vital events for the period of interest.

If one wishes to identify the specific disease that caused a person's death or determine whether or not a person is ill from a certain disease, it is necessary to specify how we know when a person has the disease. Obviously, patients seldom walk around with signs saying, "I am a case of diabetes."

Identifying a person as having a disease is accomplished by finding out the signs, symptoms, clinical history, and laboratory findings. The terms "signs" and "symptoms" have distinct clinical meanings. The SIGNS of a disease are the objective and observable clinical and laboratory findings, while the SYMPTOMS are the subjective complaints of a patient, which are not directly observable but which are still a part of the clinical picture of the disease. Some diseases carry one or more distinctive signs, which absolutely establish the diagnosis. These are termed pathognomonic signs. Koplik spots, white patches found in the mouth, are pathognomonic for measles (rubeola).

Question 4

The following are some terms frequently used to describe clinical diseases. Indicate which are signs and which are symptoms.

fever
cough
headache
malaise
fatigue
pain
hearing loss
pins and needles sensations
   (paresthesias)
wheezing
chills
giddiness, lightheadedness
anxiety
rash
coryza

hallucinations
tenderness
restricted range of motion
diminished reflexes
shortness of breath
weakness
loss of appetite
weight loss
nausea
vomiting
cramps
palpitations
jaundice
exanthema
enanthema

Question 5

Figure 5 depicts the eye pressure distributions for normal and diseased eyes in glaucoma. Assume that you are conducting a health survey. How would you define the presence of the disease, i.e., a case of glaucoma? What is the effect of raising or lowering the diagnostic criterion?

Figure 5. Intraocular pressure of glaucomatous and nonglaucomatous eyes.

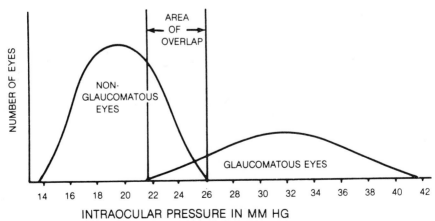

Source: Thorner and Remein, Principles and procedures in the evaluation of screening for disease, U.S. Dept. HEW, 1961.

Question 6

The following signs, symptoms, and laboratory findings are associated with different diseases. Assume that you are conducting a study of hospital records and must define the numerator (cases) for several diseases.

a.   Loss of appetite, nausea and vomiting, jaundice, dark urine, light-colored feces, abdominal pain, distaste for cigarettes, fatigue, malaise, slight fever, weakness, and elevation of the serum enzyme SGPT (a nonspecific finding in many types of liver disease) are all associated with hepatitis. Which signs or symptoms are the most suitable criteria for defining a case? In what situation might an epidemiologist have to exclude certain cases that fit within the definition of a case?

b.   Rheumatic fever is an acute inflammatory complication of streptococcal infection that may involve the joints (arthritis), brain (chorea), heart (carditis and valve disease), subcutaneous tissue (nodules), and the skin (rash). The disease rarely affects all five body systems and typically involves only one or two. A "strep throat" may be involved in the initial stages of the disease but accurate diagnosis may occur only 20% of the time. Other nonspecific findings include acute fever, elevated white blood cell count, and an increased red blood cell sedimentation rate. What criteria would you use to define a case of rheumatic fever?

c.   Review of hospital records reveals that prior to 1973, cases of sudden and unexplained infant deaths were most frequently diagnosed as interstitial pneumonitis, bronchopneumonia, or unknown or ill-defined cause, but after that date the cause of death was specifically listed as Sudden Infant Death Syndrome (SIDS, ICDA code no. 795.0 or 795.1) What steps might be taken to identify or estimate SIDS cases prior to 1973?

Question 7

Why are clear criteria and specific definitions of cases and noncases important in epidemiology?

SUGGESTED RESPONSES
Exercise 5--Classification of Diseases

1a. Nature of the etiologic agent

Micro-organisms	Chemical agents		Physical agents	Genetic inheritance
bacteria	inorganic	(vapors	cold	single gene defect
viruses	organic	{liquids	heat	autosomal or x-linked,
fungae		(solids	force	dominant or recessive
rickettsia			sound	multifactorial inheritance
protozoa			electricity	chromosome abnormality
parasites			radiation	trisomy, translocation
				sex chromosome abnor-mality

1b. Pathologic process

inflammation
ischemia or anoxia
necrosis (with or without fibrosis)
neoplasia
granuloma formation

fibrosis
demineralization (of bone)
hemorrhage
thromobosis, embolism, plaque formation, spasm or dilation of blood vessels

Developmental defects

aplasia, hypoplasia
atrophy
hypertrophy, hyperplasia

Abnormal cell growth

metaplasia
dysplasia
anaplasia

1c. Body systems

musculoskeletal
respiratory
cardiovascular
gastrointestinal
neurologic (peripheral and central)

excretory
reproductive
endocrine
defense (skin, lymphatic)
hematologic

1d. Treatment

surgical
chemical
radiologic

physical (heat, cold, exercise, manipulation)
psychic or other counselling
acupuncture (mechanism of action is not clear)

1e. Method of transmission to susceptible human

source: animals, arthropods, birds, food, water, contaminated articles, infected humans

transmission: ingestion, contact, inhalation, absorption, inoculation

1f.   <u>Method of entry and exit</u>

    entry sites: oral, nasal, on or through skin, transplacenta (in utero), urogenital

    entry methods: ingestion, inoculation, inhalation, absorption

    exit sites: oral, nasal, anal, urogenital, skin, blood, feces

    exit methods: cough, exhalation, excretion, exudation

1g.   <u>Characteristics of susceptibility or exposure</u>

age	genetic background
sex	occupation
ethnicity	personal and social habits
socioeconomic status	etc.
nutrition and diet	

1h.   <u>Degree of incapacity</u>

death
disability
discomfort
disruption of social functioning
discontent or dissatisfaction

2a.   The ICDA uses elements of different classification schemes including etiology, pathology, organ systems, and clinical symptoms.

2b.   The ICDA does not categorize all diseases from one point of view, e.g., etiology. This is both a strength and a weakness. A strength of this system is that it is very flexible. For example, many diseases are of unknown etiology. Rather than group them together the ICDA permits them to be separated on some other characteristic. A weakness of the ICDA scheme is that it forces a disease to be categorized in a way that emphasizes one characteristic of the disease over another, which might result in a stereotyped way of thinking about the disease. This weakness is recognized and corrected for by some of the steps indicated in the responses to questions 2c and 3.

2c.   The ICDA is a standardized general classification scheme that encompasses all known diseases or causes of illness grouped according to reasonably current information, which is revised every 7-10 years. The potential for revision gives the ICDA a great flexibility and resilience. Clinical and epidemiologic classifications are specific to the needs of those specialities and permit the clinician or epidemiologist to analyze the disease process using the skills or methods of their respective specialties.

2d.   In general, the disadvantage of the ICDA scheme relates to the overlap of several different types of classification used in the construction of this system. It is therefore more difficult for clinicians or epidemiologists to use the ICDA because in many situations it may not be possible to directly apply the respective techniques of these disciplines.

On the other hand, the clinical or epidemiologic systems may not be appropriate for useful classification of some (or many) diseases because the etiology, pathology, method of transmission, etc., may not be well enough understood to permit a useful separation of the diseases into different categories.

Disease classification, in order to be useful, must therefore straddle the line between being overly general and specific.

3a. The ICDA is a universally accepted system. It permits comparison of mortality and morbidity data from different places by use of a uniform and standard format. A careful set of rules (nosology) for classifying diseases from death certificates and medical records has been formulated.

3b. In order for the ICDA to be useful to epidemiologists the following considerations are important.

1. Complete reporting of cases

2. Accurate diagnosis by the physician
Steps 1 and 2 will provide numerator data for calculating rates.

3. Current and accurate census data (or special surveys) are needed to provide the estimated population at risk in the denominator, when calculating rates for nations or communities.

4. Completion of medical records and death certificates by physicians who understand that the data might be used for research purposes.

5. Medical terminology and definitions should be similar in different geographic areas.

6. Technicians who collate and process the data should be well trained in nosology.

Considering the requirements identified, you might conclude that it is almost impossible to meet the conditions stated. Any deviations from these conditions will introduce error into the data. It is difficult to know how much error occurs at each stage of the reporting and processing of the information, and the extent that the required conditions differ from one place to another. Further, it is impossible to say how much error is tolerable. One can only strive to improve the quality of data collection and processing at each stage. The major problem would seem to be training physicians about the uses and requirements of reporting systems for vital events and morbidity at an early stage of their medical education.

Despite all the errors that can potentially affect the quality of health data, the ICDA is an important tool for epidemiologic research.

3c.　It is difficult to interpret trends or to compare results of studies of incidence, prevalence, or mortality when those data were classified using different versions (revisions) of the ICDA code. Over a period of time the accumulation of new knowledge may result in a change of the definition of a disease. Frequently, a disease will be reclassified from one code number to another in subsequent revisions of the ICDA. For some diseases an investigator may be able to estimate the amount of change of incidence or prevalence resulting from differences in coding used by the newest revision of the ICDA code. However, it may not be possible to produce revised estimates for many diseases.

3d.　Interpretation of incidence and prevalence data for different time periods may be difficult. For example, an apparent increase of a disease may be due to changes in definition and better reporting practices rather than any biologic change in the host's susceptibility or exposure to the etiologic agent(s) of a disease. In a similar manner, although not related to the disease definition, other factors such as medical care and treatment might result in improved survival of patients with a disease. Thus, prevalence might markedly increase from one time period to another. Epidemiologists frequently encounter the dilemma of trying to sort out biologic from nonbiologic factors in assessing changing risk.

3e.　It depends on the problem being studied and the purpose for which the results will be used. You have been introduced to many different schemes for classification. Use whichever is appropriate to the problem under investigation.

Figure 2. Specific rates for Sasquatch fever by selected characteristics per 100 persons, 1981.

Characteristic	Incidence per 100 persons
Shape	
Diamonds	53.3
Circles	40.0
Squares	46.7
Loops	60.0
Size	
Small	55.0
Medium	45.0
Large	50.0
Angles	
None (circles, loops)	50.0
Four (diamonds, squares)	50.0
Position	
Upper 6 rows	53.3
Lower 6 rows	46.7
Total	50.0

Figure 3. Sasquatch fever by size and shape per 100 persons, 1981.

Size and Shape	Incidence per 100 persons
Small diamonds	60.0
Medium diamonds	50.0
Large diamonds	50.0
Small squares	40.0
Medium squares	30.0
Large squares	70.0
Small circles	50.0
Medium circles	40.0
Large circles	30.0
Small loops	70.0
Medium loops	60.0
Large loops	50.0
Total	50.0

Figure 4. Rank order of incidence rates of Sasquatch fever per 100 persons, 1981.

Group	Incidence per 100 persons	Group	Incidence per 100 persons
Large squares	70.0	Large size	50.0
Small loops	70.0	4 angles	50.0
Small diamonds	60.0	No angles	50.0
Medium loops	60.0	Lower rows	46.7
All loops	60.0	All squares	46.7
Small size	55.0	Medium size	45.0
All diamonds	53.3	Medium circles	40.0
Upper rows	53.3	Small squares	40.0
Medium diamonds	50.0	All circles	40.0
Large diamonds	50.0	Large circles	30.0
Small circles	50.0	Medium squares	30.0
Large loops	50.0	Total	50.0

4. | Signs | Symptoms |

Signs	Symptoms
fever	headache
cough	malaise
hearing loss (objective exam)	fatigue
wheezing	pain
chills (if shaking accompanies)	hard to hear
tenderness (pain elicited)	paresthesias
restricted motion	chills (sensation of coldness)
diminished reflexes	
shortness of breath (gasping for air)	giddiness, light-headedness
weakness	anxiety
weight loss	shortness of breath (sensation)
vomiting	
palpitations (may sometimes be observed)	weakness
jaundice	loss of appetite
hallucinations (behavior may be unusual)	nausea
coryza (runny nose, watery eyes)	cramps
enathem	palpitations
exanthem	hallucinations
rash	coryza (fatigue, aches and pains)

5. If the disease is diagnosed when examination reveals 22 mm pressure then we shall misdiagnose a large number of healthy eyes.

Raising the diagnostic criteria to 24 will reduce the number of healthy eyes that are misdiagnosed. However, there is a costly and perhaps unethical trade-off; some glaucomatous eyes will not be diagnosed.

6a.   Observable criteria usually are preferred in establishing a diagnosis because of their objective, quantifiable, and unambiguous nature.

Hepatitis would be strongly suspected upon finding an elevation of SGPT with one or more of the following: jaundice, dark urine, light-colored stools, fever.

A less severe form of hepatitis might be suspected if an elevation of SGPT was observed and the patient described symptoms of loss of appetite, fatigue, malaise, abdominal pain, nausea, and vomiting.

6b.   Diagnosis of rheumatic fever is a bit complicated. Because the disease may take many forms and affect different organ systems, the diagnosis requires the physician to have a high degree of suspicion. Diagnosis depends upon the presence of at least one and preferably two or more "major manifestations" of the disease which includes carditis, chorea, arthritis, erythema marginatum (a skin rash), and subcutaneous nodules.

In addition to the "major" manifestations there should be recent evidence of a group A streptococcal infection and the presence of "minor" manifestations of the disease such as fever and elevation of the sedimentation rate and white blood cell count.

6c.   You might have to identify all deaths diagnosed as interstitial pneumonitis, bronchopneumonia, and unknown or ill-defined cause of death from death certificates or hospital records for each year of interest prior to 1973.

The next step would be to obtain the clinical records for each of these deaths, and review the medical history, physical findings, etc., to judge whether the diagnosis of SIDS is possible.

A third step would be to obtain autopsy data and microscopic specimens of body organs to verify the death certificate diagnosis and to reassign the cause of death to SIDS when the pathologic reports suggest that reassignment is appropriate.

Interviews of surviving family members to supplement or verify medical records might be attempted and this may or may not yield usable information depending upon the emotional stress of the interview on the family member.

The task of reclassifying cases years after death occurred is obviously a difficult endeavor. There is a greater potential for error.

7a.   Definitions of cases identifies persons properly assigned to the numerator of rates. The task of specifying criteria to be used in defining "cases" and distinguishing them from "noncases" is one of the major issues addressed by epidemiologists investigating the etiology of acute as well as chronic diseases. Epidemiologists have differences of opinion about what constitutes suitable criteria for defining a case of a disease. When preparing your epidemiologic report clear definitions will establish to the event to which your report refers. Readers of this report will be free to disagree with your definition, but at least they will know how you defined your cases, and how that decision may have influenced the conclusions that you reached. Clear definitions also might be used to resolve apparent differences in results from different investigators. It might turn out that by defining the case or event in different ways, separate investigators reached widely diverse conclusions.

Clear definitions help to minimize error in classification, thereby leading to more accurate data and conclusions. Clear definitions are essential to ascertaining the aggregation of disease in defined groups of persons. These aggregations, if not due to chance or to measurement error, must be the result of increased frequency, intensity, or duration of exposure or increased susceptibility to the causative agent. Conversely, low incidence occurs because of less exposure or susceptibility. A certain proportion of mistaken diagnoses are to be expected. Thus, numerators are subject to error and misclassification of the disease state may be unavoidable.

EXERCISE 6. SCREENING FOR DISEASE

Goals

Upon completion of this exercise you should be able to (1) define the term screening and (2) explain its purpose and uses, and the properties of screening tests. You should also be able to (3) calculate the various measures used to evaluate a screening test.

Methods*

In order to achieve these goals you will need to understand

I.   DEFINITION OF SCREENING
II.   SENSITIVITY AND SPECIFICITY
III. THE EFFECT OF PREVALENCE ON SCREENING TEST RESULTS
IV.   THE EFFECT OF COMBINATIONS OF TESTS

Terms

Validity, efficiency, sensitivity, specificity, false positives and negatives, predictive value, screening by testing in parallel or series.

Suggested Readings

Thorner, and Remein, Principles and Procedures in the Evaluation of Screening for Disease, U.S. Dept. HEW, Public Health Monograph No. 67, 1961.
Galen, R.S. and Gambino, S.R.: Beyond Normality: The Predictive Value and Efficiency of Medical Diagnosis. New York: Wiley and Sons, 1975.
Cole, P., and Morrison, A.S., Basic Issues in Population Screening for Cancer. J. Nat. Cancer Inst. 64:1263, 1980.
Friedman, G. Primer of Epidemiology, 2nd ed. 1980, pp. 244-249, pp. 37-39.
Mausner, J.S., and Bahn, A., Epidemiology, Ch. 11, pp. 237-263.
Lilienfeld and Lilienfeld, Foundations of Epidemiology, 2nd ed., 1980, pp. 149-159.

I.   DEFINITION OF SCREENING

Screening is defined as "the presumptive identification of unrecognized disease or defect by the application of tests, examinations, or other procedures which can be applied rapidly to sort out those who probably have a disease from those who probably do not." A screening test is not intended to be diagnostic. The basic purpose of screening for disease is to separate from a large group of apparently well persons those who have a high probability of having the disease under study, so that they may be given a diagnostic workup and, if diseased, brought to treatment.

---

*Adapted from Thorner and Remein, reference given above.

Screening is carried out in the belief that it can alter the natural history of disease by earlier initiation of therapy in a significant proportion of those who are identified as "positives." This assumption, however, must be tested for each disease. In fact, there is very little objective evidence that the assumption is true.

A generally accepted principle is that screening should only be done if it can be integrated into the existing medical-care program. In practice, this means not only that adequate treatment, care, and follow-up must be available for those who are found to have positive results, but that the screening test's results must be acceptable to the practicing physicians in the area. Some professionals think it is unethical to screen for a disease when a follow-up treatment program is absent. Screening may sometimes be performed for research purposes, but in such an instance, the investigator should inform the study participants that no follow-up therapy will be available.

The implications and consequences of screening must be considered before starting screening programs. Is the test justified, scientifically and financially, by the resulting benefit to the community? Each proposal for screening is usually made with the belief that earlier diagnosis makes currently available therapy more efficient.

Example: Porphyria variegata is a rare inherited abnormality of the liver with an estimated prevalence of about 4 per million. If subjects with this abnormality take barbiturates or sulfonamides they run the risk of death by paralysis. Latent cases can be discovered by a biochemical test of feces costing about two dollars. If such patients are warned not to take barbiturates and sulfonamides, the incidence and the mortality of acute attacks can be drastically reduced. Let us assume that in only one in four latent cases would an attack occur, and that of those experiencing an attack only one in four is fatal.

Question 1

a. How much would it cost to save the life of a patient with porphyria variegata by population screening?

b. Given the cost, time, and anticipated benefits of saving a life, do you believe that this is a worthwhile health program?

c. On a scale of 1 (little value) to 10 (great value), what priority would you give this program?

What should be the measurement properties of the proposed screening test? A test used in screening must be relatively simple and must be acceptable to the subjects. The test should give a true measurement of the attribute under investigation (accuracy) and provide consistent results in repeated trials (precision, sometimes called reproducibility). In addition, a screening test should have high sensitivity and specificity for the disease in question.

II.   SENSITIVITY AND SPECIFICITY

Sensitivity is the ability of a test to give a positive finding when the person tested truly has the disease under study. Specificity is the ability of the test to give a negative finding when the person tested is free of the disease under study. Both are usually expressed as percentages.

The evaluation of sensitivity and specificity requires that a diagnosis for the disease under study be established or ruled out for every person tested by the screening procedure, regardless of whether the person screened negative or positive.

The results of the screening and diagnostic examinations can be examined conveniently by use of the fourfold contingency table shown below:

Figure 1.   Screening test results by diagnosis.

Screening test results	Diagnosis		Total
	Diseased	Not diseased	
Positive	a	b	a + b
Negative	c	d	c + d
Total	a + c	b + d	a + b + c + d

Note: a = diseased persons detected by the test (true positive)
        b = nondiseased persons detected by the test (false positive)
        c = diseased persons not detected by the test (false negative)
        d = nondiseased persons negative to the test (true negative)

The following measures are used to evaluate a screening test:

Sensitivity (true positive)	=	Percentage of persons with the disease who were positive to the test	=	$\frac{a}{a+c} \times 100$
Specificity (true negative)	=	Percentage of nondiseased persons who were negative to the test	=	$\frac{d}{b+d} \times 100$
False negative	=	Percentage of persons with the disease who were negative to the test	=	$\frac{c}{a+c} \times 100$

False positive $=$ Percentage of persons without the disease who were positive to the test $= \dfrac{b}{b+d} \times 100$

Predictive value
of a positive test $=$ Percentage of persons with a positive
test who have the disease $= \dfrac{a}{a+b} \times 100$

Predictive value
of a negative test $=$ Percentage of persons with a negative
test who do not have the disease $= \dfrac{d}{c+d} \times 100$

For most diseases there will be overlapping of the distributions of an attribute for diseased and nondiseased persons. When the distributions overlap it is not possible to correctly assign individuals with these values to either the normal or the diseased group on the basis of screening alone (see Figure 1). False positives and false negatives comprise the area of overlap.

The degree of sensitivity and specificity of the screening test may be varied by placing the screening criterion at different points in the area of overlap, i.e., 22-26 mm Hg. It is apparent that sensitivity is inversely related to specificity; adjusting the criterion of positivity to reduce the number of false positives increases the number of false negatives. Conversely, reducing the number of false negatives increases the number of false positives.

Ideally a screening test should establish either the presence or the absence of a disease in every individual screened. Both sensitivity and specificity would then equal 100%. Unfortunately, this is generally impossible to achieve in practice because there is usually overlap between the distributions of the ill and nonill populations.

Question 2

a. If the screening criterion to detect glaucoma shown in Figure 2 is set at 22 mm Hg, what happens to the sensitivity and specificity of the test?

b. If the screening criterion is then set at 26 mm Hg, how do the sensitivity and specificity change?

Figure 2. Hypothetical distribution of intraocular pressures in glaucomatous
and nonglaucomatous eyes, measured by tonometer.

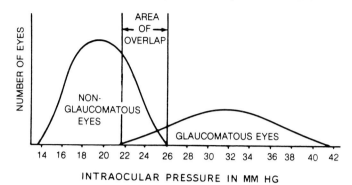

INTRAOCULAR PRESSURE IN MM HG

Source: Thorner and Remein, Principles and procedures in the evaluation
of screening for disease, U.S. Dept. HEW, 1961.

c.   What general principle does this example illustrate?

d.   Where would you establish the criterion if this screening test were to be
used?

III. THE EFFECT OF PREVALENCE ON SCREENING TEST RESULTS

One important problem in screening concerns the relationship between sensitivity, specificity, and prevalence of disease. When the prevalence of a
disease is low (in the order of 1.0 or 2.0%), as it is for many chronic diseases, most of the population will be free of the disease, and the positive
results, even for a highly sensitive and highly specific test, will include a
large number of false positives. A small decrease in the specificity of a test
will greatly increase the number of false positives, and unless this is offset by
a large gain in sensitivity, the proportion of positives that are false will increase or, at least, remain high. The effect of various screening criteria on
test results should be carefully considered before a screening project is undertaken, especially when prevalence is low.

With a given sensitivity and specificity, a small increase in prevalence (1.0 or
2.0 percent) results in a negligible reduction in the number of false positives
for the same number of tests, but the yield of new cases increases in proportion to the increase in prevalence. As a result, the proportion of false positives among persons screening positive is reduced.

By directing his screening efforts toward high prevalence groups that have been previously defined by epidemiological studies, the administrator can increase the yield of the screening test. For example, he can limit a diabetes screening program to persons over 40 and make special efforts to screen obese persons and persons with a family history of diabetes. Screening becomes a two-stage process in which selection of a high prevalence group is the first stage and application of the screening test is the second.

Question 3

What effect does a two-stage screening procedure have on the yield of true positives?

Question 4

The prevalence of undetected diabetes in a population to be screened is approximately 1.5% and it is assumed that 10,000 persons will be screened. The screening test will measure blood serum sugar content. A value of 180 mg percent or higher is considered positive. The sensitivity and specificity associated with this screening are 22.9 and 99.8%, respectively.

a.   Set up a fourfold table with the appropriate numbers in each cell of the table.

Calculate the following values:

b.   The percentage of false positives.

c.   The percentage of false negatives.

d.   The predictive value of a positive test.

e.   The predictive value of a negative test.

f.   How many false positives and negatives will occur if 100,000 people are screened?

Question 5

To observe the effect of increasing sensitivity, assume a blood sugar screening level of 130 mg percent, with a sensitivity of 44.3% and a specificity of 99.0%. Set up a fourfold table with the appropriate numbers in each cell. Calculate the following values when the number of persons screened is 10,000 and the prevalence of undetected diabetes is 1.5%:

a.   The percentage of false positives.   <u>Space for calculation</u>

b.   The percentage of false negatives.

c.   The predictive value of a positive test.

d.   The predictive value of a negative test.

e.   How many false positives and false negatives will occur if 100,000 people are screened?

f.   Summarize the effects of increasing the sensitivity, observed from your calculations for Questions 4 and 5.

g.   If you were the director for the diabetes screening program would you prefer to screen at 130 mg or 180 mg percent?

Question 6

The previous problem looked at the effect of varying sensitivity when the disease prevalence was unchanged. Next, let us assume a situation in which the blood sugar distributions are similar to example 5, but prevalence is 2.5% instead of 1.5%. The screening level remains at 130 mg percent, 10,000 persons are screened, sensitivity is 44.3%, and specificity is 99.0%. Set up a fourfold table with the appropriate numbers in each cell.

Calculate the following values:

a.   The percentage of false positives.   Space for calculation

b.   The percentage of false negatives

c.   The predictive value of a positive test.

d.   The predictive value of a negative test.

e.   What general principle do the data from Questions 5 and 6 illustrate?

f.   If 100,000 persons were screened how many false positives and negatives would occur?

IV. THE EFFECT OF COMBINATIONS OF TESTS

One method for enhancing the sensitivity or specificity of screening is to combine several different tests or to repeat the same test. The combination of tests may be used in "parallel" or in "series." When used in parallel, a screenee is considered positive (+) if he tests positive (+) to any one of the tests. He is considered negative (-) if he tests negative (-) to all tests. In series, the screenee must be positive (+) to each successive test to be considered positive (+); if he is negative (-) to any of the tests he is considered to have screened negative (-).   A schematic diagram is shown below.

tests done in	test 1 result	test 2 result	interpretation
parallel	+	+	+
	+	-	+
	-	+	+
	-	-	-
series	+	+	+
	+	-	-
	-	not necessary	-

When used in parallel, some diseased persons whose values would lie close to the cutoff point may test positive to one but not the other test, resulting in detection of a higher proportion of diseased persons by the combination of tests, i.e., increased sensitivity, decreased specificity.

A combination of tests in series enhances the specificity of the testing but reduces the sensitivity, because some diseased persons whose values lie close to the cutoff point may test positive on one but not the other test.   Also, if the first test result is negative, they do not have the possibility of testing positive on the second.

Consider the hypothetical data in Figure 3, assuming the test population was screened for diabetes using a blood sugar test and a urine sugar test.

Figure 3.   Screening results of blood and urine tests for diabetes mellitus.

Test results	Diabetic	Not diabetic
Positive to urine test, negative to blood	7	3
Positive to blood test, negative to urine	23	11
Positive to both tests	45	7
Negative to both tests	124	7,620
Total	199	7,641

Source: Thorner and Remein, 1961.

Question 7

Calculate the sensitivity and specificity for: <u>Space for calculation</u>

a.   blood sugar test:

b.   urine sugar test:

c.   in parallel, both urine sugar and blood sugar tests performed:

d.   in series, urine test and then blood test performed:

e.   How do the sensitivity or specificity of each combination of the tests change when compared with single tests?

f.   Assuming you are the director of a large diabetes screening program, which test or combination of tests would you prefer to use?

Question 8

Remembering that screening tests are not diagnostic, what effect might occur to a patient who is incorrectly classified as a case of:

a.   breast cancer.

b.   diabetes mellitus.

Question 9

State your opinion on the ethics involved in screening where your test fails to detect a probable case of:

a.   breast cancer.

b.   diabetes mellitus.

Question 10

What do you think ought to be the properties or characteristics of a good screening test?

Question 11

What role does the laboratory or the person making the observation have in determining the accuracy or precision of a screening test? How might the test itself affect this determination?

Question 12

State your opinion concerning the use of screening tests, when there is no effective treatment for the disease or when there are limited medical services available to treat persons who screen positive.

SUGGESTED RESPONSES
Exercise 6--Screening for Disease

1a. Incidence is 4 latent cases per million people. Only 1 in 16 cases is fatal. We must screen 4 million people to save one person's life. At $2 per test the cost is $8 million.

1b. On a cost-benefit basis it is hardly worth it. This program would have low priority if it was competing for limited health funds.

1c. If it is your life it is a 10. If someone else's life, maybe a 1 or 2.

2a. 100% sensitivity but the specificity is below 100% because of a large number of false positives.

2b. 100% specificity but sensitivity decreases below 100% because some glaucomatous eyes will be false negatives.

2c. Sensitivity and specificity are usually inversely related and, therefore, one may be increased only at the expense of the other.

2d. The point at which the distributions intersect is frequently used because it will generally minimize the false positives and false negatives when both are considered important.

The decision on the screening criterion used is ultimately a reasoned judgment about the number of false positives and false negatives that are tolerable to the population and to the provider of the screening service. This judgment should be based on the severity of the disease, the cost of the test, the time taken to administer it, and the advantages and probability of obtaining early treatment.

3. It increases the yield of true positives and it is a very efficient technique.

4b. False Pos. $= \frac{20}{9,850} \times 100 = 0.2\%$

4c. False Neg. $= \frac{116}{150} \times 100 = 77.3\%$

4d. Pred. Pos. $= \frac{34}{54} \times 100 = 63.0\%$

4e. Pred. Neg. $= \frac{9830}{9946} \times 100 = 98.8\%$

4f. False Pos. = 200 persons
    False Neg. = 1160 persons

4a. Table for Question 4

		Disease		
		+	-	Total
Test	+	34	20	54
	-	116	9,830	9,946
Total		150	9,850	10,000

5a.   False Pos. $= \dfrac{98}{9850}$ X 100 = 1.0%

5b.   False Neg. $= \dfrac{84}{150}$ X 100 = 56.0%

5c.   Pred. Pos. $= \dfrac{66}{164}$ X 100 = 40.2%

5d.   Pred. Neg. $= \dfrac{9752}{9836}$ X 100 = 99.1%

Table for Question 5

Test	Disease +	Disease -	Total
+	66	98	164
-	84	9,752	9,836
Total	150	9,850	10,000

5e.   False Pos. = 980 persons; False neg. = 840 persons

5f.   Increasing the sensitivity to 44.3% reduces specificity from 99.8 to 99%.
      False positives increase from 0.2 to 1.0%
      False negatives decrease from 77.3 to 56.0%
      Pred. power of positives decreases from 63.0 to 40.2%
      Pred. power of negatives increases from 98.8 to 99.1%
      The number of false positives would increase from 200 to 980 persons
      The number of false negatives would decrease from 1160 to 840 persons.

5g.   The test yielding more false positives and fewer false negatives (130 mg%)
      would be preferable; otherwise one misses a lot of people who might be
      diabetic. However, a different decision might be made depending upon
      the resources of the program, or other administrative or political consid-
      erations.

6a.   False Pos. $= \dfrac{97}{9750}$ X 100 = 1.0%

6b.   False Neg. $= \dfrac{139}{250}$ X 100 = 55.6%

6c.   Pred. Pos. $= \dfrac{111}{208}$ X 100 = 53.4%

6d.   Pred. Neg. $= \dfrac{9653}{9792}$ X 100 = 98.6%

Table for Question 6.

Test	Disease +	Disease -	Total
+	111	97	208
-	139	9,653	9,792
Total	250	9,750	10,000

6e.   With the sensitivity remaining constant,
      the gain in yield of new cases is pro-
      portional to the gain in prevalence.

6f.   False positives = 970, false negatives = 1390. With a given sensitivity,
      any increase in prevalence results in a proportional increase in the num-
      ber of false negatives.

7a.   Blood

      Sensitivity $= \dfrac{23 + 45}{199}$ X 100 = 34.2%

      Specificity $= \dfrac{3 + 7,620}{7,641}$ X 100 = 99.8%

7b.   Urine

Sensitivity $= \dfrac{7 + 45}{199} \times 100 = 26.1\%$

Specificity $= \dfrac{11 + 7,620}{7,641} \times 100 = 99.9\%$

7c.   In parallel

Sensitivity $= \dfrac{7 + 23 + 45}{199} \times 100 = 37.7\%$

Specificity $= \dfrac{7,620}{7,641} \times 100 = 99.7\%$

7d.   In series

Sensitivity $= \dfrac{45}{199} \times 100 = 22.6\%$

Specificity $= \dfrac{3+11+7,620}{7,641} \times 100 = 99.9\%$

7e.   In parallel

Sensitivity (37.7%) is increased, in comparison with single test results for: urine = 26.1%; or blood = 34.2%. Specificity = 99.7%, which is about the same as each test performed individually.

In series

Sensitivity (22.6%) is decreased, in comparison with single test results for urine = 26.1%; or blood = 34.2%. Specificity = 99.9%, which is about the same as each test performed individually.

7f.   The choice would be influenced by your operating budget and size of your staff, the availability of follow-up or treatment, and your judgment concerning the relative importance of false positive or false negative results.

8a.   Effects might occur with regard to follow-up treatment and psychologic reactions. Identifying a healthy woman as a potential breast cancer case might cause psychologic problems to the woman and might subject her to unnecessary surgical or x-ray procedures. By raising the possibility that she had breast cancer the woman would probably never feel completely secure again.

8b.   Therapy for early diabetes is usually limited to modification of diet and so treatment even if not necessary, is not likely to be harmful. Subsequent examinations are relatively easy to do, do not require surgery or radiation and are not terribly expensive. Although there is a possibility of psychologic reaction on the part of the patient, diabetes is not as terrifying a disease to contemplate as cancer.

9a.   Inability of the test to correctly identify a true positive might result in missing potential early cases of disease. A successful screening test raises expectations for early detection leading to treatment and cure. A test with a high percentage of false negatives might reassure patients and physicians but would not produce the desired improvement in the public's health if women believing themselves to be free of disease developed cancer and did not seek treatment.

9b.   Diabetes mellitus is an illness with a long and progressive course. There is no evidence that early detection and treatment prevents the development of the disease, although the incidence of many of the severe manifestations such as diabetic acidosis and coma have been reduced. Thus, inability to detect probable cases of diabetes in an early stage is not as troubling as missing a potential case of cancer. As diabetes progresses, signs and symptoms will appear and effective treatment can be initiated. Also, the screening test is fairly crude and not necessarily limited to detection of diabetes.

10.   A good screening test should have the following properties:

1.   high sensitivity⎫
2.   high specificity⎬ (accuracy)
3.   easy to perform
4.   clearly defined test results
5.   low cost
6.   reproducible results (precision)
7.   acceptable to the person screened (e.g., painless and not invasive)
8.   no side effects or undue risk of complications or disease from the test

Unfortunately, there are no screening tests currently available that can meet all these criteria.

11.   Screening procedures can involve direct determination of some attribute of the screenee such as height, weight, visual acuity, or blood pressure. Screening procedures can also involve determination of some attribute from body tissues such as blood, wine, skin, hair, or cells taken from smears or biopsy. No matter what the source, all of the test results will be subject to a certain error. Some errors are measurable and stated, for example, a piece of laboratory equipment may measure some specimens to less than 1% error while other specimens have 10-20% error.

In addition there can be errors attributable to the person reading, recording, or interpreting the test result. Some of these are termed digit preference, in which an observer will round off the number to some convenient one, for example, 2, 4, 6, 8, or 0; or may round off to every

5 or 10 units. When the observer doesn't indicate that this was done, it may be difficult to reproduce that person's observations and to compare those results to those of a different observer.

Another type of observer error occurs when the test has no clearly evident endpoint. For example, if a liquid must change from red to colorless and goes through a continium involving pink, the exact point when one color begins and ends cannot be determined without some subjective judgment. Different observers would be likely to have different opinions about when the color changed. Moreover, the same observer would also be likely to read a test result in different ways on separate occasions.

Finally, some test results require a subjective determination, e.g., observers may be required to classify results as 1+, 2+, 3+, 4+, or judge when a chemical solution changes from pink to colorless. Different observers might disagree as to the concentration of chemical or degree of cellular abnormality defined by these categories, or when the endpoint of the test was reached.

In summary, an epidemiologist who contemplates using a screening test must carefully consider the potential sources of error that might arise in the laboratory or through an observer's reading or recording of the test result.

12. The use of screening tests raises the expectation of follow-up care for diagnosis or treatment of persons who are positives. While availability of diagnostic and therapeutic services is not included among the criteria of what makes a good screening test, their availability is implied when screening tests are employed. The use of screening tests if further diagnostic or therapeutic services are not available should not be encouraged. When limited services are available there will be competition among the positive screenees to receive further diagnostic tests or therapy. We do not know of any procedures to help decide in a fair and equitable way who shall receive and who shall be denied the additional care or services.

PART III.   EPIDEMIOLOGIC STRATEGY

Part III consists of Exercises 7-9, which will demonstrate the strategy epidemiology employs in searching for the causes of disease and the measures taken to prevent or control ill health in human populations.

EXERCISE 7.   INVESTIGATION OF AN EPIDEMIC

One of the major applications of the epidemiologic method is the strategy for investigation of epidemics in human populations.   The exercise provides an opportunity to learn the principles of the investigative approach.

Goals

Upon completion of this exercise you should be able (1) to determine if an epidemic has occurred; (2) to use the epidemic curve to distinguish the type of epidemic; (3) to determine the information needed to carry out a case investigation; (4) to understand the purpose and sequence of the different stages of an investigation; and (5) to make a reasonable judgment about the source of an outbreak after review of the collected epidemiologic facts pertaining to that disease outbreak.

Methods

In order to achieve these goals, you will need to understand

I.   TYPES OF EPIDEMICS

    A.   Common-source epidemics
    B.   Propagated epidemics

II.   MODE OF TRANSMISSION
III. CONTROL MEASURES FOR EPIDEMICS
IV.   OUTLINE FOR EPIDEMIC INVESTIGATIONS

Following these sections, you will have the opportunity to apply some of the concepts and techniques learned in Exercises 1-6.

V.   INVESTIGATION OF A FOOD-BORNE EPIDEMIC

    A.   Preparation of graphs, tables and rates to permit determination of groups that were ill or at risk of being ill
    B.   Formulation of hypotheses of causation

VI.   DESIGN OF EPIDEMIOLOGIC RECORD FORMS

Terms

Common-source, propagated, and point-source epidemics, epidemic curves, median incubation period, infection and disease, subclinical or inapparent infection, herd immunity, high risk groups.

Suggested Readings

Standard texts are not specifically concerned with the sequence of steps employed in the analysis of epidemics.

Last, J.M. (Ed.). Maxcy-Rosenau Public Health and Preventive Medicine, (11th Ed.) (pp. 9-85). New York, Appleton-Century Crofts, 1980.
Dack, G.M. Food Poisoning, Ed. 3 (pp. 2-11). Chicago, University of Chicago Press, 1956.
Meyer, K.F. Food poisoning. New England J. Med. 249:804-812 and 843-852, 1953.
Feig, M. The investigation of food-borne outbreaks of acute gastroenteritis. Am. J. Pub. Health 42:1535-1541, 1952.
Hobbs, B.C. Food Poisoning and Food Hygiene (4th Ed.), Chapters 3 and 6. London: Edward Arnold, 1978.
International Association of Milk and Food Sanitarians, Inc. Procedure for the Investigation of Food-borne Disease Outbreaks. Shelbyville, Ind., Intern. Assoc. of Milk and Food Sanitarians, 1957.
American Public Health Association. Control of Communicable Diseases in Man, Ed. 13. New York: Am. Pub. Health Assoc., 1980.

I.   TYPES OF EPIDEMICS

The pattern of a disease over time can give clues about the source or etiology of the disease. An unusual occurrence of cases is termed an epidemic. There are two major types of epidemics: common-source (or common exposure) and propagated or progressive epidemics (person-to-person transmission). A graph of the distribution of epidemic cases over time is called the epidemic curve. The shape of the curve may sometimes permit us to distinguish between common-source and propagated epidemics.

A common-source epidemic occurs when a group of people are exposed to the same causative agent. If the period of exposure to the agent is brief and essentially simultaneous for all persons contracting the disease, the epidemic is called a point-source epidemic. Common-source epidemics are frequently but not always due to exposure to an infectious organism. They can result from common exposure to noxious agents in the environment, e.g., children who swim in a chemically polluted river, workers exposed to extreme heat or volatile chemicals, persons whose water might be contaminated by a nearby waste disposal site, or cholera organisms.

Propagated epidemics are most often of infectious origin and result from the transmission of an infectious agent from one susceptible host to another.

Transmission of the infecting organism continues until the number of susceptibles is depleted or susceptible individuals no longer are exposed to infected
persons or intermediary vectors.

The incidence of epidemic cases can be depicted graphically by plotting the
date of the onset of illness over time. The resulting graph is termed the
epidemic curve. The shape of the epidemic curves will usually vary for several reasons, including the number of susceptible individuals who are exposed
to the disease agent, and the duration of the incubation period.

The incubation period is the time between exposure to (and infection with) a
pathogenic agent and the onset of clinical illness. The incubation period
varies for different infectious agents; illness may occur within hours (e.g.,
salmonella infection after eating contaminated food) or weeks or months (e.g.,
hepatitis infection after receiving contaminated blood in a transfusion) after
exposure. For each infectious agent the incubation period may be expected to
vary depending upon the amount of the agent present in the infecting dose,
the agent's pathogenicity, and the host's susceptibility. Every disease agent
has a minimum incubation period before which no illness occurs. Also of
interest is the median incubation period (the time required for 50% of the cases
to occur following exposure). Inspection of the shape of the epidemic curve
will frequently enable an epidemiologist to determine the time of exposure to
the epidemic agent. Incubation periods for the important infectious diseases
may be found in the APHA handbook, Control of Communicable Diseases in
Man.

A.   COMMON-SOURCE EPIDEMICS

These depend upon exposure to a common source, but exposure may occur
either repeatedly or be prolonged over a long period of time. Because exposure is over an extended time period, the occurrence of cases is also prolonged. The shape of the epidemic curve will vary depending upon the disease agent; size of the population exposed; the type of source and its distribution or extent of use, or contact with the susceptible population. A typical
common source outbreak epidemic curve is illustrated below. The London
cholera outbreak (see Exercise 8) and the Guillain-Barre syndrome outbreak
(see Exercise 2) are actual examples.

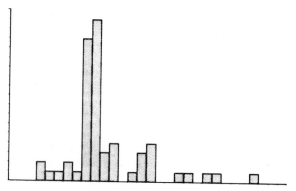

Point-source epidemics are a subset of common-source epidemics in that the cases are all exposed to the same source in a brief period of time. The source may be infectious agents contaminating foods or liquids, or exposure to a non-infectious agent contaminating the environment, such as the air pollution in the London fog incident. Whatever the source, cases occur in clusters that usually are very closely related in time and space. The curve rises and falls abruptly within hours or days of exposure depending upon the incubation period of the responsible agent. The curve has a characteristic shape (a log-normal curve) usually with one peak as shown below. Exceptions to this shape may occur if more than one disease agent (each with a different incubation period) is involved or if secondary cases (person-to-person transmission) follow exposure to the original point source. Examples of a point-source epidemic are the influenza outbreak aboard an airliner and the mortality due to air pollution during the London fog episode (see Exercise 2).

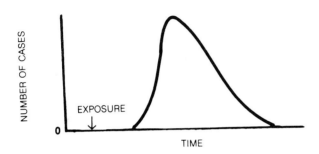

B.   PROPAGATED EPIDEMICS

Propagated epidemics involve person-to-person transmission. The shape of the epidemic curve reflects several factors, including the population size and composition, the proportion of susceptibles in the population, the number of cases at the start of the epidemic, the contact rate between infected and susceptible individuals, the infectivity or pathogenicity of the disease agent, and the incubation period of the disease.

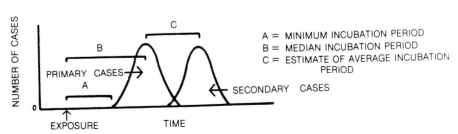

The disease may continue to spread until there are few susceptibles remaining or until susceptibles no longer come in contact with infected persons or vectors. An epidemiologist must be aware of the distinction between <u>infection</u> and disease. Both infected and diseased persons harbor the organism but only the diseased person becomes ill, i.e., exhibits signs and symptoms and is diag-nosed as a clinical case. The term <u>subclinical</u> <u>cases</u> refers to infected persons who do not develop clinical illness (<u>disease</u>); however, they may show a rise in antibody titer or the presence of antibody.

Occasionally, diseases of uncertain etiology and incubation period, e.g., leukemia, Hodgkins disease, and lymphomas, have been reported to show an unusual time-place clustering. It is exceedingly difficult to determine if these clusters represent an epidemic having a common source or mode of occurrence, or whether they comprise a rare aggregation of unrelated events.

Figure 1. Distribution of cases of infectious hepatitis by week of onset, Sharpsburg, Maryland, 1966.

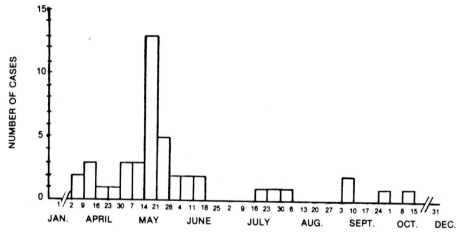

Source: Whatley, T.R., Comstock, G.W., Garber, H.J., Sanchez, F.S., A waterborne outbreak of infectious hepatitis in a small Maryland town, Am. J. Epidemiol. 87(1):138, 1968.

<u>Question 1</u>

a.   Figure 1 shows the epidemic curve of an outbreak of infectious hepatitis in Maryland. The incubation period of hepatitis ranges from 2 weeks to 2 months. What type of epidemic is suggested by this curve?

b.   How would you explain the occurrence of late cases?

Population Immunity and Individual Protection

For a propagated epidemic to occur and spread in a population, susceptible persons must be exposed to infectious cases. Since an individual's risk of disease is determined by his own susceptibility and chance of exposure, anything which reduces the risk of exposure offers protection for the individual. As the number of recovered (immune) persons increases, the susceptibility of the population to that disease decreases, and the opportunity for further spread will also decline. The protection from an epidemic accruing to a community because of the decreased likelihood of exposure of susceptible individuals to infectious cases is called <u>herd immunity</u>. Herd immunity occurs when a population has a large proportion of immune individuals that serves as a buffer to decrease the probability of exposure of susceptible individuals to infected cases.

The proportion of the population that must be immune to prevent an epidemic is not fixed but varies with the disease, the density of the population and other factors influencing exposure. In some situations an epidemic will not occur even if a relatively low percentage of the population is immune, while in others an epidemic will occur even if a very high percentage of the group is immune. The important point to remember is that 100 percent immunity is not necessary in a community to prevent an epidemic. The population immunity may be an important factor in the dynamics or the periodicity of some of infectious diseases.

Question 2

Plot the following data of two epidemics of infectious hepatitis. Use the x axis to denote time and y axis for the number of cases. What type of epidemic does each appear to be?

Figure 2. Date of onset of two epidemics of infectious hepatitis, city x, 1978 and 1979.

Epidemic Number 1

Cases of hepatitis by date of onset, Aug-Sept 1978

Date	Cases	Date	Cases
1978 Aug 21	1	1978 Sept 3	13
22	0	4	12
23	1	5	11
24	0	6	11
25	0	7	3
26	0	8	1
27	2	9	3
28	4	10	3
29	0	11	2
30	2	12	0
31	7	13	2
Sept 1	7	14	0
2	13	Total	98

EPIDEMIC 1

Epidemic Number 2

Cases of hepatitis by week, June 1978-April 1979

1978	Jun	7	0	1978 Nov 15	6
		14	0	22	6
		21	2	29	5
		28	0	Dec 6	4
	Jul	5	0	13	4
		12	0	20	2
		19	1	27	4
		26	0	1979 Jan 3	5
	Aug	2	0	10	10
		9	0	17	5
		16	1	24	8
		23	1	31	2
		30	0	Feb 7	3
	Sept	6	1	14	3
		13	1	21	1
		20	2	28	8
		27	2	Mar 7	1
	Oct	4	0	14	1
		11	0	21	2
		18	4	28	3
		25	12	Apr 4	2
	Nov	1	5	11	1
		8	0	18	0
				Total	118

Source: MMWR, Center for Disease Control.

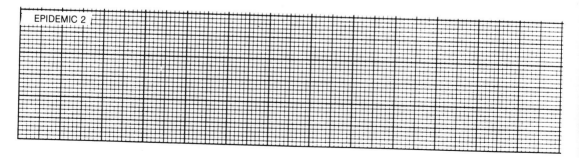

EPIDEMIC 2

An Outbreak of Measles

Question 3

a. Plot the following data for a measles epidemic. Use the x axis to denote
    time and y axis for the number of cases.

Figure 3. Cases of measles by week, U.S., November 1970 - May 1971.

Week Ending	Number of Cases	Week Ending	Number of Cases
1970 Nov 28	1	Feb 27	91
Dec 5	2	1971 Mar 6	81
12	11	13	94
19	3	20	92
26	4	27	31
1971 Jan 2	11	Apr 3	42
9	15	10	44
16	17	17	38
23	37	24	28
30	29	May 1	19
Feb 6	51	8	11
13	82	15	2
20	87	22	0

Source: MMWR, Center for Disease Control.

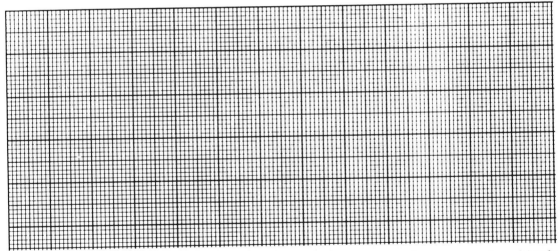

b. The incubation period of measles is 8-14 days. What type of epidemic
    does this appear to be?

c.   What possible explanations can you give for the abrupt decline in the number of cases (in terms of exposure and susceptibility)?

II.   MODE OF TRANSMISSION

Question 4

a.   An agent responsible for causing an illness must reach susceptible hosts. List the mechanisms by which infectious diseases can be transmitted.

b.   Epidemics of disease or clusters of health problems not caused by infectious agents may also occur. List the mechanisms by which these can be transmitted or occur.

III.   CONTROL MEASURES FOR EPIDEMICS

Epidemiologists are frequently called in to investigate an epidemic when the peak of the outbreak has already occurred, the epidemic curve is on the decline, and little active intervention is required. In situations where the epidemic is still a public health problem, epidemiologists would attempt to apply certain principles leading to the CONTROL of the current problem and the PREVENTION of subsequent outbreaks.

Question 5

What general principles apply to the control and prevention of epidemics?

Question 6

a.   What are the actual measures that can be taken to control an epidemic of an infectious disease?

b.   What measures can the epidemiologist take or recommend to control or prevent epidemics of noninfectious etiology?

Question 7

What is meant by the term "high-risk group"?   Why are they important to identify?

Question 8

If you, as the City Health Commissioner, decided that an immunization campaign was necessary to control an epidemic of an infectious disease:

a.   What percentage of the community would you attempt to immunize?

b.   Do you think it would be possible or necessary to have all persons immunized?   Why?

IV. OUTLINE FOR EPIDEMIC INVESTIGATIONS*

The investigation of an epidemic of infectious disease in a community is an exciting and challenging experience for the epidemiologist. The purpose of this outline is to provide a guide to the steps to be taken in such investigations, an understanding of the rationale for each procedure, and an appreciation of the variety of considerations that precede preparation of a report that neatly summarizes, but that oversimplify the complexity or problems actually encountered in performing the investigations.

A. BASIC PRINCIPLES USED TO STUDY THE DISTRIBUTION OF AN INFECTIOUS DISEASE IN A POPULATION.

1. The occurrence of a disease in a population follows a PREDICTABLE PATTERN, which is specific for that disease and which is determined by the characteristics of the etiologic agent, the host population, and the environment.

2. Differences in the risk of contracting illnesses are not randomly distributed but are INFLUENCED BY VARIATIONS IN THE EXPOSURE AND SUSCEPTIBILITY of individual members of a population.

3. Exposure and susceptibility as biologic variables are closely related to and INFLUENCED BY ONE OR MORE CHARACTERISTICS OF PERSONS in a community, such as race, sex, occupation, age, length of residence, nutritional status, or immunity status.

4. Factors of EXPOSURE AND SUSCEPTIBILITY OF A POPULATION RARELY CAN BE MEASURED, INFERRED, OR OBSERVED DIRECTLY, especially with reference to events that have already occurred. In other words, the epidemiologist rarely is present to observe critical events at the time they occur. However, the PROBABLE CONDITIONS OF EXPOSURE AND SUSCEPTIBILITY CAN BE RECONSTRUCTED FROM INDIRECT EVIDENCE. A simple example would be:

> Fifteen cases of measles have occurred within the past 5 days in a population of 100 children in a mental institution. The population of the institution is evenly distributed between ages 5-15, and all cases have been in the age group 5-9. The epidemiologist knows these cases were exposed to a source of infection, an ill person, within the past 2 weeks; new cases were not immune (had not had measles before); the older children, who have escaped clinical disease, either were not exposed or have had the disease before and are immune; and another group of new (secondary) cases is expected to develop their disease onsets within the next two weeks, if there are additional susceptibles in the population.

*Adapted from Smith, C.E., and Reeves, W., the University of California, School of Public Health, Dept. of Epidemiology.

In this extremely simple example, the epidemiologist:

a.   Characterized the pattern of disease by selected measurable qualities of the population (age distributions), which gave an indirect measure of the population's exposure and susceptibility.

b.   Used knowledge of the disease process (infection source, incubation period, and probable clinical response).

c.   Used knowledge of the relationship of the population to its environment (infectiousness and respiratory transmission).

d.   Made a series of LOGICAL INFERENCES THAT WOULD EXPLAIN THE OCCURRENCE of the event and predict future events.

5.   The validity of the epidemiologic information depends on the thoroughness, care, and precision of the investigator.

6.   BEFORE AN HYPOTHESIS TO EXPLAIN THE OCCURRENCE OF DISEASE IN A POPULATION IS ACCEPTED, IT MUST FIT THE PATTERN OF EVENTS IN THE INVESTIGATION AND EXCEPTIONS TO THE PATTERN MUST BE MINIMAL OR NONEXISTENT AND MUST BE BIOLOGICALLY EXPLAINABLE.

B.   APPROACHES TO AN EPIDEMIOLOGIC INVESTIGATION.

1.   Historically, all cultures, in their folklore, have used a form of epidemiology because of concern with diseases in their populations. Thus, certain rules or taboos were developed to govern the habits of the people and to minimize their risk of disease. These actions most frequently were based on experience and unorganized observations, and generally were not subject to scientific evaluation.

Epidemiology became a science when a few highly motivated and well-disciplined physicians developed a concern with the problem of why certain of their patients had a given disease and other persons did not. These physicians observed that groups of patients with a single disease shared certain common events or characteristics different from those of other persons without disease, and that this would explain an increased risk of the disease.

Such observations preceded knowledge of the specific nature of infectious agents or other causative factors, yet, in these classical studies, the causative factor was almost precisely defined. Examples are included in your reference list in Appendix 2. Among the finest are Snow on cholera, Budd on typhoid, Panum on measles, Goldberger on pellagra, and Potts on scrotal cancer.

Many early epidemiologic studies have been called "shoeleather" epidemiology,* because the investigator went from case to case, to study the disease, to determine the exposures, and to observe the environment of cases. The accumulated data allowed the investigator to infer a pattern of behavior and experience unique to his cases, one that definitely explained the cause and distribution of the disease. These data also permit us to explain the distribution of absence of disease.

2. Modern day epidemiology frequently is characterized by the team or multidisciplinary approach, rather than the individual investigator.

The skills of a wide variety of scientists and technicians from different fields can be focused on current health problems. Physicians, nurses, dentists, and veterinarians from the clinical and public health fields are frequently involved, but epidemiologic investigations may also require the participation of individuals from other fields, some of which are

biostatistics	psychology
computer science	anthropology
genetics	ecology
microbiology	social work
zoology	industrial hygiene
virology	traffic and safety management
bacteriology	hospital administration
biochemistry	engineering
nutrition	meteorology
sanitation	laboratory technology

It is the responsibility of the epidemiologist to know what disciplines are necessary to complement the investigation of the particular disease in question, and to correlate and interpret the information collected.

C. STEPS IN A DESCRIPTIVE EPIDEMIOLOGIC STUDY OF AN EPIDEMIC

Specific steps are usually taken in response to a reported outbreak of a health problem in a population. Consideration of these steps will provide you with a useful approach, which can be applied to a variety of situations, although it is not intended to be a "cookbook recipe" that will cover any and all situations.

Imagine yourself as an epidemiologist in a state health department who has just received a telephone call from a local health officer who reports an epidemic and requests your assistance in its investigation.

1. PRIOR TO INITIATING A FIELD INVESTIGATION, THE EPIDEMIOLOGIST WOULD DESIRE SOME OF THE FOLLOWING INFORMATION AND MIGHT OBTAIN IT IN THE INITIAL TELEPHONE CONTACT. THE INFORMATION

---

*B. Roueche has written many intriguing accounts of shoeleather epidemiology, listed in the bibliography in Appendix 1.

MIGHT, OF NECESSITY, BE TENTATIVE, AND UNCONFIRMED. IF UN-AVAILABLE FROM THE REPORTING HEALTH OFFICER, OTHER SOURCES MAY NEED TO BE USED.

a.   The probable diagnosis, including symptomatology and laboratory data available to confirm the diagnosis. The disease may be known at the onset of the study or it could be a new disease.

b.   Confirm that an epidemic has actually occurred by determining:

(1) The number of known cases in order to establish a preliminary estimate of the magnitude of the problem.

(2) The distribution of the cases with regard to person, place, and time of onset. These considerations are important as they indicate the magnitude of the problem, distances to be covered, number of agencies or other health jurisdiction potentially involved, and type of background information needed to evaluate the expected incidence of the disease.

(3) Preliminary estimates of rates calculated after obtaining denominator data from census records or other appropriate sources.

(4) The trend of this disease in the area. Inquiry should be made concerning the occurrence of similar episodes in the past or whether cases of similar illness have been observed in neighboring areas.

c.   Determine the local facilities that are available to aid in the investigation, such as personnel, field and laboratory equipment, office space, and cars.

d.   Obtain from the reporting person a clear notion of what help is required and what assistance is being requested of you.

e.   Finally, the epidemiologist may need to review new and background literature on the subject to become up to date, and arrange for diagnostic laboratory support before initiating a field study. In addition, he may need to obtain general literature on the disease, data reporting forms, and equipment.

2.   THE SECOND STEP IS TO GO TO THE SCENE OF THE EPIDEMIC. ON ARRIVAL:

a.   Identify yourself to the necessary authorities, health officer, hospital administrator, local medical society, etc., and coordinate your activities with them.

b.   Establish a basis for the confirmation of diagnosis of the disease or diseases to be investigated. This will entail a personal visit to examine cases if the epidemiologist is a physician, or arrangement for proper consultation with competent physicians if there are any questions or problems. The bases for confirmation of diagnoses are

(1) Complete clinical characterization of the cases. Criterion for inclusion as a case must be <u>clear</u> <u>and</u> <u>explicit</u> for present and future reference.

(2) Establish and document clear procedures for collection and processing of diagnostic specimens if a laboratory confirmation test is used. In some situations where potential for litigation may exist, you might need to institute <u>chain</u> <u>of</u> <u>custody</u> <u>procedures</u> to assure that specimens would be admissible in a court of law.

(3) Collect diagnostic specimens for the investigation with a proper explanation of their intended use and limitations. The initial concentrated effort will be on persons currently ill (particularly cases with recent onset), as they are the most promising sources of determining etiologic agents, and it is still possible to demonstrate diagnostic rises in their antibody titers.

(4) A laboratory confirmation of the diagnosis is important, if possible, to eliminate misdiagnosis and confusion, particularly when there is overlap of symptoms of the disease of interest and other diseases that may be similar.

c. Know what diseases are occurring in the area at the same time. When a group of diseases has overlapping clinical syndromes, one of them may be the popular (and sometimes mistaken) diagnosis at a particular time. The same biologic conditions may be favorable for transmission of several diseases.

d. Determine if cases of the same disease are occurring concurrently in adjacent or geographically related areas. The epidemic may not be restricted to one county or health jurisdiction.

e. At this stage (or earlier) in the investigation, you will have to answer the question, "Is this an epidemic?" Evaluation of the degree to which the usual or expected frequency of disease is exceeded was discussed in Exercise 1. Certain factors make the determination difficult:

(1) A marked and recent increase or decrease in the population may increase or decrease the number of cases, even though the attack rate remains constant.

(2) There may be gross exaggeration of the number of cases due to misdiagnosis or duplicate reporting by hospitals, physicians, and schools.

(3) A new health officer, recent legislation, or a newly developed diagnostic procedure may stimulate increased completeness of reporting, or may lead to reporting of old chronic cases as new cases. The incidence versus prevalence of cases may require clarification.

(4) The normal seasonal variation in occurrence of a disease may give the impression of an epidemic when no or few cases occurred until recently. Comparison with the incidence of cases during the same season in prior years will reveal the expected frequency of disease and clarify whether the observed frequency is unusual. It is possible to sometimes underestimate as well as overestimate the magnitude of an epidemic because of fluctuation in the cyclical or secular trend of the particular disease over several years.

(5) A simple numerical comparison of the number of cases in different time periods is risky, as was indicated in (1). The use of population based rates is preferable. An increase in rates, however, can reflect either increased completeness of reporting [points (2) and (3)] or an actual increase in disease.

(6) Special surveys and efforts to find missed cases and inapparent infections (cases in whom infection occurred, but no clinical disease was evident, also called subclinical cases) will inevitably increase numerator data as compared with normal reporting of the disease. This can lead to the so-called "manufactured epidemic."

3. INCIDENCE DATA WILL BE THE MOST CRITICAL TO THE INVESTIGATION AND USUALLY WILL BE BASED ON INFORMATION ACCUMULATED FROM A SERIES OF CASE HISTORIES THAT THE INVESTIGATOR MUST OBTAIN AND ORGANIZE. A CASE HISTORY FORM INCLUDES:

Name
Age
Period of residence in the community
Sex
Race
Address (home, business, school, etc.)
Occupation
Description of the illness and basis for diagnosis
Outcome of illness
Dates of onset, hospitalization, recovery, and/or termination (death)
Roster of family or resident associates and their age, sex, occupation, and current illnesses
History of travel, contact with other known cases, exposure to food sources, milk and water supply, insects, etc., which may be the source or mode of transmission depending upon the type of disease under study

4. IN ORDER TO DETERMINE WHETHER THE CASE GROUP TRULY DIFFERS FROM THE REMAINDER OF THE POPULATION, AND TO EXPRESS THE DIFFERENCE QUANTITATIVELY, COMPARABLE INFORMATION MUST BE OBTAINED FROM PERSONS WHO ARE NOT ILL

    a.   Some data, especially age, sex, and race distributions may be available from census tabulations.

    b.   A probability sample of the base population is the most accurate means of describing that population.

    c.   Comparison subjects may be drawn and matched to the case group for some one or several characteristics.

    d.   Among the persons sharing a common event, the total group of noncases is often compared with the cases.

5. ANALYSIS OF HOST CHARACTERISTICS TO IDENTIFY FACTORS THAT ARE COMMON TO THE CASES AND DIFFERENTIATE THEM FROM THE UNAFFECTED POPULATION. ONCE FACTORS OF SIMILARITY WITHIN THE CASE SERIES ARE IDENTIFIED, THERE WILL BE A BASIS FOR FORMULATION OF HYPOTHESES TO EXPLAIN THE SEQUENCE OF EVENTS THAT CAUSED THE EPIDEMIC.

    a.   The analysis might start with a comparison of the simplest types of variables that can be examined to reveal significant differences between the ill and not ill populations. If possible, the analysis should consist of rates of illness in the population at risk, distinguished by characteristics of person, place, and time, such as:

    Age   Length of residence
    Ethnicity, race, color   Sex
    Eating and drinking histories   Attendance at a function having a
    Recent activities   large number of persons present
    Occupation

    Establishing these categories is done to detect any increased risk of illness in persons of different characteristics or with different prior experiences. The importance of such differences, epidemiologically, can be appreciated by a brief consideration of several examples:

        (1) Why is an analysis of the age of cases as compared with the general population important?

        You might get an indication of selective exposure to the cause and this would lead you to the source.

        The age distribution of cases may reflect the prior experience of the total population with that disease, particularly when immunity controls susceptibility.

Severity of disease may vary with age for certain diseases. Clusters of cases in a restricted age group may reflect that only the severely ill are in the series. A careful study of small groups of contacts in other age groups may reveal milder or inapparent infections, and show the complete spectrum of the disease.

(2) An analysis of the length of residence of cases in contrast to age distribution can be useful in the study of diseases having limited or even focal geographic distribution. Thus, populations that live in endemic areas are at risk while others are not. That portion of the population that migrates into such an area is unusual in that all members regardless of age are at equal risk of infection in the absence of immunity. Thus, all members of a family are of equal age in terms of prior experience and susceptibility.

(3) A cluster of cases in an occupational group, or in residents exposed to the environment of a particular industry, or the accumulation of cases predominantly in one sex, or ethnic group has obvious implications in determining the source of a disease because of the potential for selective exposure.

The purpose of this type of analysis is to study the differences between cases and noncases in the hope that they will lead to clues as to the probable source or sources of infection or exposure. With adequate numerator and denominator data, the comparison can be made of attack rates or percent distributions. The simplest analysis usually is by means of a fourfold table.

6. ANALYSIS OF THE DISTRIBUTION OF CASES GEOGRAPHICALLY, TO IDENTIFY EXPOSURE OF CASES TO A COMMON LOCATION OR LOCATIONS DIFFERENT FROM THAT OF THE GENERAL OR THE NONILL POPULATION. THIS MAY PROVIDE A CLUE AS TO THE SOURCE OF INFECTION.

a. The most common procedure is to spot the cases on maps by

> Place of residence
> Place of employment
> Place of onset
> Areas of recreation
> Other possible exposures in schools, restaurants, etc.
> Distinguishing between primary and secondary cases by place and time allocations.

b. The most common sources of maps and the information provided are

> County engineers: roads, rivers, cities, sewers, terrain, elevation, water supply.
> Air photo or geodetic surveys: terrain and physical features.

Tax assessor: real estate property by city blocks.
Post office: rural routes, street maps of urban areas.
Political ward; precinct; U.S. Census; Chamber of Commerce: population distribution.
School district: urban and rural school location.
County agricultural service: farms.
Soil conservation service : soil types.
Forest service and national parks: human occupation or primitive sites and watershed areas, animal ecology.
Fire department: houses and building locations.
Real estate developers: residential areas, roads, subdivision lay-outs.
Demographic maps from municipal government: population distribution.
Military: special purpose maps.
Food and milk distribution routes.
Library: recent or out-of-date maps, reference material.

With the distribution of cases demarcated, it is possible to recognize clusters. However, it is essential to know the distribution of the general population because the cases may be distributed proportionately to the population distribution.

7. ANALYSIS OF THE DISTRIBUTION OF THE CASES ON A TIME SCALE TO OBTAIN A PICTURE OF THE SEQUENTIAL DEVELOPMENT OF THE EPIDEMIC (THE EPIDEMIC CURVE). IN THIS INSTANCE, THERE ARE NO DENOMINATOR DATA.

a. To appreciate the problems of interpreting the relationship between a disease and the distribution of the cases in time one must visualize the sequence of events that may occur. They include:

Exposure → Incubation → Onset → Diagnosis → Death or Recovery.

(1) When describing the occurrence of an infection in time, several dates may be of interest. Each of the dates has its limitations for use in describing the case series.

The date of exposure or infection would be ideal. However, these dates usually are unknown and are major items to be determined in the epidemiologic study.

The date of onset is the most commonly used date. However, the disease may not be recognized in its early stages and onset dates will vary for persons exposed simultaneously because of variations in incubation period. Generally, however, if certain signs and symptoms are established as basic criteria for the onset of the clinical syndrome, this is the most consistently available time marker for all cases.

The date of diagnosis may be the day a physician first sees the case. However, great variation exists in this date, depending on the need of the patient to see a doctor early or late in the disease, and the ease of diagnosing the disease. The date of diagnosis may depend on the patient's economic status, the severity of illness, the availability of a doctor, or merely when the doctor makes up his mind or changes it.

The date of reporting may vary widely, as does diagnosis. The physician may let cases accumulate before reporting or may await the results of laboratory confirmatory tests.

A date of hospitalization may be the only one available for some diseases or cases. It is of limited use because only a few cases may be severe enough to require hospital care.

The dates of death, recovery, or development of a chronic state have the disadvantages of the other alternatives. Moreover, they may be so far separated from the date of exposure that they have little epidemiologic value.

(2) Interpretation of the epidemic curve depends upon certain features of the epidemic.

One abrupt rise usually means one exposure but, due to the element of dosage and different defense mechanisms of individuals, the incubation period of cases will vary. The curve is also influenced by the amount of the infecting dosage and the susceptibility of individuals exposed.

A series of waves usually indicates that the force causing the epidemic has operated more than once, that a second source of infection has evolved, that carriers are at large, or that the original cases may be spreading the disease. It is possible to have concurrent epidemics with different causes.

Missed, unrecognized, and unreported cases may distort the true picture of onset dates.

Overreporting and secondary cases may distort the true picture of the decline of the epidemic, causing a tailing out of the curve, one skewed to the right.

The period of time between the onset and peak of the epidemic may vary because of the number of contacts, the vehicle of infection, the number of cases in the epidemic, the severity of cases, etc.

The decline may indicate the removal of the source of infection, the reduction of susceptibles in the population, the introduction of control measures, etc.

Prolongation of the epidemic may indicate prolonged exposure to the initial source or to carriers and contacts in the population such as ambulatory patients, secondary cases, or some other vehicle of transmission.

It is fallacious to assume at the onset of a study that there can only be one source of infection available for the case series. Unusual symptom complexes or peculiar epidemic curves (e.g., bimodal or double peaked curves) should suggest the involvement of a second disease agent.

(3) Spot maps or pin maps may also be used to indicate the distribution of cases by place. By using different colored spots or pins for different times of onset, the geographic spread of the disease over time can be visualized. Graphs are especially valuable in indicating time relationships.

8. THE ANALYSIS OF THE CASES AND THEIR CONTACTS WITH THE ENVIRONMENT.

a.   Widespread origin of food sources, and the ease of travel to far off places frequently requires consideration of remote and recent exposures. The importance of such considerations will depend on the incubation period of the disease being investigated, the mobility of the population, the origin of food and water supplies, etc.

b.   If the probable source of infection is man or animal, be alert to the possibility that the source may not have been ill. It may be necessary to use special techniques to uncover inapparent infections and missed cases that occurred. Some of the methods used are:

(1) Immunologic surveys to elicit responses to skin tests or to determine antibody presence in serologic tests.

(2) Search for etiologic agents by isolation of viruses, bacteria, or other microorganisms from cases.

(3) X-ray or other screening test surveys.

(4) Questioning people or reexamining medical and hospital records to uncover actually ill cases that were not previously counted.

9. A FINAL POINT IN THE EVALUATION OF AN EPIDEMIC MAY BE TO CLASSIFY ITS SEVERITY. THE USUAL PROCEDURE IS TO MEASURE THE CASE-FATALITY RATE.

a.   An unusually high case-fatality rate may have several epidemiologic explanations.

(1) The organism may be unusually virulent.

(2)   The dosage of the agent may have been unusually high.

(3)   There may be many mild cases not reported or diagnosed.

(4)   Cases of another and more severe disease may have been mis-diagnosed as the disease under study.

(5)   A superimposed secondary infection may increase mortality.

(6)   The nutritional level or other resistance factor was unusually low in the population.

(7)   There was a lack of proper treatment.

(8)   The pathogen has developed resistance to a previously effective drug.

b.   An unusually low case-fatality rate suggests the reverse of any of the above factors, or the introduction of a new treatment that is effective.

10.   CONSTRUCTION OF THE HYPOTHESIS

a.   Contrasts between data analyzed for the case series and the total population (or a selected control population), should identify characteristics or experiences that the case series share that differ from those of nonill persons.

b.   Once significant differences are detected that distinguish the case series from the control or total population, it may be possible to construct an hypothesis or alternative hypotheses that will explain the circumstances of exposure, unique to the case series.

c.   To test the hypothesis critically, it may be necessary to obtain additional data concerning specific foods or liquids consumed, contact with a specific individual or location, etc.

d.   A hypothesis must be examined critically in relation to all available facts and CANNOT BE CONSIDERED ACCEPTABLE IF IT WILL NOT EXPLAIN THE OCCURRENCE OF ALL OR, IN SOME INSTANCES, THE VAST MAJORITY OF CASES IN THE EPIDEMIC. Hypotheses that cannot meet this criterion should be rejected in favor of a more reasonable explanation.

11.   THE FINAL STEP IN THE INVESTIGATION WILL BE TO WRITE A REPORT AND, IF POSSIBLE, TO MAKE RECOMMENDATIONS TO PREVENT FURTHER OUTBREAKS.   A REPORT OF AN INVESTIGATION OF AN EPIDEMIC OUTBREAK WOULD INCLUDE:

a.   Title
b.   Author and affiliation

    c.   Background and introduction statement of the problem
    d.   Methods
    e.   Results:
        Symptomatology
        Incubation period
        Distribution of cases by various characteristics
        Vehicle of transmission
        Laboratory evidence
    f.   Discussion:
        Probable etiology
        Vehicle of transmission
        Source of vehicle contamination
        Conclusiveness of findings
    g.   Summary
    h.   Recommendations
    i.   Acknowledgments
    j.   Summary morbidity report form for State Health Department
    k.   References
    l.   Appendices (master tables and data)

V.   INVESTIGATION OF A FOOD-BORNE EPIDEMIC*

One approach to the epidemiologic classification of diseases is to characterize diseases by the portion of the body affected as discussed in Exercise 5. In many instances, the affected body part reflects the portal of entry and/or exit of the pathogenic agent. Enteric disease is one of the major epidemiologic disease groupings. The following problem concerns an epidemic affecting the gastrointestinal tract. It will take you through the sequence of considerations in the investigation of an epidemic.

Background Information on the Epidemic

For 40 years a Home Week gathering has been observed annually at the Congregational Church in a small city in eastern Massachusetts. About 200 persons, present and former residents of the town, attended the gathering on Sunday, July 27, 1981. Some did not remain after the noon services, while others attended only the luncheon, which began at noon.

Within the next few days a considerable number of persons had become ill, and preliminary inquiry indicated that the luncheon was probably the common source of infection. On July 30 the local health officer called in a state health department epidemiologist to study the outbreak and submit a report. The

---

*Source: Getting, V.A., S.M. Wheeler, and G.E. Foley, Am. J. Pub. Health 33:1217, 1943. Data from this article were used as a teaching exercise at the Harvard University School of Public Health. It was later revised for use at The Johns Hopkins University and University of California Schools of Public Health. The present form is adapted from the California version.

health officer indicated that insofar as his staff had been able to determine, there had been no unusual community-wide prevalence of the type of illness characterizing this outbreak.

If you were the epidemiologist assigned to this study, what steps would you take to investigate the outbreak? Keep in mind that your principal objectives are to:

1. Describe the situation and occurrence.
2. Determine the specific nature of the infection or contamination, i.e., etiology.
3. Determine the source, i.e., the responsible meal and the food item or items responsible for the outbreak.
4. Determine the method and source of contamination, i.e., "whodunit" and how.
5. Recommend steps to prevent further spread of the agent, if infectious, and recurrence of similar episodes.

When you have organized your thoughts on the above points, proceed to the next section.

DATA ON THE CASES, POPULATION, AND LUNCHEON

No register was kept of the people attending the luncheon, but the pastor and his wife made a list from memory, aided by the women who had served refreshments. Epidemiologic follow-up of this list yielded records on 128 people, 83 ill and 45 nonill. These 128 people must serve as the population available for study. Many records were incomplete because of difficulty in contacting out-of-town residents or failure of participants to remember details.

Question 9

What was the attack rate in the population studied?

The menu at the church luncheon included minced ham sandwiches, several kinds of homemade cakes, and coffee. Data from the individual epidemiologic records of ill and nonill persons are shown in Figures 4 and 5. These records provide information about age, sex, symptoms, their time of onset and foods eaten by persons at the luncheon. Information on the preparation of the food will be furnished when you have completed the following preliminary steps in the investigation.

Examine the data in Figures 4 and 5, and then complete Figures 6 and 7.

Figure 4.   Summary of case histories of 83 ill persons.

Case No.	Age	Sex	Symptoms[1]						Time of onset[2]		Ate[3]		
			NV	D	GI	ST	R	O			SA	CA	CO
1	59	F	+			+		+	Mo.	am	+		+
2	?	F	+	+	+	+				?	+		
4	?	F				+			Tu.		+	+	+
9	11	F	+	+					Su.	pm	+	+	
13	73	M	+	+		+			Su.	pm	+	+	+
16	46	M	+						Mo.	4pm	+		
19	57	F	+	+		+	+		Su.		Ham[4]		+
21	74	F	+	+	+				Su.	3pm	+		
25	34	F				+		+	Tu.	2am	+	+	+
26	9	F	+			+	+		Su.	3pm	+	+	
27	7	F	+			+	+		Su.	3pm	+	+	
28	10	F	+			+			Su.	4pm	+	+	
29	3	M	+		+	+	+		Mo.	pm	+	+	
30	72	F			+				Su.	2pm	+	+	
31	5	F	+			+	+		Su.	7pm	+		
32	10	M	+			+	+		Su.	pm	+		
33	32	F	+	+		+	+		Su.	7pm	+		
34	61	M				+			Tu.	pm	+	+	+
35	36	F			+				Mo.	3am	+		
36	59	F	+			+			Su.	6pm	+		+
37	74	F	+	+					Su.	5pm	+	+	
38	50	F				+		+	Mo.	pm	+	+	
39	56	M	+	+	+	+			Su.	pm	+	+	+
40	?	F				+				?	+		
42	?	F	?	?	?	?	?	?	Su.	4pm	+		
43	39	F				+	+		Tu.	4pm	+	+	+
45	44	M		+		+		+	Mo.	noon	+	+	+
46	39	F	+	+					Su.	pm	+		
47	?	F				+			We.	pm	+		
48	40	F	+	+					Su.	4pm	+	+	+
49	87	F				+			Mo.	am	+	+	+
50	57	M	+	+		+			Su.	6pm	+		
56	12	M	+			+			Su.	3pm	+	+	
58	13	M	+	+		+	+		Su.	4pm	+	+	
59	60	F				+			Tu.	am	+	+	+
62	?	F				+		+	Mo.		+	+	+
63	63	F				+		+	Mo.	4pm	+		
64	81	F	+			+		+	Su.	3pm	+	+	
65	57	F	+	+		+		+	Su.	6pm	+		
68	32	F				+			Tu.	6am	+	+	+
70	71	M				+			Mo.	9pm	+	+	+
72	75	F	+						Su.	2pm	+	+	+
74	39	F	+	+		+	+		Mo.		+		
75	70	F				+			Mo.		+	+	
76	70	F	+			+		+	Su.	6pm	+		
79	48	F	+	+					Su.	6pm	+	+	
80	6	M	+		+		+		Su.	4pm	+		
81	7	F	+			+	+		Su.	3pm	+		
82	40	F				+		+	Mo.	6pm	+		+
83	19	M	+		+				Tu.	8am	+	+	+

Figure 4. (continued)

Case No.	Age	Sex	Symptoms[1]						Time of onset[2]		Ate[3]		
			NV	D	GI	ST	R	O			SA	CA	CO
84	58	M		+		+			Su.	pm	+		
86	?	F				+			Su.		+		
87	41	F						+	We.		+		+
89	55	F		+		+			Su.	5pm	+		+
91	13	M		+		+		+	Tu.	am	+		
92	15	M	+	+		+	+	+	Tu.	noon	+	+	
93	42	F		+		+			Tu.	am	+		
94	5	?	+			+	+		Tu.		+		
95	12	M	+			+	+		Tu.		+		
96	33	M	+			+	+	+	Mo.	9pm	+	+	+
97	65	M	+						Su.	5pm	+	+	+
98	13	F	+						Su.	10pm	+	+	
99	10	M	+						Su.	8pm	+	+	+
101	?	F	+						Su.	5pm	+		
102	88	F	+						Su.	7pm	+		
103	50	M				+	+			?	+		
105	?	M	+	+					Su.	pm	+	+	+
107	17	M				+			Tu.		+	+	+
108	81	M	+	+		+		+	Su.	7pm	+	+	+
109	70	F	+	+		+			Mo.		+		
111	33	M				+	+		We.	5pm	+	+	+
112	60	F				+			Mo.		+		
113	50	F				+		+	Mo.	am	+	+	+
114	48	M			+	+		+	Su.	2pm	+	+	+
116	?	F				+			?		+		
117	?	M			+	+			?		+		
118	?	F			+	+			?		+		
119	13	M				+	+		?		+		
121	19	F				+	+		?		+		
122	?	F				+			?		+		
123	?	M				+			?		+		
125	?	F	+			+			?		+		
128	?	M				+			?		+		

1. CLINICAL SYMPTOMS: NV=nausea and/or vomiting; D=diarrhea; GI= gastrointestinal symptoms such as borborygismus and cramps; ST=sore throat; R=rash; O=other symptoms such as fever, chills, adenitis, head- ache, malaise. 2. TIME OF ONSET: Onset of earliest symptoms. 3. ATE: SA=sandwiches; CA=cake; CO=coffee. 4. Ate ham on Saturday before luncheon.

Figure 5. Summary of histories of 45 persons not ill.

Person no.	Age	Sex	Food ingested		
			Sandwich	Cake	Coffee
3	?	F		+	+
5	35	M	+	+	+
6	6	F	+	+	+
7	8	M	+	+	+
8	8	M	+	+	+

Figure 5. (continued)

Person no.	Age	Sex	Food ingested		
			Sandwich	Cake	Coffee
10	9	F	+	+	
11	32	F	+	+	
12	49	F	+	+	+
14	?	M	+	+	+
15	?	M	+?	+?	+?
17	13	F	+	+	
18	43	F	+		
20	56	M	+	+	+
22	?	F	+	+	+
23	?	M	+	+	+
24	34	F	+	+	+
41	?	M	Ham[1]		
44	41	M	+	+	+
51	?	F	Ham[1]		
52	4	?	Ham[1]		
53	5	?	Ham[1]		
54	54	F	+		+
55	57	M	+		+
57	22	F	+	+	+
60	10	F	+	+	+
61	?	M	+	+	+
66	67	M	?	?	?
67	?	F		+	+
69	45	F		?	?
71	23	M	+		
73	74	F	+	+	
77	?	M	+	+	+
78	?	F	+	+	+
85	?	F	?	?	?
88	15	F	+	+	
90	60	M	+	+	+
100	41	F	+	+	
104	?	F	+	+	+
106	13	M	+	+	+
108	18	F	+	+	+
115	?	M	+		
120	?	M	+		
124	?	F	+		
126	?	M	+		
127	72	F	+		

[1]Ate ham on Friday before luncheon.

Question 10

a. Complete Figure 6 by calculating the frequency of occurrence of various symptoms in the 83 cases. Use Figure 4 to obtain information on symptoms.

b. Graph the time of onset for each case shown in Figure 4.

Figure 6. Occurrence of symptoms among 83 ill persons.

Symptom	Number of persons with each symptom	Percent of symptoms among all symptoms	Percent of symptoms among all cases
Nausea and/ or vomiting (NV)			
Diarrhea (D)			
Other gas- trointestinal (GI)			
Sore throat (ST)			
Rash (R)			
Other (O)			
Total			

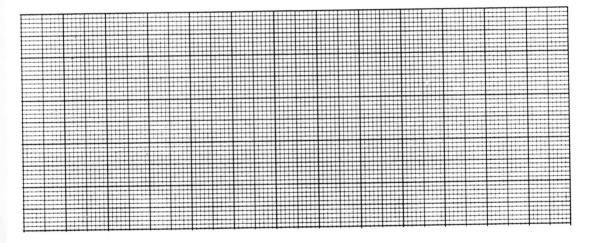

c. Graph the onset times for symptoms using information from Figure 7.

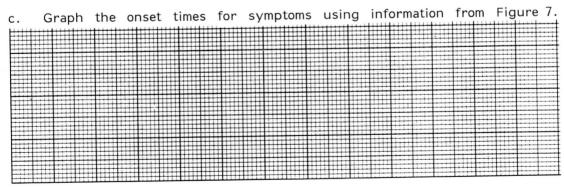

Figure 7. Time of onset of symptoms following church luncheon.

Day	Time of onset of illness	Type of symptoms during illness					
		NV	D	GI	ST	R	O
Sunday	2 - 3 p.m.	7	1	3	6	3	2
	4 - 5 p.m.	7	4	1	3	2	0
	6 - 12 p.m.	11	5	0	7	2	3
	Not specified	7	7	1	6	2	-
Monday	A.M.	1	1	0	3	0	2
	P.M.	3	1	1	7	2	5
	Not specified	2	2	0	5	1	1
Tuesday	A.M.	1	2	1	5	0	2
	P.M.	1	1	0	3	2	1
	Not specified	2	0	0	4	2	0
Wednesday	P.M.	0	0	0	2	1	0
	Not specified	0	0	0	0	0	1
Total	Known onset	42	24	7	51	17	17
	Onset not specified	2	1	3	12	3	0
TOTAL		44	25	10	63	20	17

d.   What do the two graphs suggest?

e.   What is meant by the term incubation period and how can it be used when investigating an epidemic?

f.   Does the variation in distribution of onset times, i.e., the incubation period of the various symptoms, offer any further clues as to etiology?

Question 11

Why do the symptoms shown in Figure 7 and your graphs offer clues as to the etiology of the outbreak? Why are there more "persons with symptoms" than there are cases?

Question 12

How would you define a case?

Question 13

The sex distribution was known for 125 persons in the population of 128; 49 were male and 76 were female. Of the cases 30 were male and 52 were female.

a. What were the sex-specific attack rates?

b. How would you explain a difference in attack rates by sex in this outbreak?

Question 14

The distribution of population and cases by age is summarized in Figure 8.

a. Calculate and enter the age-specific attack rates in Figure 8.

b. What would explain high attack rates by age in a food-borne outbreak?

Figure 8.   Age-specific attack rates per 100.

Age	Population	Cases	Attack rate per 100
0-9	13	7	
10-19	19	14	
20-29	2	0	
30-39	12	9	
40-49	13	8	
50-59	14	11	
60-69	7	5	
70-79	11	9	
80+	4	4	
Unknown	33	16	
Total	128	83	

c.   Tabulate the symptoms from Figure 4 by age (use groups designated 0-9, 10-19, etc.   Do any of the symptoms appear to prevail in any particular age groups?

Figure 9.   Symptoms by age group.

Age	NV		D		GI		ST		R		O		Total	
	%	no.	%	no.	%	no.	%	no.	%	no.	%	no.	%	no.
0-9														
10-19														
20-29														
30-39														
40-49														
50-59														
60-69														
70-79														
80+														
Unkn														
Total														

= Number of individuals reporting symptom in each age group.

At this point, you have completed the preliminary phase of the analysis of this epidemic by describing the pattern of disease in the exposed population. Further analysis is necessary to determine the agent and the source of contamination by investigating the foods eaten by cases and noncases.   To accomplish this analysis, organize pertinent data from the summaries of the 83 cases (Figure 4) and 45 persons who were not ill (Figure 5) to complete Figure 10.

d.   Figure 10.   Consumption of luncheon foods by clinical status.

Food	Number ill			Number not ill			Totals		
	Eaten	Not eaten	Not known	Eaten	Not eaten	Not known	Eaten	Not eaten	Not known
Sandwich									
Cake									
Coffee									
Total people	83			45			128		

e.   Calculate the attack rates for those eating and not eating particular foods by completing Figure 11.

Figure 11.   Attack rates by exposure status to luncheon foods.

Food	Persons who ate			Persons not eating		
	No.	No. ill	Attack rate per 100	No.	No. ill	Attack rate per 100
Sandwich						
Cake						
Coffee						

Question 15

a.   What did you do with unknowns in calculating percentages?

b.   Set up a fourfold table of illness and exposure for each food--sandwich, cake, coffee--using Figure 10 and calculate the relative risk of illness for each food.

c.   What food do you believe was the vehicle?

d.   Which items of information were most important in suspecting a food as the source of infection?

e.   Which food would be most susceptible to contamination and most likely to serve as a medium for the growth and multiplication of an infectious organism?

f.   What food or foods would you have sent to the laboratory for analysis?

In the course of the investigation, the following information was obtained on food preparation:

The coffee was prepared from a standard commercial vacuum-packed brand in a coffee urn used repetitively each week. Cans of condensed cream were opened at the time of serving and placed on the tables.

The cakes were made by about 20 persons, and they included at least the varieties below. Very few of the epidemiologic records specified the kind of cake eaten at the luncheon. A number of participants had eaten two or three different kinds of cake.

Chocolate
Yellow with green frosting
White with pink frosting
White with white frosting

White with chocolate frosting
White with orange frosting
Sponge cake

The hams were cooked at home by two women. Mrs. D, case 38, cut her ham in two pieces as it was too large for her kettles. She put the pieces in two aluminum kettles with water to cover and boiled them from 9:30 a.m. to 3:30 p.m. on Friday, until the meat fell off the bones. The ham was removed and the water discarded. It was cooled and put in the icebox. The grinding took about half an hour. The food chopper had not been used for about a week. Mrs. D also bought 25 loaves of bread, which were not unwrapped until the sandwiches were made on Saturday.

Mrs. B, case 19, has cooked a ham for the meeting for at least 8 years. Her husband bought two 18 pound hams from a local meat-processing establishment. The hams had been cured in St. Louis and shipped from Boston in covered barrels to the local concern, where they were kept frozen for about a week, then thawed and smoked for 30 hours. They were cooled for 2 hours and sold to the church committee.

Mrs. B used a covered Army Cannon boiler placed on an asbestos pad over a bottled gas flame. She covered the ham with water, brought it to a boil, and then turned the gas down so the water simmered. The ham cooked from 8:15 a.m. to 12:30 p.m., then she pulled a small bone out of the ham as a test of proper cooking and turned off the gas. The ham was left in the water all night and removed about 7:30 a.m. on Saturday. It was drained and dried and her husband ground it in a chopper that they have had for 6 or 8 years. The meat was then packed into two bowls and taken to the church about 2 p.m.

Mrs. B's ground ham was much lighter and moister than Mrs. D's, so a spoonful of each was used on each sandwich. Commercial dressing was spread on the bread. Mrs. B assisted in preparing the sandwiches, her duties being to cut the sandwich in triangles and pack two sandwiches in waxed paper. They were put into boilers and left at room temperature until about 1 or 2 p.m. the next day. The maximum and minimum temperatures on Saturday were 89°F and 64°F, and on Sunday, 86°F and 57°F. Those who assisted in preparing sandwiches at the church are case numbers 18, 19, 38, 63, 131, 133, and 144.

Question 16

Are the data on food preparation supportive to your hypothesis concerning the probable vehicle of transmission?

Question 17

Trace the most probable single food source through the preparation process. Where do you think contamination occurred and how would you prevent a reoccurrence?

In the course of investigation, additional information was obtained about persons who prepared food and on additional cases in the community who did not eat lunch at the church on Sunday:

Case
no.

The D family:

38 Mrs. D ate a sandwich on Saturday noon, made from the ham she had cooked. She also ate sandwiches and one piece of cake at the church luncheon. On Monday night and Tuesday morning, she had a sore throat and right cervical adenitis (swollen lymph nodes located at the junction of the jaw and the side of the neck).

39 Mr. D ate one large mouthful of the ham his wife cooked on Friday, while it was cooling. On Saturday noon he had a sandwich of the same ham. At the church luncheon he ate two sandwiches, two or three pieces of cake with coconut frosting, and coffee with cream and sugar. On Sunday at 3 p.m., he had borborygmus (rumbling sensations of the stomach), and at 10 p.m., diarrhea and nausea. Later he had a sore throat.

Mrs. D's son-in-law, Neil had two large mouthfuls of ham Friday night while it was cooling, one of these from the same fork Mr. D used. He was not ill.

41 Mrs. D's son David also ate a large mouthful of ham while it was cooling. He was not ill.

Question 18

What information would you like to know about Neil and David?

Question 19

Now that you have had a chance to work through the investigation, go back and reflect on the methodology involved. Be sure you understand the sequence of steps in the investigative process. List the steps you performed.

Question 20

What recommendations would you make to avoid further outbreaks in this population?

The following pages will provide you with basic information on construction of records for epidemiologic study.

VI. DESIGN OF EPIDEMIOLOGIC RECORD FORMS*

General

In epidemiologic work, whether for the investigation of an epidemic or for research purposes such as a serologic survey or a case-control study, record forms are a necessity. They constitute a tool that, if well designed, can facilitate the work greatly. In an emergency the back of an old envelope may have to suffice, but it is a poor substitute for a well-designed form.

There are two principal types of epidemiologic records. One is a case record--i.e., a form for recording pertinent information about a person who has, or is suspected of having, a disease that requires some sort of investigation; in other words, a numerator person. The other is a survey or census record--a repository for the usually much briefer information to be secured on each member of a population that is surveyed or in some other fashion ascertained--in other words, the denominator people.

The record form has two basic purposes: (a) to remind the investigator of the questions that he should routinely ask, and their proper sequence; and (b) to provide a repository for the answers so that they will be available for later analysis. The first purpose could be adequately met by a checklist of questions to which the investigator can refer while taking the history or securing the other data needed, and occasionally this is the best procedure. For the second purpose, a form with a list of entries, and space provided opposite each entry for the answer, is the most practicable solution.

In constructing record forms, the use to which they are to be put must be kept in mind. Is it, for example, to find out the source

*Source: Sartwell, P.E. (Ed.), Maxcy-Rosenau, Preventive Medicine and Public Health, 10th Edition, New York: Appleton-Century-Crofts, copyright 1973. Reproduced by permission of the publisher.

and mode of transmission of infection merely to identify cases, so that statistical data of general interest about the disease can later be assembled? Or, is it to be used as a tool in a preplanned research study? Often the record will have multiple purposes, but failure may result from an attempt to make a single record form serve too many purposes.

The training and background of the personnel who are to fill in the entries must be considered. Obviously, the forms will be constructed differently, depending upon whether they are to be used by the health officer, the attending physician, a public health nurse, a lay interviewer, or the patient.

Too great complexity and detail in records is a common fault. The inclusion of items just because they may conceivably be of some value once in a while makes for records that are so long and difficult to use, that they either will not be made out at all, or will be filled in hastily and inaccurately, probably with an unflattering comment about health department red tape and bureaucratic methods. On the other hand, the omission of a crucial item can be fatal to a study unless the investigator is able to go back and get it on a second visit (which is frequently impossible).

Records should be so constructed as to discourage equivocal or uninterpretable answers. A useful device applicable to certain questions is to print a choice of answers, the appropriate answer to be checked.

The number of persons who will misinterpret entries in a record, especially in a questionnaire to be filled in by the subject, is remarkable. The author of a questionnaire should ask himself, not "Is the question clear?" (to which he will usually answer "Yes," since he knew what he wanted to ask even before he wrote it down), but "Is there any possibility that anyone could misinterpret the meaning of this question?" Then if there is time, he should use the questionnaire in a pilot study and revise it to correct the faults which will inevitably be found.

In most agencies, record forms may be found that were never really needed, were poorly designed, and have outlived whatever purpose they may originally have had. Records have a kind of obdurate immortality.

Epidemiologic Case Record

Most epidemiologic records are obtained from cases of acute communicable disease for the purposes of case identification, determination of sources of infection and modes of transmission, and to assist in developing general control measures. Records should include the following items:

1. Identification (name, age, sex, address, occupation, etc.)

2. Name of physician who reported the case, and hospital where the case was treated.

3. Dates of onset, report, hospitalization, release from isolation, or death.

4. Essential clinical or laboratory findings, which show the degree of confidence with which the diagnosis has been established.

5. Items of epidemiologic importance. These will depend on the particular disease and purpose of the investigation. In typhoid, for example, they might include sources of water and food, household sanitation, names of household associates and their vaccination status, history of contact with other cases, or travel within 30 days prior to onset. If a total population survey is to be undertaken, this information should be collected for everyone.

6. Further entries and remarks including space for unforeseen information, which often proves of great importance.

Epidemiologic Survey Records

Although case-finding programs may yield epidemiologic information and epidemiologic surveys may incidentally identify cases, their primary purposes are distinct. Epidemiologic surveys are studies of a population group or sample for the purpose of determining the distribution and frequency of a disease not routinely reported, or of some attribute or test result which is related to a disease. The test may be a physical diagnostic procedure, a laboratory test, or any combination of a number of procedures. Inquiries concerning medical history, symptoms or hygienic practices (e.g., immunization status or smoking history) constitute another type of survey.

The tests selected for a survey should be as reliable and unequivocal as possible, and applicable for mass use. Much attention will have to be paid to the sampling design and to the preparation of the population so as to obtain maximal cooperation.

Survey records may either take the form of lists or case cards. When lists are employed, each subject is entered on a separate line, and the appropriate entries are made in columns under headings for the variables under study (e.g., age, sex, race, blood pressure).

This works well for recording data where only a few simple items of information are needed for each individual, but it is very cumbersome for analysis. Usually a separate case card for each individual is advantageous.

The record form should be based on a clear concept of the aims of the survey and the type of information obtainable with the least amount of scope for subjective errors. It usually includes the minimum identifying information, plus such items as are easily obtained and relevant to the particular condition, and the result of the test.

When a large number of subjects is involved, it is frequently useful to provide from the outset a record card precoded for transfer of information to mechanical punch cards, which will later greatly facilitate analysis of the findings. A list of intended tabulations prepared in advance will point out superfluous as well as missing items of information.

Mechanical Aids to Analysis of Data

In the simplest situations, the data on the case cards can be put into tabular form merely by hand-tallying the cards. For more complex situations, the common practice is to design a code for transferring the data to standard 80-column IBM cards. It is often helpful to employ record forms on which one can precode the data, thus obviating the preparation of a code sheet. This will save time and may prevent errors.

Between these extremes, in cases where the number of subjects and number of variables to be studied are relatively small, marginal punch cards are useful. Their chief utility is in situations where they serve as the primary case record, that is, where the original entries are made in writing on the face of the cards as the observations are made. They require no expensive or cumbersome equipment and no skilled operators. The epidemiologist can take them into the field and fill out, code, punch, and sort them unaided, if necessary. They are unsuited to large research studies and unnecessary in very small ones.

The functions of data processing systems are to facilitate the recording, storage, retrieval, and presentation of information. They cannot compensate for bad study design or biased or inaccurate observations, and they cannot relieve the investigator of his responsibility to plan the analysis and interpretation of data. They can only facilitate mechanical procedures. To the extent that the user of such systems is tempted not to bother to look at the raw data, they may actually be a deterrent to good work. When complex tabulations from large numbers of records are to be made, they are a practical necessity.

Whatever technique is adopted for processing data, the <u>classification</u> <u>of</u> <u>the</u> <u>raw</u> <u>data</u> <u>into</u> <u>appropriate</u> <u>groupings</u> <u>is</u> <u>the</u> <u>most</u> <u>important</u> <u>step</u>. Upon this rests the development of a code for translating the data into categories which may be punched on a card. With some items this is just a matter of "yes-no," or "positive-negative," etc. For items on a quantitative scale there is a choice between punching the exact value or grouping. The choice will depend on the purpose, on the accuracy of the measurement, and on the method used in processing the data. Grouping should usually be done, because it facilitates subsequent sorting and is more economical of the space on the card. When working with electronic computers it is often more desirable to punch exact data onto the cards and allow the machine to do whatever grouping is subsequently desired. However, when dealing with marginal punch cards, where the retrieval process is slow and the space for coding limited, it is usually desirable to group data prior to punching onto the cards. For example, it is often better to classify subjects by age groups and punch the age group rather than the exact age. In coding the information collected in the field it is always helpful to reserve space for "not done," "no information," "specimen lost," etc., because not all of the individuals included in the study may be represented in each of the individual measurements. The immediate identification of persons from whom data on one or more measurements are not available facilitates the computation of the denominator for individual tests.

As early as possible in any investigation, it is important to try to visualize the form in which the findings will be presented. Usually the best way to do this is to draw up blank tables showing the variables that are to be examined, and the way you expect to relate them to each other. Such blank tables often help to sharpen the questions that are to be answered, and to show the population subgroups that are critically important. They will also help the investigator visualize the appropriate grouping of data, prior to the development of a code. Once the cards are punched, it is very troublesome to change the groups that have been defined by the code.

Summary of Essential Points of Data Processing

Where feasible, draw up blank tables in advance.
Don't leave designing of record forms to a subordinate.
Arrange entries in the order in which the data are normally available.
Don't include entries you can't justify.
Precode where feasible, if machine processing is anticipated.
Always pretest a new record form.
Use the data processing method best adapted to your needs and circumstances: number of records, their complexity, facilities available, etc.

Question 21 (Optional)

Try your hand at design of a record form for a hypothetical study:

a.   to determine the source of an infectious disease outbreak of hepatitis.

b.   to describe the smoking history of persons with lung cancer.

SUGGESTED RESPONSES
Exercise 7--Investigation of an Epidemic

1a. Figure 1 depicts a point-source epidemic.

1b. Cases occurring later than June may be explained in several ways. They might be secondary cases (person-to-person transmission) or occur because of later exposure to the original source of the epidemic; they may also represent endemic disease in the community, unrelated to the epidemic.

2. Figure 2. Epidemic curves, infectious hepatitis

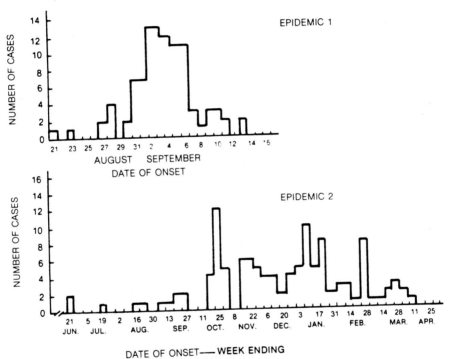

Epidemic 1 is a point-source epidemic. Epidemic 2 is a propagated epidemic.

3a. Graph is shown on next page.

3b. Figure 3 (below) suggests a propagated epidemic because of the presence of several peaks separated in time but within the incubation period of measles.

3c. The number of susceptibles is decreasing or there is insufficient contact (exposure) between susceptibles and infected cases.

3a.   Figure 3.   Cases of measles by week of onset, U.S., May 1970-May 1971.

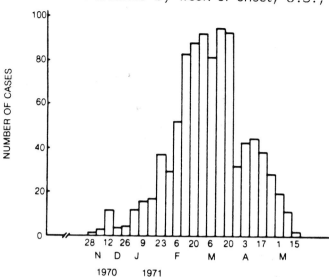

4a.   The mechanisms have been previously covered in Exercise 5, Classification of Diseases (Question 1).

4b.   Contamination of the environment (air, water, or soil) by industrial chemicals or pollutants, e.g., Minamata disease in Japan.

Disease due to medication or treatment by physicians. Disease occurring in this way is termed IATROGENIC illness (physician induced), e.g., Thalidomide (a tranquilizer) induced congenital defects in babies. Diethylstilbestrol (a hormone) may have caused vaginal cancer in the children of some women treated for threatened abortion early in pregnancy.

Sudden and dramatic change in one's environment, e.g., travellers diarrhea caused by infectious agents or altitude sickness (headache, fatigue, digestive disturbances) when travelling to places located at high altitudes.

Hysteria and stress. Unusual experiences or symptoms related to mob psychology, e.g., certain instances of UFO sightings, conversion reactions, and faith healing centers. Also, attributing coincidental illness to a perceived evil, e.g., a local industrial polluter is blamed for all varieties of illness among local residents.

Noxious physical agents. Neurologic or gastrointestinal symptoms induced by excess or prolonged noise, extreme heat, or strobe lights.

Natural disasters, fire, accidents, war, etc., can be the cause of unusual clustering of disease or health problems.

A cluster of deaths or injuries due to violent crime, e.g., the Boston strangler, Jack the Ripper, the Los Angeles Freeway killer, murder of young boys in the Houston-Galveston area; these crimes generally followed a similar pattern for each killer.

5. Reduce exposure of susceptibles to infected persons. Reduce the number of susceptibles. Eliminate the disease agent, its reservoir, or its vectors. Promote factors known to have a beneficial effect with respect to the disease. For example, if tuberculosis is found to be associated with poor nutrition and overcrowding, then one of the long-term preventive measures might be devoted to health education or development of economic policies leading to improved nutrition; second might be a public policy to reduce slums, ghettos, and barrios.

6a. Specific measures include:

    (1) Quarantine (isolation) of cases.
    (2) Immunization of contacts.
    (3) If immunization is not feasible then diagnostic procedures leading to early treatment, if necessary, of infected contacts.
    (4) Remove the source of infection. If water or food are suspected vehicles, then they must be eliminated or removed from public consumption.
    (5) Immunization of high-risk groups.
    (6) If a vector such as mosquitos is known for the disease, then chemical spraying of the air or elimination of stagnant water sources that are mosquito breeding grounds may be necessary.

6b. (1) Testing and evaluation of industrial processes, products, and environments. Testing and evaluation of pollution control equipment.
    (2) Sufficient testing of new drugs or therapeutic techniques prior to commercial marketing or widespread use.
    (3) Encourage and participate in programs to improve public awareness.
    (4) Consultation and assistance to lawmakers who draft legislation to protect the public's health.

7. Persons known to be exposed to or potentially susceptible to a disease agent because of their occupation (doctors and nurses--tuberculosis; dentists--hepatitis B); age; sex; ethnicity (poor and minority groups known to have deficient immunization records against diphtheria; pregnant women without a history of rubella); presence of coexisting illness (elderly patients with cardiovascular and advanced respiratory illness susceptible to influenza); genetic inheritance (Blacks have sickle cell anemia); and personal habits or lifestyle (smokers and physically inactive persons develop heart disease). Identifying high-risk groups may be useful in preventing epidemics in which the disease agent is known and when a preventive or control measure is available. A health agency can use its limited resources more efficiently, i.e., it might prevent or control more illness for a given amount of money when efforts are concentrated in high-risk groups.

8a.   There is no fixed percentage or magic number. The number necessary depends upon the disease, the number of susceptible individuals, and the likelihood of contact between susceptible and infected individuals.

8b.   It is rarely possible, feasible, or practical to immunize all persons in a population. An epidemic can be prevented or controlled by reducing the number of susceptibles, for example, by an immunization campaign aimed at high-risk persons. Or a major outbreak of illness can be prevented by immunizing a sufficient proportion of the population to minimize the probability of contact between susceptible and infected individuals. Herd immunity would play a role.

Investigation Of A Food-Borne Epidemic

9.   83/128 x 100 = 64.8 per 100

10a. Figure 6.   Occurrence of symptoms among 83 ill persons.

Symptom		Number of persons with each symptom	Percent of symptoms among all symptoms	Percent of symptoms among all cases
Nausea and/ or vomiting	(NV)	44	24.6	53.0
Diarrhea	(D)	25	14.0	30.1
Other gas- trointestinal	(GI)	10	5.6	12.1
Sore throat	(ST)	63	35.2	75.9
Rash	(R)	20	11.2	24.1
Other	(O)	17	9.5	20.5
Total		179		

Notes: Nausea per 100 symptoms = 44/179 ×100 = 24.6 per 100.   Nausea per 100 cases = 44/83 x 100 = 53.0 per 100.

10b. Figure 4a.   Time of onset of earliest symptoms following luncheon.

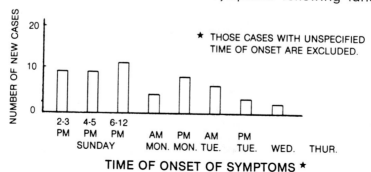

★ THOSE CASES WITH UNSPECIFIED TIME OF ONSET ARE EXCLUDED.

TIME OF ONSET OF SYMPTOMS ★

10c. Figure 7a. Time of onset of symptoms for cases with known symptoms.

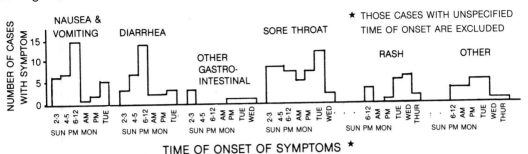

TIME OF ONSET OF SYMPTOMS *

10d. Figure 4a shows that many cases occurred within 6 hours of the meal, declined Sunday night and Monday A.M., but showed a second peak Monday P.M. Excluded cases might have affected the curve of onset times.

Figure 7a shows the distribution of symptoms among cases by their time of onset. There appear to be differing symptom complexes occurring early and late after exposure to the meal. Presentation of the data is somewhat arbitrary. If you had different time periods designated on the time axis, your graphs would be different.

10e. Incubation period refers to the period of time between exposure to the etiologic agent and the onset of illness. The most commonly used measure is the median incubation period, which is the amount of time necessary for 50% of the cases to develop illness. The incubation period of infectious diseases may also be expressed as a range, specifying the minimum and maximum incubation periods for this disease. The incubation period can be used to estimate when exposure to the epidemic agent occurred.

10f. Yes, perhaps there are 2 different pathogens; #1 produces nausea, vomiting, or diarrhea within 12 hours; #2 produces sore throat, rash, and other symptoms within 48 hours. A second explanation would be that there is a single pathogen which has both immediate effects and later toxic effects. Laboratory results of microorganisms from the throats and feces of cases might be helpful in answering this question.

11. Yes, different pathogens can cause different symptoms. Also, the incubation period for onset of symptoms is specific to the causative organism. Each case can have more than one symptom.

12. Your idea. Defining a case may be difficult because the symptoms and signs are rather general. It is difficult to actually name a responsible organism because of the absence of specific or pathognomonic findings. A case may be defined by the presence of one or more of the signs and symptoms.

13a. Males = 30/49 × 100 = 61.2 per 100; Females = 52/76 × 100 = 68.4 per 100. One case could not be determined and is not included in the rates.

13b. Women prepare food and might sometimes taste it raw or partially cooked.

14a. Figure 8. Age-specific attack rates.

Age	Population	Cases	Attack rate per 100
0-9	13	7	54
10-19	19	14	74
20-29	2	0	0
30-39	12	9	75
40-49	13	8	62
50-59	14	11	79
60-69	7	5	71
70-79	11	9	82
80+	4	4	100
Unknown	33	16	48
Total	128	83	65

14b. (1) Preference for foods (exposure).
     (2) Amount eaten (dose).
     (3) Susceptibility to the disease agent.

14c. Figure 9. Symptoms by age group.

INFORMATION WORKSHEET

Age	NV		D		GI		ST		R		O		Total	
	%	no.	%	no.	%	no.	%	no.	%	no.	%	no.	%	no.
0-9	32	7	0	0	9	2	27	6	32	7	0	0	100	22
10-19	30	10	12	4	3	1	30	10	18	6	6	2	100	33
20-29	-	0	-	0	-	0	-	0	-	0	-	0	-	0
30-39	17	3	17	3	0	0	28	5	28	5	11	2	100	18
40-49	19	3	25	4	6	1	25	4	-	0	25	4	100	16
50-59	20	6	20	6	3	1	37	11	7	2	13	4	100	30
60-69	14	1	-	0	-	0	71	5	-	0	14	1	100	7
70-79	33	7	24	5	10	2	29	6	-	0	5	1	100	21
80+	33	3	11	1	-	0	33	3	-	0	22	2	100	9
Unkn	17	4	9	2	13	3	57	13	-	0	4	1	100	23
Total	25	44	14	25	5	10	35	63	11	20	9	17	99	179

= Number of individuals reporting symptom in each age group.

NV in 0-19, 50-59, 70-79
D in 50-59, 70-79
GI in Unkn., 0-9, 70-79
ST in Unkn, 50-59, 10-19
R in 0-9, 10-19, 30-39
O in 50-59, 40-49

0-9   had NV, R, ST
10-19 had NV, ST
30-39 had ST
40-49 had O, ST, D
50-59 had ST
60-69 had ST
70-79 had NV, ST
80+   had NV, ST

NV appears to be less frequent in middle-aged groups, but higher in young and old (>70 years). Sore throat appears in all age groups, but more often in older children and adults. This analysis demonstrates the effect of age on the pattern of disease. If one organism was responsible for this epidemic, it produces different symptom complexes in different age groups. If two organisms were responsible, the data show the selection of different age groups to develop different diseases.

14d. Figure 10. Consumption of luncheon foods by clinical status.

Food	Number ill			Number not ill			Totals		
	Eaten	Not eaten	Not known	Eaten	Not eaten	Not known	Eaten	Not eaten	Not known
SA	83	0	-	39	3	3	122	3	3
CA	39	44	-	28	13	4	67	57	4
CO	30	53	-	24	17	4	54	70	4
	Total ill = 83			Total not ill = 45			Total = 128		

14e. Figure 11. Attack rates by exposure status to luncheon foods.

Food	Persons who ate			Persons not eating		
	No.	No. ill	Attack rate per 100	No.	No. ill	Attack rate per 100
SA	122	83	68	3	0	0
CA	67	39	58	57	44	77
CO	54	30	56	70	53	76

15a. Leave them out of the calculations. For this phase of the analysis there are not a large number of unknowns, and so the rates are not much affected. In some disease investigations or for certain parts of the analysis the number of unknowns may be so great that a clear conclusion cannot be reached, as you noted for the time of onset of cases.

15b. Sandwiches.

		ILL	NOT ILL	TOTAL
(Exposed)	ate	83	39	122
(Not exposed)	didn't eat	0	3	3

Incidence rate in exposed   = 83/122 x 100 = 68.03 per 100
Incidence rate in not exposed = 0/3 x 100   = 0 per 100
Relative risk   = 68.03/0   = infinity

Similar tables can be set up for cake or coffee.

Relative risk for cake   = 0.75
Relative risk for coffee = 0.74

15c. Probably the sandwiches. Cake and coffee are not likely vehicles because the relative risk is less than 1. But if one ate sandwiches, the risk was high.

15d. Symptoms suggest ingestion of something. Many enteric pathogens have a short incubation period; plus the fact that this sort of thing occurs frequently.

15e. Ham sandwich.

15f. Bread, ham, milk, cake, mayonnaise, and water are frequent sources of contamination and should be investigated if specimens are still available. Cultures can also be obtained from containers and serving dishes.

16.   Yes. They do not rule out the food-borne hypothesis.

17.   Adequate heat during cooking and proper refrigeration for storage will usually prevent such events.

18.   Did they eat the ham at the church supper or only at home? If they did not go to the church supper, it may suggest that the ham was not con- taminated at the time they ate it, since neither became ill.

19.   The steps in investigation are

a.   Determine characteristics of person-place-time for known cases. Obtain background information and calculate the appropriate rates to verify that an epidemic has occurred. Cases of the disease must be defined.

b.   Develop working (and alternative) hypotheses to explain the source, the vehicle or the mode of transmission of the outbreak. Alternative hypotheses are necessary in the event that your first (or second) impressions are incorrect.

c.   Develop your data collecting instrument.

d.   Obtain case histories which may identify potential sources to which cases were exposed prior to the onset of disease, and during the interval defined by the minimum and maximum incubation periods of the suspected agent.

e.   Obtain physical evidence--blood, throat cultures, fecal specimens--as necessary from cases. Obtain food, water, or other specimens for bacterial, viral, or other studies if available.

f.   Obtain history and specimens from persons who were not ill for appropriate examinations and comparisons to cases.

g.   Perform data analysis by comparing rates, relative risk, etc., for characteristics and exposure histories of ill and nonill persons. Use all available data to confirm or reject your working hypothesis.

20.   We are fairly sure about how the epidemic occurred. You would try to educate the food preparers about correct procedures for cooking and storing food. The cause of the outbreak was β streptococcus and the disease was scarlet fever.

21a. Your questionnaire or data form should include date of birth; sex; ethnicity; occupation; area of residence; date of onset of illness; signs and symptoms occurring with the illness; contacts with known cases of hepatitis; eating raw fish, especially oysters and shellfish; exposure to hemodialysis clinics; drinking unchlorinated surface water (especially in rural areas); recent blood transfusion, injections or tattoos; recent hospitalization; recent contact with prostitutes or homosexuals. There are 3 types of viral hepatitis, types A, B, and nonA/nonB. The incubation periods range from 2-8 weeks for type A, 2-26 weeks for type B, and somewhere between for nonA/nonB. Your data collection form should include exposures occurring within the incubation period for whichever type is being investigated.

21b. Your questionnaire or form might include date of birth; sex; ethnicity; age at first smoking experience; years smoked; periods in which person was a nonsmoker; type of tobacco used; amount smoked daily at different points in the smoking history; current smoking habits; smoking habits with regard to inhaling and whether or not the entire cigarette (cigar or pipe) is smoked. Occupation and duration of occupation are also important characteristics because lung cancer is associated with many substances that may be encountered in the workplace (asbestos, chromium, etc.).

EXERCISE 8.   ETIOLOGY OF DISEASE

Goals

The exercise demonstrates additional examples of the strategy epidemiologists use to investigate the etiology of a disease. You should note that controlling a disease need not require identifying the actual disease agent.

Methods

Epidemiologic strategy will be illustrated by data from the investigations of two actual disease outbreaks.

I.   BLINDNESS X, A NONINFECTIOUS DISEASE[†]

II.   CHOLERA IN LONDON, 1854[§]

Terms

In utero development, descriptive study, gestation, experimental study, biologic trigger, statistical significance, p value.

Suggested Readings

A list of pertinent references will be provided at the conclusion of Section I.

I.   BLINDNESS X, A NONINFECTIOUS DISEASE

A.   IDENTIFYING AND DESCRIBING THE PROBLEM.

An outbreak of blindness X was first described in 1942. New cases of the disease occurred until the mid-1950s. Epidemiologists were involved in observing the distribution of cases and developing and testing hypotheses to account for those distributions. Through the following data you will see the epidemiologic strategy for determining the cause of this disease. The first task of an epidemiologist consists of identifying the existence of a health problem. Findings of case reports or other observations by epidemiologists, clinicians, or public health workers may suggest that a problem exists. The epidemiologist would, at the earliest possible time, define the cases in terms of person, place, time.

[†]Adapted from an exercise by Dr. M.M. Henderson, Department of Social and Preventive Medicine, University of Maryland.

[§]Adapted from an exercise by Dr. M. Terris, Editor of the Journal of Public Health Policy, Burlington, Vermont.

Blindness X was first described in 6 infants born prematurely in the U.S. Symptoms developed slowly over the first 3-6 months of life. Similar cases were soon identified in all states and in a number of foreign countries, mostly in larger citites. Cases were spread uniformly over the year, paralleling the occurrence of births. Trends over time in different places were similar to those depicted in Figures 1 to 4.

Figure 1.   Secular trends of blindness X in New York State, 1940-1954.

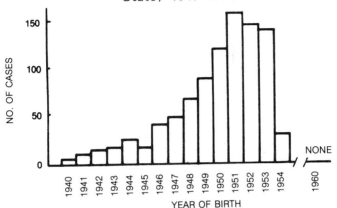

Source: Ingalls, T.H., reprinted by permission of New England J. Med., 251: 1017, 1954.

Figure 2. Annual births, and trends in blindness among preschool children in 11 States, 1937-1950.

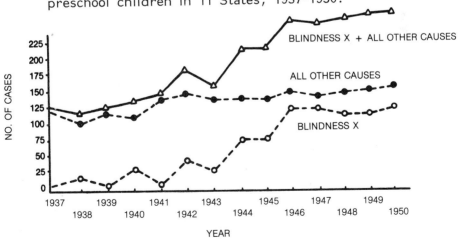

Source: Kerby, C.E., Sightsaving Review, 24:15, 1954.

284

Exercise 8-3

Figure 3.   Incidence of blindness X by cause, 1927-1950.

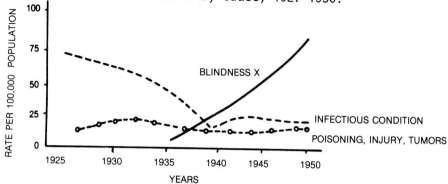

Source: Ingalls, T.H., reprinted by permission of New
England J. Med., 251:1017, 1954.

Figure 4. Incidence of blindness X in three centers in England, 1946-1951.

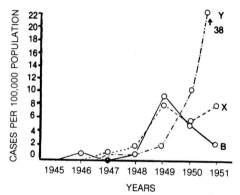

Source: Henderson, M.M., unpublished.

<u>Question 1</u>

What is the trend of this disease over time?

<u>Question 2</u>

Based on Figures 1-4, state reasons for believing that the increase of cases
might be due to:

a.   Better case finding

b.   Actual increase in blindness X.

c.   Which is more likely to have occurred, better case finding or an increase
in the disease?

B.   INITIAL ASSOCIATIONS AND PRELIMINARY EXPLANATIONS

After reviewing the initial data, epidemiologists and/or clinical physicians will
propose various explanations that fall in one or more of the categories of
disease etiology you considered in the exercise on "Classification."   Before its
etiology was actually discovered, blindness X was attributed at different times
to each of the categories of disease listed in Question 3.

Question 3

Assuming the reported cases in Figures 1-4 represent a new disease, how
might the following explain blindness X?

a.   Genetic inheritance or genetic defect

b.   Infectious disease

c.   Trauma

d.   Dietary deficiency/excess

e.   Environmental hazard/toxin

f.   Medication/therapy.

C.   SEARCHING FOR CAUSES.

As data became available, certain explanations became untenable and others more feasible.

Question 4

As additional descriptive evidence became available it was used to support or discredit some of the explanations considered in Question 3.   The following data will provide additional clues to the etiology of this disease.   In the space below each illustration, write your impression of the idea(s) presented.

Figure 5.   Prematurity rates in New York State, 1945-1954.

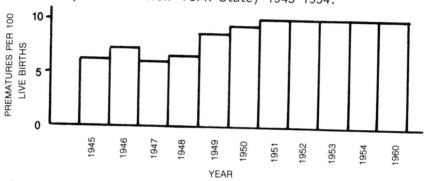

Source: New York State, Dept. Vital Statistics Publications, 1945-1950, Vital Statistics of the U.S., 1950-1960.

Conclusions:

Because of the age of cases at the time of disease onset, factors relating to the in utero and newborn environment were investigated.

Maternal Studies

Figure 6.   Age of mother, Boston Lying-in Hospital, 1949.

Maternal age in years	No. of births	No. normal children	No. children with blindness X	Percent with blindness X
16-25	103	89	14	13.6
26-35	173	146	27	15.6
36-45	62	52	10	16.1
Unreported	13	11	2	15.4
Total	351	298	53	15.1

Source: Kinsey, V.E., and Zacharias, L., JAMA 139:572, 1949. Copyright 1949, American Medical Association.

Conclusions:

Miscellaneous Findings

Comparisons of mothers of prematures with and without blindiness X showed no differences in the frequency of Rh incompatibility, operative deliveries, anesthesia and analgesia administered during delivery, prenatal X-ray, maternal infections during pregnancy, the causes of prematurity, the percentage of illness among males and females, and whether the infants were fed with cow or breast milk. Other early descriptive studies of person, place, time; or host, agent, and environment revealed:

Figure 7.   Occurrence by city, hospital type, and color.

City	Hospital type	Whites		Non whites	
		No. of prematures	No. with blindness X	No. of prematures	No. with blindness X
New Orleans	Charity	90	0	210	0
	Private	100	9	·31	0
New York	Voluntary (fee for service, some charity)	1541	188	759	2
Chicago	Municipal (some fee for service, mostly public asistance)	600	2	600	2
	University	100	35	30	3
Providence	Voluntary	115	10	67	0
Total		2446	244	1697	7

Source: M and R Pediatric Research Conference, 1951.

Conclusions:

Exercise 8-7

Figure 8. Incidence of blindness X by quality of hospital care, Maryland, 1952.

Hospital by rank	Percent blindness X by birth weight in grams							
	Under 1,001		1,001-1,500		1,501-2,000		Total	
	No.	percent	No.	percent	No.	percent	No.	percent
Upper 10%	4	50	64	26.6	176	3.4	244	10.2
Others (15% sample)	8	25	61	9.8	358	1.4	427	3.0

Source: Rothmund, H.I.M., Rider, R.V., and Harper, P., Pediatrics, 14: 455, 1954. Copyright, American Academy of Pediatrics, 1954.

Conclusions:

Figure 9. The incidence rate of blindness X in premature infants born at the Providence Lying-in-Hospital, 1938-1947.

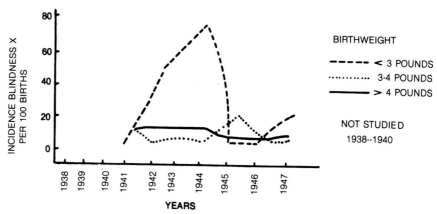

Source: Kinsey, V.E. and Zacharias, L., JAMA 139:572, 1949. Copyright 1949, American Medical Association.

Conclusions:

Figure 10. Incidence of blindness X by birth weight, Maryland, 1952.

Birth weight in grams	Number of infants	Percent blindness X
under 1,001	12	33.3
1,001-1,500	129	17.8
1,501-2,000	548	2.0

Source: Rothmund, H.I.M., Rider, R.V., and Harper, P., Pediatrics, 14:455, 1954. Copyright, American Academy of Pediatrics, 1954.

Conclusions:

Figure 11. Incidence of blindness X by gestational age, 1950-1952.

Age of premature in weeks*	Total	Stage of disease					
		Active[†]		Residual[†]		Irreversible	
		No.	Percent	No.	Percent	No.	Percent
31 or more	51	29	57	6	12	1	2
30 or less	42	28	67	15	36	6	14

*Weight at 30 weeks is approximately 1500 grams or 3 pounds, 5 ounces.
†Categories not mutually exclusive. Infant may have active and residual disease at the same time.

Source: Engle, M.A., et al., Amer. J. Dis. Child., 89:399, 1955. Copyright 1955, American Medical Association.

Conclusions:

Figure 12. Gestational age and severity of blindness X, Boston, 1951-1952.

Eye examination findings	Mean gestational age in weeks
Normal	33.3
Mildly abnormal	31.8
Moderately to severely abnormal	30.8

Source: Zacharias, L., et al., published with permission from Amer. J. Ophth., 38:317, 1954. Copyright by Ophthalmic Publishing Company.

Conclusions:

Figure 13. Percentage of blindness X by birth weight and age, Maryland, 1952.

Birth weight in grams	Age of infant							
	Stillborn		Under one week		One week to one month		Over one month	
	No.	percent blindness X	No.	percent blindness X	No.	percent blindness X	No.	percent blindness X
Under 1,001	--		--		--		12	33.3
1,001-1,500	2	0	11	0.0	66	16.7	45	26.7
1,501-2,000	54	0	182	0.5	254	2.8	40	7.5

Source: Rothmund, H.I.M., Rider, R.V., and Harper, P., Pediatrics 14:455, 1954. Copyright, American Academy of Pediatrics, 1954.

Conclusions:

Additional Findings

1. Blindness X was common in pairs of twins and in triplets.

2. One study showed that prematures with blindness X stayed in the hospital nursery for an average of 56 days while other prematures had an average stay of 46 days.

Hospital records revealed that several aspects of the therapy for premature babies had been recently changed.

Summarize the findings that you have observed. Try to formulate a single explanation that uses all the data. Explanations that cannot explain all or most of the facts will be discredited by your colleagues!

D.   TESTING THE HYPOTHESES

Based upon the initial reports and descriptive evidence, epidemiologists formulate theories and hypotheses to link together the available data.   The hypotheses are then tested to see if they are consistent with the available data or
with other data that will be collected specifically to investigate an hypothesis.
Studies were conducted to determine whether or not the incidence of blindness
X was correlated with certain popular modes of therapy shown in Figures 14-17.

Figure 14. Methods of treatment vs. blindness X, 3-4 lb prematures, 1938-1947.

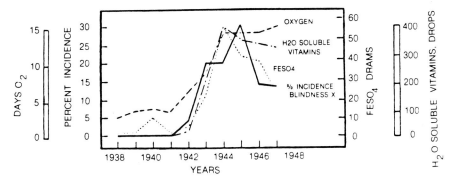

Source: Kinsey, V.E. and Zacharias, L., JAMA 139:572, 1949.   Copyright
1949, American Medical Association.

<u>Conclusions</u>:

Figure 15. Vitamin therapy and blindness X, 1946-1950.

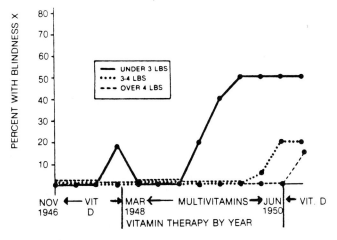

Source: Dancis, J. et al., New Eng. J. Med. 245:402, 1951.   Reprinted by
permission of New England Journal of Medicine.

Figure 16. Effect of vitamin E supplements on the incidence of blindness X in premature infants.

Vitamin E supplement	No. of infants	No. with blindness X	Percent blindness X
Yes	23	1	4.4
No	78	17	21.8

Source: Owens, W.C., and Owens, E.V., published with permission from Am. J. Ophth., 32:1631, 1949. Copyright by Ophthalmic Publishing Company.

Conclusions:

The relation between oxygen and blindness X was also studied.

Figure 17. Incidence of blindness X in single births and multiple births according to duration of oxygen therapy.

Duration of oxygen in days	Incidence of blindness X in percent			
	Single births		Multiple births	
	Number blindness X	Incidence	Number blindness X	Incidence
0	93	1.1	19	0.0
1-2	130	5.4	42	4.8
3-5	86	3.5	25	28.0
6-10	52	3.8	13	23.1
11-20	43	14.0	6	50.0
21 or more	68	13.2	9	44.4

Source: Kinsey, V.E., and Hemphill, F.H., Arch. Ophth., 56:481, 1956. Copyright 1956, American Medical Association.

What do these data suggest about oxygen therapy and blindness X?

Conclusions:

E. EXPERIMENTAL EVIDENCE

Epidemiologists and clinicians continued to gather data describing the characteristics of ill infants, performed studies comparing ill and nonill infants to
determine the relative risk and attributable risk of many of the above implicated factors in order to assess the validity of the hypotheses regarding the
etiological mechanism.

THE CLINICAL TRIAL

Believing that the etiologic agent for disease X had been identified, epidemiologists and clinicians planned to test the validity of the theory. A clinical
trial, i.e., a carefully conducted human experiment was planned. All babies
between 1000 and 1850 grams and under 12 hours old on admission to the
premature nursery of Bellevue Hospital, New York were allocated at random
into one of two groups:

Group 1. High oxygen therapy: 69 percent O_2 for at least 2 weeks.

Group 2. Low oxygen therapy: O_2 given only for cyanosis; concentration
of about 38 percent. O_2 discontinued at least once daily.
Same care, otherwise, as Group 1 infants.

Figure 18.   Incidence of residual blindness X by oxygen administration.

Oxygen therapy	Number of infants	Percent with blindness X
High - 69%	36	22
Low - 38%	28	0

Source: Lanman, J.T., et al., JAMA, 155:223, 1954.
Copyright, 1954, American Medical Assoc.

A second clinical trial was performed to further test the validity of the O_2 hypothesis. Kinsey and Hemphill (Arch. Ophth., 56:481, 1956, copyright 1956,
American Medical Association) reported results from a cooperative epidemiologic
study involving 18 hospitals in the United States. Prematures of 1500 grams
or less birth weight were divided into unequal groups on a random admission
basis. A high-oxygen group received only 50 percent O_2 for 28 days, and
curtailed-oxygen group received O_2 only for a clinical emergency. Death rates
did not differ between the two groups. The incidence of blindness X was as
follows (weight and gestation did not differ):

Conclusions for Figures 18 and 19:

Figure 19.   Incidence of blindness X by oxygen dose and type of birth.

Oxygen therapy	Single-birth blindness X			Multiple-births blindness X		
	Number	Cases	Percent	Number	Cases	Percent
High O_2	47	33	70.2	6	5	83.3
Curtailed O_2	425	133	31.3	108	45	41.7
			p < 0.01*			p < 0.05*

*NOTE: A "p" value <0.01 or <0.05 means that results differing to the observed degree would be expected to occur by chance less than 1 in 100 times or less than 5 in 100 times.   Differences of this magnitude are said to be <u>statistically significant</u>.   In most cases, an investigator whose results are statistically significant would argue that the differences may be attributed to the biologic effect of the independent variable.   In this case, the independent variable of differing oxygen concentrations was proposed to explain the dependent or outcome variable of blindness X.   While an investigator's inclination is to believe that the biologic plausibility of his study is proved by the statistical tests, one should be aware that in any given situation an extreme result (p <0.01 or p <0.05) will occur by chance occasionally.   This is analogous to the situation in which a coin tossed in the air, sooner or later, will fall either face or back side up 100% of the time, even if the number of flips is quite large.   In biologic research, statistically significant results that cannot be consistently replicated by other studies raises the possibility that results of the original study may have occurred by chance; or they may be due to errors in the study design or in the methods used to collect the data.   These subjects will be covered in Exercises 10-12.

In the search for causes of disease, epidemiologists often will utilize the work of researchers in other fields, who may contribute important information. Frequently, animal or laboratory experiments provide a clue; the missing piece in the puzzle, which enables us to tie together many of the demographic, epidemiologic, and clinical observations.   Janerich has used the term <u>biologic trigger</u> to describe the physiologic mechanism that explains the disease.   The biologic trigger is usually the last piece in the puzzle and will clarify and help resolve the scientific debate, if the previous existing data had led to confusion.

EXPERIMENTAL STUDIES IN ANIMALS

1.   It was shown that kittens have retinal blood vessel development during the first few weeks of life comparable to that of the human fetus during the terminal months of intrauterine life and therefore comparable to that of a premature baby.

2.   Kittens a few days old were exposed to 60-80 percent oxygen for several days.

3.   Oxygen in these concentrations had a severe damaging effect on the retina of the kittens.   Some litter mates used as controls did not experience damage to the retina.

4.   When the kittens were removed to air, some but not all of the vessels reopened.

As a result of these studies, the etiologic agent of blindness X was identified, and the use of O_2 therapy of premature infants was modified. Incidence of blindness X showed a marked decrease beginning in the early 1950s.

Question 5

Review the epidemiologic and demographic evidence describing the distribution of blindness X from Figures 1-13. Explain why blindness X had the observed distributions given that O_2 therapy was the real cause.

EPILOGUE

The disease was named retrolental fibroplasia (RLF) meaning that fibrous tissue, scars, occurred behind the lens of the eye in susceptible newborns. It was caused by oxygen therapy, which was used to prevent the death of premature newborns, many of whom have impaired respiratory function. The unintended result of the therapy was blindness X. However, the problem of infant blindness was not resolved completely by eliminating O_2 therapy! Examine the data shown in Figures 20 and 21.

Subsequent studies of hyaline membrane disease of the newborn (the most common cause of death in newborns) and of spastic diplegia (a type of cerebral palsy) revealed:

Figure 20. Mortality of premature infants from hyaline membrane disease in two decades.

Birth weight in grams	High oxygen therapy common 1944-48						High oxygen therapy reduced 1954-58					
	White			Black			White			Black		
	Births	Deaths #	Deaths %	Births	Deaths #	Deaths %	Births	Deaths #	Deaths %	Births	Deaths #	Deaths %
1000-1499	38	14	36.8	55	25	45.0	44	25	56.8	108	63	58.3
1500-1999	86	8	9.3	124	21	16.9	117	26	22.2	190	31	16.3
2000-2499	355	11	3.1	494	16	3.2	379	22	5.8	654	19	2.9
TOTAL	479	33	6.9	673	62	9.2	540	73	13.5	952	113	11.9

Source: Avery, M.E., and Oppenheimer, E.H., J. Pediatrics, 57:553, 1960.

Figure 21. Therapy vs. disease in premature infants.

Median duration of O₂ therapy in days	No. of premature infants	Percent spastic diplegia	Percent RLF
0-1	23	17.4	8.7
5-8	102	15.7	9.8
10-17	69	5.8	21.7
Total	194	12.4	13.9

Source: McDonald, A.D., Arch. Dis. Childhood, 38:579, 1963. Re-printed with permission from New England J. Medicine.

Question 6

Describe the relationship between spastic diplegia, infant mortality, and oxygen therapy.

Recommended reading on Retrolental Fibroplasia:

Terry, T.L., Extreme prematurity and fibroblastic overgrowth of persistent vascular sheath behind each crystalline lens. I. Preliminary report. Am. J. Ophthalmol., 25:203,1942

Patz, A., Retrolental fibroplasia, Survey of Ophthalmology, 14:1:1, 1969.

Owens, W.C., and Owens, E.U., Retrolental fibroplasia in premature infants, Am. J. Ophthalmol., 32:1, 1949.

Kinsey, R.E., and Hemphill, F.M., Etiology of retrolental fibroplasia and preliminary report of cooperative study of retrolental fibroplasia. Trans. Amer. Acad. Ophthalmol. Otolar., 59:15, 1955.

In the next section you will be introduced to John Snow's work on cholera. It is one of the classic stories in epidemiology. There was no defined field called epidemiology in Snow's time, no school that taught him the basic principles. The beauty of his study is in his logical pursuit of the causal association and his use of various techniques to relate events visually and factually. He utilized the spot map, capitalized on a natural experiment, and tried to instigate control measures based on his findings.

II.   CHOLERA IN LONDON, 1854*

Epidemiology at any given time is something more than the total of its established facts. It includes their orderly arrangement into chains of inference which extend more or less beyond the bounds of direct observation. Such of these chains as are well and truly laid guide investigation to the facts of the future; those that are ill made fetter progress ....

A nearly perfect model is John Snow's analysis of the epidemiology of cholera which led him to the confident conclusion that the specific cause of the disease was a parasitic microorganism, conforming in all essentials of its natural history to what is now known of the Vibrio cholerae. His central conclusion [today] lies within the boundaries of direct observation; it is now reached by a shorter and easier path than that which he was obliged to follow. But his argument has the permanence of a masterpiece in the ordering and analysis of a kind of evidence which enters at some stage and in some degree into every problem in epidemiology.

... His account should be read once as a story of exploration, many times as a lesson in epidemiology.

Wade Hampton Frost, from his
Introduction to <u>Snow</u> <u>on</u> <u>Cholera</u>

The Broad Street Pump Outbreak*

The most terrible outbreak of cholera which ever occurred in this kingdom is probably that which took place in Broad Street, Golden Square, and the adjoining streets, a few weeks ago. Within two hundred and fifty yards of the spot where Cambridge Street joins Broad Street, there were upwards of five hundred fatal attacks of cholera in ten days. The mortality in this limited area probably equals any that was ever caused in this country, even by the plague; and it was much more sudden, as the greater number of cases terminated in a few hours. The mortality would undoubtedly have been much greater had it not been for the flight of the population. Persons in furnished lodgings left first, then other lodgers went away, leaving their furniture to be sent for when they could meet with a place to put it in. Many houses were closed altgether, owing to the death of the proprietors; and, in a great number of instances, the tradesmen who remained had sent away their families so that in less than six days from the commencement of the outbreak,

*Passages quoted from Snow, J., <u>Snow</u> <u>on</u> <u>Cholera</u>, Hafner Publishing Co., 1936, used by permission of Harvard University Press.

the most afflicted streets were deserted by more than three-quarters
of their inhabitants... I requested permission, therefore, to take a
list, at the General Register Office, of the deaths from cholera,
registered during the week ending 2nd September, in the subdistricts of Golden Square, Berwick Street, and St. Ann's, Soho, which
was kindly granted.

Figures 22 and 23 illustrate how John Snow made use of information on the
time sequence and geographical location of cases. A black dot for each death
is placed at the location of the house in which a fatality occurred.

Figure 22. Asiatic cholera and the Broad Street pump, London, 1854.

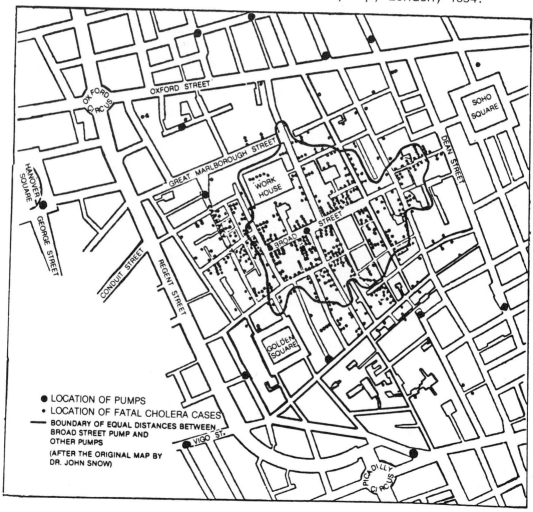

Question 7

Describe the geographical distribution of cases.

Question 8

List the factors that may have determined this distribution.

Question 9

What conclusions would you draw from this map with regard to:

a.   possible agent

b.   source(s)

c.   means of spread or contact.

Question 10

If you were John Snow, working at that time, what further steps would you take to confirm your hypothesis of transmission and the likely source of the infection?

Question 11

a.   Draw a graph of the dates of onset of fatal attacks using the data from Figure 23. Graph paper is provided.

Figure 23.   Cases of cholera by date of onset, London, 1854.

Date	No. of fatal attacks	Deaths	Date	No. of fatal attacks	Deaths
August 19	1	1	September 11	5	15
20	1	0	12	1	6
21	1	2	13	3	13
22	0	0	14	0	6
23	1	0	15	1	8
24	1	2	16	4	6
25	0	0	17	2	5
26	1	0	18	3	2
27	1	1	19	0	3
28	1	0	20	0	0
29	1	1	21	2	0
30	8	2	22	1	2
31	56	3	23	1	3
September 1	143	70	24	1	0
2	116	127	25	1	0
3	54	76	26	1	2
4	46	71	27	1	0
5	36	45	28	0	2
6	20	37	29	0	1
7	28	32	30	0	0
8	12	30	Date unknown	45	0
9	11	24	Total	616	616
10	5	18			

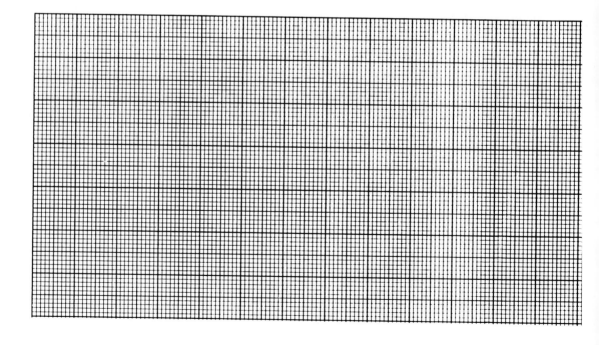

Question 11 (continued):

b.   What was the date of onset of the epidemic?

c.   What type of epidemic curve is suggested by the distribution of cases?

d.   What are the possible reasons for the termination of the epidemic?

> On proceeding to the spot, I found that nearly all the deaths had taken place within a short distance of the pump. There were only ten deaths in houses situated decidedly nearer to another street pump. In five of these cases the families of the deceased persons informed me that they always sent to the pump in Broad Street, as they preferred the water to that of the pump which was nearer. In three other cases, the deceased were children who went to school near the pump in Broad Street. Two of them were known to drink the water; and the parents of the third think it probable that it did also. The other two deaths, beyond the district this pump supplies, represent only the amount of mortality from cholera that was occurring before the eruption took place.
>
> I had an interview with the Board of Guardians of St. James' parish, on the evening of Thursday, 7th September, and represented the above circumstances to them. In consequence of what I said, the handle of the pump was removed on the following day... .

Question 12

What effect do you think that the removal of the handle of the pump played in the decline of the outbreak?

To further confirm his hypothesis of the mode of transmission of cholera, Snow turned his attention to making a study of a more widespread outbreak that had occurred earlier.

London had been without cholera from 1848 to 1853 when the disease appeared in the southern part of the city. Many parishes south of the Thames were involved in 1853, and cases were still occurring in the latter part of 1854 when Snow started his investigation there. After looking over the death records for these parishes for 1853, and comparing the geographical distribution of cases with that of the water supplies, Snow became convinced of a relation between the incidence of cholera and the type of water consumed.

The results of this epidemiological survey are presented in Figure 24. In the areas served by the two water companies, the pipes of both companies went down all the streets, and each household was supplied by one or the other of the companies, according to the decision of the owner or occupant.

Figure 24.   Deaths from cholera by subdistrict, South London, 1853.

Subdistrict	1851 population at risk	Number of cholera deaths	Death rate per 100,000	Water Supply
1 Battersea	10,560	11	104.17	*
2 Borough Road	15,862	26	163.91	* +
3 Brixton	14,610	2	13.68	* +
4 Camberwell	17,742	9	50.73	*
5 Christchurch (Southwark)	16,022	7	43.69	* +
6 Clapham	16,290	10	61.39	* +
7 Dulwich	1,632	0	0	+
8 Kennington (1st part)	24,261	12	49.46	* +
9 Kennington (2nd part)	18,848	6	31.83	* +
10 Kent Road	18,126	37	204.13	* +
11 Lambeth Church (1st part)	18,409	9	48.89	* +
12 Lambeth Church (2nd part)	26,784	11	40.07	* +
13 Leather Market	15,295	23	150.38	*
14 London Road	17,836	9	50.46	* +
15 Norwood	3,977	0	0	+
16 Peckham	19,444	7	36.00	*
17 Putney	5,280	0	0	*
18 Rotherhithe	17,805	20	112.33	*
19 St. George	15,849	6	37.86	* +
20 St. James	18,899	21	111.12	*
21 St. John	11,360	7	61.62	*
22 St. Mary Newington	14,033	5	35.63	* +
23 St. Mary Magdalen	13,934	27	193.77	*
24 St. Olave	8,015	19	237.06	*
25 St. Peter	29,861	23	77.02	* +
26 St. Savior	19,709	45	228.32	*
27 Streatham	9,023	0	0	+
28 Trinity	20,922	11	52.58	* +
29 Wandsworth	9,611	3	31.21	*
30 Waterloo (1st part)	14,088	1	7.10	* +
31 Waterloo (2nd part)	18,348	7	38.15	* +
Total	482,435	374	77.52	

± Subdistricts supplied by Lambeth Water Company
* Subdistricts supplied by Southward and Vauxhall Co.

Question 13

a.   Calculate the death rates for each subdistrict and its water supply.   Is there an association evident?

b.   What interpretations do you make of these data?

c.   What additional information could you, as an epidemiologist, have sought at that time to further investigate the source of this outbreak?

The experiment, too, was on the grandest scale.   No fewer than 300,000 people of both sexes, of every age and occupation, and of every rank and station, from gentlefolks down to the very poor, were divided into two groups without their choice, and in most cases, without their knowledge; one group being supplied with water containing the sewage of London, and, amongst it, whatever might have come from the cholera patients, the other group having water quite free from such impurity.

To turn this grand experiment to account, all that was required was to learn the supply of water to each individual house where a fatal attack of cholera might occur.   I regret that, in the short days at the latter part of last year, I could not spare the time to make the inquiry; and, indeed, I was not fully aware, at that time, of the very intimate mixture of the supply of the two water companies, and the consequently important nature of the desired inquiry.

When the cholera returned to London in July of the present year, however, I resolved to spare no exertion which might be necessary to ascertain the exact effect of the water supply on the progress of the epidemic, in the places where all the circumstances were so happily adapted for the inquiry.   I was desirous of making the investigation myself, in order that I might have the most satisfactory proof of the truth or fallacy of the doctrine which I had been advocating for five years.   I had no reason to doubt the correctness of the conclusions I had drawn from the great number of facts already in my possession, but I felt that the circumstance of the cholera-poison passing down the sewers into a great river, and being distributed through miles of pipes, and yet producing its specific effects, was a fact of so startling a nature, and of so vast importance to the community, that it could not be too rigidly examined, or established on too firm a basis.

The inquiry was necessarily attended with a good deal of trouble. There were very few instances in which I could at once get the information I required. Even when the water rates are paid by the residents they can seldom remember the name of the water company till they have looked for the receipt. In the case of working people who pay weekly rates, the rates are invariably paid by the landlord or his agent, who often lives at a distance, and the residents know nothing about the matter. It would, indeed, have been almost impossible for me to complete the inquiry, if I had not found that I could distinguish the water of the two companies with perfect certainty by a chemical test. The test I employed was founded on the great difference in the quantity of chloride of sodium contained in two kinds of water, at the time I made the inquiry. On adding solution of nitrate of silver to a gallon of the water of the Lambeth Company, obtained at Thames Ditton, beyond the reach of the sewage of London, 2.28 grains of chloride of silver were obtained, indicating the presence of 0.95 grains of chloride of sodium in the water. On treating the water of the Southwark and Vauxhall Company in the same manner, 91 grains of chloride of silver were obtained, showing the presence of 37.9 grains of common salt per gallon. Indeed, the difference in appearance on adding nitrate of silver to the two kinds of water was so great, that they could be at once distinguished without further trouble. Therefore, when the resident could not give clear and conclusive evidence about the water company, I obtained some of the water in a small phial, and wrote the address on the cover, when I could examine it after coming home. The mere appearance of the water generally afforded a very good indication of its source, especially if it was observed as it came in, before it had entered the water-butt or cistern; and the time of its coming in also afforded some evidence of the kind of water, after I had ascertained the hours when the turncocks of both companies visited any street. These points were, however, not relied on, except as corroborating more decisive proof, such as the chemical test, or the company's receipt for the rates....

Figure 25. The proportion of deaths to 10,000 houses, during the first seven weeks of the epidemic, in the population supplied by the Southwark and Vauxhall Company; and that supplied by the Lambeth Company; and in the rest of London.

Water supply	Number of houses	Deaths from cholera	Deaths in each 10,000 houses
Southwark and Vauxhall Co.	40,046	1,263	315
Lambeth Co.	26,107	98	37
Rest of London	256,423	1,522	59

The mortality in the houses supplied by the Southwark and Vauxhall Company was therefore between eight and nine times as great as in the houses supplied by the Lambeth Company...

Question 14

a.   What questions might be raised concerning the "proof" of Snow's findings?

b.   Are you satisfied with this experimental proof?   Explain.

Duration of Epidemic and Size of Population

There are certain circumstances connected with the history of cholera which I admit of a satisfactory explanation according to the principles explained above, and consequently tend to confirm those principles. The first point I shall notice, viz., the period of duration of the epidemic in different places, refers merely to the communicability of the disease, without regard to the mode of communication. The duration of cholera in a place is usually in a direct proportion to the number of the population. The disease remains but two or three weeks in a village, two or three months in a good-sized town, whilst in a great metropolis it often remains a whole year or longer. I find from an analysis which I made in 1849 of the valuable table of Dr. Wm. Merriman, of the cholera in England in 1832, that fifty-two places are enumerated in which the disease continued less than fifty days, and that the average population of these places is 6,624. Forty-three places are likewise down in which the cholera lasted fifty days, but less than 100; the average population of these is 12,624. And there are, without including London, thirty-three places in which the epidemic continued one hundred days and upwards, the average population of which is 38,123; or if London be included, thirty-four places, with an average of 78,823....

There was a similar relation in 1849 between the duration of the cholera and the population of the places which it visited; a relation which points clearly to the propagation of the disease from patient to patient; for if each case were not connected with a previous one, but depended on some unknown atmospheric or telluric condition, there is no reason why the twenty cases which occur in a village should not be distributed over as long a period as the twenty hundred cases which occur in a large town....

Question 15

What factors could account for the observed relationships between the duration of an outbreak and the size of the population?

Question 16

a.   Summarize Snow's strategy to prove the vehicle of the epidemic.

b.   What epidemiologic principle regarding disease prevention or control is illustrated by Snow's discovery of the disease vehicle?

This concludes the exercise based on Snow's work. The following essay on the Broad Street Pump reveals the bizarre story of the aftermath of the cholera epidemic. Regrettably, as in Snow's era, epidemiologists of the modern day are also not always successful in their endeavors to change the social customs and political practices in the interests of improved health.

JOHN SNOW: THE BROAD STREET PUMP AND AFTER
(Source: Chave, S.P.W., The Medical Officer,
13th June 1958, 99; 347-349)

On 19th June, 1858, the following notice appeared among the announcements of deaths in The Times: "On the 16th inst., at his residence 18 Sackville Street, Piccadilly, John Snow, M.D., of apoplexy, aged 45." For some weeks prior to his last illness Snow had been working on his book "On Chloroform and Other Anaesthetics." According to his friend Benjamin Ward Richardson, he was drafting the concluding paragraph and was actually writing the word "exit" when he was seized with a stroke from which he died ten days later.

It was nine years before his untimely death that Snow had first put forward his theory concerning the spread of cholera by polluted water. This he did in a small pamphlet of about 30 pages which was published at his own expense. But this first essay in the field of infectious diseases received only scant attention at the time. Five years later, in 1854, when cholera was sweeping across the country for the third time, he carried out his classic researches in South London. This investigation, which remains to this day a model of scientific inquiry, established beyond all reasonable doubt that cholera is a waterborne disease. Snow incorporated the substantial body of new evidence which he had gathered in the course of this inquiry into his much enlarged volume of 162 pages: the so-called "second edition" of his book "On the Mode of Transmission of Cholera" which was published early in 1855. In the next three years only 56 copies of the book were sold, and in return for an outlay of £200 incurred in its preparation, the author was reimbursed with the princely sum of £3,12s. 0d.

Snow's theory ran counter to the prevailing view of his time, which attributed infectious diseases like cholera to the effluvia arising from filth and putrefaction. It is hardly to be wondered, therefore, that at first there were few who were disposed to accept this new explanation. In 1849, a reviewer commenting in the Lancet on Snow's first pamphlet on cholera wrote, "The arguments adduced by the author against emanations causing the disease are not by any means conclusive." Following the cholera epidemic of 1853-4, the Royal College of Physicians set up an investigation into its causes under Drs. William Baly and William Gull. They considered Snow's theses and rejected it outright. "The theory as a whole is untenable," they reported and added, "The matter which is the cause of cholera increases and finds the conditions for its action under the influence of foul or damp air." So, too, the medical inspectors appointed by the General Board of Health in 1854 to inquire into the Soho outbreak, having examined Snow's views upon it, commented, "We see no reason to adopt this belief." The principal objections raised against Snow's theory were that it did not account either for the sudden onset or for the decline of the epidemics as satisfactorily as the current explanation in terms of miasmata.

In 1856, John Snow visited Paris with his uncle, Mr. Empson, of Bath. Empson, a dealer in curios, was known personally to the Emperor, and Ward Richardson records that "on this occasion special imperial favours were shown to him in which the nephew participated." While in Paris, Snow entered his book at the "Institut de France" for a prize which was offered for the most outstanding contribution towards the prevention or treatment of cholera. Ward Richardson reports that no notice was taken of Snow's researches by the Institute. On the other hand Sir D'Arcy Power, the medical historian, writing of Snow in the Dictionary of National Biography, states that "his essay upon the mode of communication of cholera which was first published in 1849 was awarded by the Institute of France a prize of £1.200." In reply to a recent inquiry made by the writer, M. Pierre Gauja, the present Archivist of the Institute, confirmed that Snow did not in fact receive this award. It would appear that his theory was no more acceptable abroad than at home, for about the same time Max Pettenkofer in Germany also rejected it.

In England two men of note, William Budd and William Farr, were almost alone in voicing their approval of Snow's thesis during his lifetime. In 1849, shortly after Snow had published his first paper on cholera, Budd brought out a pamphlet of his own on the same subject. He put forward a theory of causation and transmission of the disease similar to that of Snow's published work. In all his subsequent writings on cholera Budd stressed the water-borne nature of the disease and was at pains to give full credit to Snow for having first made this discovery.

William Farr at the General Register Office gave a more qualified support to Snow's theory. He himself had noted the high mortality from cholera which occurred in those districts of London whose water supplies were drawn directly from the sewage-laden reaches of the Thames. In the Report of the Registrar General for 1852 he discussed Snow's findings and reached the conclusion that the facts "lend some countenance to Dr. Snow's theory." Farr presented a long and detailed statistical account of the cholera epidemic of 1853-4. He concluded as follows: "It is right to state that Dr. Snow by his hypothesis and researches and by his personal inquiries; that the Registrar General by procuring information and by promoting inquiry; as well as the Board of Health [in its] Report, have all contributed in various ways to establish the fact that the cholera matter, or cholerine, when it is most fatal, is largely diffused through water as well as through other channels."

The report to which Farr referred was that made to the President of the General Board of Health by John Simon, in which he expressed the cautious view that "fecalised drinking water and fecalised air equally may breed and convey the poison." Simon remained for long an adherent of the old theory of the miasmata, and his acceptance of Snow's thesis came only gradually and after many years. In the month of Snow's death in 1858, he referred to Snow's "peculiar doctrine as to the contagiousness of cholera" and commented somewhat patronizingly that whatever may be the worth of the theory, it has been of use in contributing to draw attention to the vast hygienic importance of a pure water supply." Sixteen years later he had changed his opinion, and in a report to the Local Government Board he remarked, "Indeed, with regard to the manner of spread of the enterozymotic diseases generally, it deserves notice that the whole pathological argument which I am explaining grew amongst us in this country out of the very cogent facts which our cholera epidemics supplied, and to which the late Dr. Snow 25 years ago had the merit of forcing medical attention, an attention at first quite incredulous, but which at least for the last 15 years as facts have accumulated has gradually been changing into conviction." Later still, in 1890, in his "English Sanitary Institutions," Simon, looking back over the years to Snow's discovery, could write that it "may probably still be counted the most important truth yet acquired by medical science for the prevention of epidemics of cholera." This appreciation of Snow's work was handsome if somewhat belated.

The 30 years which followed the publication of Snow's book witnessed a plethora of new books on the subject of cholera. A perusal of 12 of these volumes disclosed no mention at all of Snow in six of them (Johnson, 1855; Jameson, 1855; Shrimpton, 1866; Jencken, 1867; Parkes, 1873; Macpherson, 1884). Chapman (1866) rejected Snow's "far-fetched doctrine," Bellew (1855) found it "untenable," as did Boyd Mushet (1885). Only three of these writers expressed their agreement with Snow's conclusions: Macnamara (1872), Blanc (1873), and Wendt (1885). These examples indicate how tardy and gradual was the general acceptance of Snow's theory.

In 1884 Koch announced his discovery of the cholera vibrio to the Berlin Conference and ten years later an English translation of his papers on cholera was published in this country. Koch made no mention of Snow, although he fully accepted the water-borne nature of the disease. William Gairdner, Professor of Medicine at Glasgow, contributed an Introduction to the English edition in which he paid a fitting tribute to John Snow:

> Since Dr. Snow's researches were published and adopted by the Registrar General in England there has never been much doubt among us as to the water-communication of the choleraic infection, the evidence of which seemed to go on accumulating as the incidence of the disease, in respect of particular places, was more and more studied, and the severity of local epidemics was found to be strictly in accordance with the presence of dangerous impurities in the water supply.

The discoveries of the bacteriologists finally dethroned the doctrine of emanations, and served both to underline the soundness of John Snow's observations and to confirm the truth of his deductions.

The Broad Street Pump

The name of John Snow is invariably associated with the Broad Street pump and with the outbreak of cholera which centered upon it. The story of this old pump forms an interesting chapter in the history of public health. Just when it was set up in Broad Street is not known. The houses in this part of Soho were built between 1700 and 1740 and it is likely that the well was sunk about the same time. The district was a suitable one for shallow wells, for water could be obtained at a depth of about 20 feet almost everywhere. As a result wells were plentiful. There were at least 12 pumps within a radius of a quarter of a mile of Broad Street.

By 1850 two private companies--the New River and the Grand Junction--were supplying piped water to all the houses in the area. At that time these supplies were intermittent, the water being turned on for about two hours daily except on Sundays. Each household had to install a butt or cistern which was filled whenever the main supply became available. These storage butts were notoriously bad. They were usually uncovered, rarely if ever cleaned, and as a result the water drawn from them was generally dirty and often unsavoury.

By contrast the water from the well in Broad Street was clear, bright, and sparkling, albeit through the presence of carbonic acid and nitrates, the end-products of organic contamination. Throughout the district around Golden Square its waters, always available and invariably cool and palatable, were most highly regarded. Not only did householders close at hand make extensive use of it, but many people living at a distance preferred to draw their water from Broad Street in preference to their local wells. It was commonly the duty of the children to fetch the water from the pump, and old people living alone bemoaned the fact that they had no one to fetch water for them. The pump-handle had a ladle attached to it from which the children were accustomed to drink, although we know that some parents disapproved of this practice. Many of the small workshops in the locality kept butts filled with the well water to be used for drinking purposes, especially in summer. The water was also used for mixing with spirits in all the taverns round about and it was suppled to customers in the coffee shops which used to bottle the water, add a little effervescent powder, and sell it as "sherbet" drink.

Perhaps the most striking testimony to the attractions of this water comes from Snow's account of the widow of Hampstead. This lady, whose husband had formerly owned the percussion-cap factory in Broad Street, had a bottle of the well water brought to her by a cart which travelled each day to St. James. This was to prove her undoing, for in the cholera epidemic she alone of the inhabitants of Hampstead contracted the disease and died.

The month of August, 1854, was hot and dry and when cholera broke out in Broad Street it spread through the little neighbourhood like fire in a rickyard. Within ten days the population was literally decimated. It was without doubt, and John Snow himself described it, "the most terrible outbreak of cholera which ever occurred in this kingdom." At the time Snow was living on Sackville Street, about half a mile from the affected area, and although he was already fully engaged in his investigation in South London he hastened to the scene of this new outbreak. His suspicions quickly fell on the well in Broad Street and these were strengthened when he discovered that "nearly all the deaths had taken place within a short distance of the pump." He was able to establish that almost all the people who had died had consumed water from the pump." After pursuing his inquiries further, Snow recorded, "I had an interview with the Board of Guardians of St. James's parish on the evening of Thursday, 7th September, and represented the above circumstances to them. In consequence of what I said the handle of the pump was removed on the following day."

It is interesting to note that the Minutes of the Board of Guardians and of the Vestry contain no reference to Snow's intervention. It is probable that he made his representation to the sanitary committee which had been set up by the Guardians to act during the epidemic, and that it was this body which ordered the pump to be taken out of use. By the morning of 8th September the epidemic had already declined sharply and the closure of the well did little to affect its course, although it may well have prevented a fresh outbreak. The removal of the handle was not by any means the end of the Broad Street pump, for within a short time it was brought into service again.

Two further associates of John Snow enter the story at this stage--one a doctor and the other a clergyman. The doctor was Edwin Lankester, who in the following year became the first medical officer of health of St. James; the clergyman was Henry Whitehead, the young curate at St. Luke's church in Berwick Street. Lankester was a member of the Vestry and at his instigation a local inquiry into the epidemic was ordered to be carried out at the expense of the parish. Both John Snow and Henry Whitehead were co-opted onto the committee which brought a triumphant confirmation of his hypothesis. This was the elucidation of the way in which the well had become polluted.

Whitehead discovered that a baby living at 40 Broad Street, the nearest house to the pump, had died from what is described as "exhaustion following diarrhea" and that the child's illness immediately preceded the onset of the cholera epidemic. From his inquiries at the house he learned that the baby's discharges had been disposed of into a cesspool which was less than three feet from the well. An immediate inspection revealed conspicuous evidence of the percolation of faecal matter from the ill constructed cesspool through the decaying brickwork which lined the well. The chain of evidence incriminating the pump was now complete. Yet even this disclosure did not secure its final removal. Instead, the well was closed six weeks while the brickwork was renewed, it was then pumped out completely three times after which it was opened for use by the public once more. In the following year, 1856, Edwin Lankester was appointed Medical Officer of Health of St. James's parish under the Metropolis Management Act. One of the first matters to which he gave his attention was the water supply of the district. It was his aim to get rid of the numerous shallow wells in the area, and in his first annual report to the Vestry he complained that "the most impure water in the parish is that of the Broad Street pump, and it is altogether the most popular." This comment is all the more striking when it is recalled that it was made within two years of the great epidemic. Lankester went on to report that a chemical analysis had revealed that this water contained more inorganic salts (chlorides and nitrates) derived from organic pollution than the common sewer.

The Vestry appear to have been unmoved by these revelations, so in the following year Lankester wrote to every one of his fellow medical officers of health in the Metropolitan area asking their opinions about surface wells. Their replies, which he published in full, showed that the general consensus of opinion was in favor of closure. This seems to have led to a minor victory, for at the beginning of 1858 all the shallow wells in the parish were closed by order of the Vestry. Lankester's success was shortlived, however, for in his report for that year he grumbled "You did not think it advisable to continue the closing of the pumps." And so, after an interval of four months all the wells were in use again.

Four years later Lankester took up the cudgels once more. In his customary forthright manner he informed the Vestry that all the wells in the parish were unsafe, with the single exception of the artesian well near the church in Piccadilly. He reminded them that St. James was now lagging behind most other districts for "with the exception of our own parish these surface well-pumps have nearly all been closed throughout London." He spoke of "offering the public the filtered sewage of these pumps." This seems to have prompted the Vestry to take some action, for in 1864 Lankester was able to report that "the wells in the parish are gradually being abandoned--seven only remain." But the Broad Street pump was among them. He remarked that drinking fountains had largely replaced wells in popular esteem but that St. James had fewer of them than any other London parish.

It was in the next year that the threat of cholera returned to this country once again. Lankester thereupon urged the Vestry to lock the remaining pumps as a safety precaution, reminding them of the part that impure water, especially from surface wells, had played in the spread of cholera in the past. His warning went unheeded. The threatened outbreak materialized in the summer of 1866 when cholera broke out in the teeming slums of East London. Lankester promptly submitted to the Vestry a special report on the state of the wells which still remained in service in the area. This revealed abundant chemical evidence of organic contamination, and once again he drew special attention to the Broad Street pump. Further support now came from another and perhaps unexpected source, for on 31st July a letter headed "The Broad Street Pump" appeared in The Times. Signed by Dr. W. Allen Miller, of King's College Hospital, and Prof. E. Frankland, of the Royal College of Chemistry, it deplored the fact that the old pump was still in use and commented on the unfitness of its waters. The writers concluded with a solemn warning that the whole area could be infected "by a single case of cholera occurring within the drainage area of the pump."

Three days later a case of cholera was reported in No. 30 Broad Street. Lankester now sounded a note of alarm. He warned the Vestry yet again of the dangers of spreading the disease through the pollution of water, "this can occur in no other way than by our pumps." He pronounced the wells to be dangerous. "I dare not take the responsibility of remaining quiet while these pumps are open, and, at the risk of offending you by my pertinacity, I implore you to order the pumps to be shut."

This appeal seems to have been successful in bringing about, at long last, the final closure of the Broad Street Pump. There are no further references to its use from that time.

Edwin Lankester died in 1874 and was succeeded as medical officer of health by James Edmunds. In his annual report for 1884, eight wells were mentioned by name, including the one in Broad Street which was said "to have been covered but not filled in." The rest is silence: Broad Street remained but its pump had passed into history.

Today, 120 years after the death of John Snow, the student of public health can still visit many of the places associated with his career. Bateman's Buildings, the little back street in Soho, where in 1836 Snow rented a room following his long walk to London to study medicine; Great Windmill Street, where a plaque on the wall of the Lyric Theatre marks the site of the Hunterian School of Medicine in which Snow was a student from 1836 to 1838; Frith Street, Soho, where in 1838 he "nailed up his colours" and started his first practice; 18 Sackville Street, which was his home from 1852 until his death, and Brompton Cemetery, where stands a replica of the original monument erected to his memory by his friends. But perhaps it is fitting that the pilgrimage should end in Broad Street--now Broadwick Street, W. 1--and at the old tavern, which 25 years ago was renamed in honour of John Snow. For, below the inn-sign which bears his portrait, a tablet on the wall draws the attention of the passer-by to a red granite stone at the curbside. "This stone marks the site of the Broad Street pump."

SUGGESTED RESPONSES
Exercise 8--Etiology of Disease

1. There were a few but relatively constant number of cases reported (identified) between 1940 and 1945. There was a decided increase beginning in 1946 and continuing until it reached a peak in 1951. A slight decline, but a continued large number of cases began in 1952-1953 and a rapid sudden decline occurred in 1954. We are able to discern a trend (pattern) of disease with three distinct periods of risk identified between 1940-1951. There is approximately a 7-fold excess of cases for the period 1951-1953 compared to the period 1940-1945.

2a. In the early years of its appearance, a reasonable proportion of new cases might be attributed to better case finding, improved diagnosis or more complete reporting. It takes some time for the medical community to become familiar with a potentially new disease. When most physicians are aware of a new disease, they may be more likely to diagnose it, when previously they had no such choice. In addition, the trend for new blindness from all causes tends to parallel the increasing birth rate. As blindness X increases, other causes of blindness show a relative decrease.

2b. Between 1948 and 1949 there was an increase in blindness X in the three centers that may be related in part to both better case finding and actual increase in the disease. However, in 1950-1951 the incidence and trend of disease differed in the 3 centers. It is not likely that differences in methods of case finding would differ so markedly between centers X, Y, and B because the disease was already well known to the medical community. Also, from Figure 3, we note that the rate of infectious and other causes of blindness remained stable after 1940, but there was a tremendous increase in the rate from blindness X.

2c. An actual increase in disease was likely.

3. Better case finding/improved diagnostic methods may of course be responsible for the awareness/appearance of some new disease. These possibilities must be investigated before one accepts the hypothesis of the new disease/syndrome. Let us assume that these explanations are not relevant, and the reported cases do in fact represent a new disease.

3a. Genetic mutation may occur randomly or it might be induced by environmental hazards such as radiation (atomic bombs were first used in the 1940s) or increased chemical air pollution due to automobile exhausts.

3b. There might be a new virus or an altered strain of an existing organism introduced into the population. Increased disease incidence in different geographic areas may represent the spread (seeding) of the organism through person-to-person contact. The organism might have been introduced to the U.S. by servicemen returning from WW II.

3c. Disease in early infancy may result from slow deterioration of vision over several months, secondary to birth trauma.

3d. Changes in mothering practices: less breast feeding/more use of formula and prepared baby foods. Premature babies may be most susceptible to some factor in cow's milk or the formula. New diets may provide excess or deficient amounts of necessary nutrients.

3e. Mothers may be smoking more. Neurotoxic chemicals from cigarettes may pass to infants in utero. Developing baby may be susceptible to a chemical agent either early or late in gestation. Disease is a slowly developing one.

3f. Numerous examples of medications capable of producing developmental defects are available. For example, thalidomide (a mild tranquilizer) caused severe developmental abnormalities of the arms and legs of newborns when the mother ingested it at a critical time in the fetus' development.

4. Figure 5. Percentage of premature births per year did not change appreciably between 1945-1960. The increase in blindness X is unlikely to be due to changes in prematurity incidence.

   Figure 6. There is a small increase in blindness X associated with older maternal age. These differences are not statistically significant.

   Figure 7. The distribution of blindness X may be related to the type of hospital. In particular, hospitals that primarily care for private patients seem to have more disease than hospitals where private patients are not predominant. The disease is primarily found in white babies but non-whites do have some reported cases.

   Figure 8. A higher percentage of the disease is found in the upper class hospitals. There is also an inverse relationship between birthweight and blindness X, which is evident in upper- and lower-class hospitals.

   Figure 9. There is higher incidence in babies < 3 pounds. The risk fell dramatically in 1945 but began to rise again in 1946.

   Figure 10. There is an inverse relation between birthweight and the disease. This study was done in a different setting and supports the evidence of other studies.

   Figure 11. There is also an association between short gestation and blindness X. Shorter duration of gestation was associated with more severe disease.

   Figure 12. In the previous figure gestational age was independent and disease was the dependent variable. Figure 12 shows eye findings (independent variable) and the gestational age as dependent. The correlation supports the previous findings.

Figure 13.   The inverse relation to birthweight is noted.   The disease incidence increases with age after birth.   This suggests that environmental exposure after birth may be an important consideration.

Figure 14.   Several modes of therapy show an increase in usage parallel to the appearance and increase of blindness X.   Iron sulfate curve is most similar to the blindness curve.

Figure 15.   Vitamin therapy (including iron in multivitamins) does not show a clear association with the occurrence of blindness X.   The rise in percent with blindness X does not occur until long after the initiation of these treatment modalities.   The association of the disease with low birthweight may be an indirect association, i.e., low-birthweight babies received vitamins plus something else that caused the disease.

Figure 16.   Vitamin E supplements may confer protection against blindness X.   While this is a promising lead, subsequent studies did not corroborate the finding.   The finding may be invalid due to errors or misclassification resulting from the selection of case and comparison groups; the finding may be valid but not reproducible in other populations; or the differences may have occurred by chance and no gross methodologic errors were committed.

Figure 17.   The data suggest a dose response (not clearly stepwise) between duration of exposure to oxygen and development of blindness X in both single/multiple births.

Figures 18, 19 further support the notion that oxygen was causally related to blindness X (RLF).   The clinical trial of Kinsey and Hemphill provides strongly supportive evidence, because infants exposed to the high dose of the suspected causal agent developed a higher rate of disease than those receiving the low dose.   The relative risk is about 2.

5.   The disease was related to the ability to pay for the new technique of oxygen/incubators for infants at high risk of death (prematures, twins, etc.).   Consequently, upper-class hospitals with private, mostly White patients, showed higher rates of disease than other hospitals.   Teaching and university hospitals produced RLF in White and non-White patients, because they provided free care to indigent patients who may have been admitted for teaching purposes.   The appearance of disease in different places at different times relates to the time necessary for the newer therapy to become an accepted/popular form of therapy in the medical community.

6.   The data from Figures 20 and 21 demonstrate the difficult decision facing a medical doctor.   Obviously, there is a trade-off in terms of death, mental retardation, and retrolental fibroplasia.   The frequency of each of these diseases in part depends upon the concentration and duration of exposure of newborns to oxygen during the neonatal period.   In cases of prematurity/multiple births, where the risks of the above unhappy consequences may occur, how does one decide what is the correct decision?

Part II. Cholera in London, 1854

7.   Cases were concentrated in the area around the Broad Street pump.

8.   Crowding, sanitation, common source in area, susceptible population.

9.   a.   The agent may be in the drinking water or a common food source.
     b.   Wells, pumps, or food shops may harbor the agent.
     c.   Ingestion of contaminated food or water by a susceptible host.

10. Stop pump use and see if it affects incidence. Your investigation might compare cases outside the area, noncases in the area, and cases in the area of the Broad Street pump with regard to their daily activities and what they eat or drink. Demonstration of feces in the water of cases would be useful evidence in supporting a fecal-oral route of transmission.

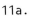

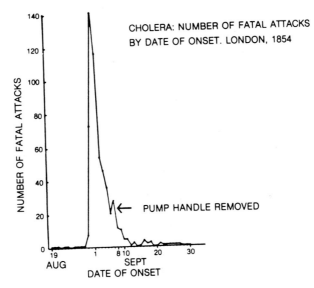

11b. August 30.

11c. A common-source, highly communicable epidemic that has a short incubation period.

11d. Deaths, many susceptibles fled, the supply of susceptibles was markedly reduced. By the time the pump handle was removed the epidemic had begun to subside.

12. Not much, but perhaps it prevented a new outbreak.

13a. Lambeth (182/314,781) = 57.82 per 100,000; Southwark-Vauxhall (374/467,803) = 79.95 per 100,000; total (374/482,435) = 77.52 per 100,000. Yes, there is an association as evidenced by the higher death rate for districts that use Southwark-Vauxhall water.

13b. Southwark-Vauxhall does something that Lambeth does not. Transmission of the disease by water is a possibility.

13c. Where do the companies get water? Are the Southwark-Vauxhall and Lambeth served populations different in other important ways? What about noncases? Why do persons served by the presumably clean water supply get the disease?

14a. In consideration of whether or not Snow's work constitutes proof of the association between water and cholera consider the following points:

Which variables were eliminated from consideration due to the "natural experiment" circumstances of the investigation?
Was there random possibility that people were using a particular water supply?
Was Snow able to completely enumerate cases of the disease and the population at risk?
How accurate was Snow's method for grouping people by their water source?
How much possibility was there for misdiagnosis of cases or misclassification of the source of exposure for the population at risk?
Could inapparent infections have affected the distribution?
Were families systematically selected in order to perform the salt test? Might this have affected Snow's ability to test his hypothesis?

14b. Snow's proof is indirect but quite plausible. It was substantiated years later when the cholera organism was discovered. The criteria that epidemiologists use to infer causation will be covered in Exercise 9. Snow's work illustrates the application of several of these criteria.

15. The number of susceptibles is larger in a big population; there is a greater probability of contact with contaminated water or a large dose of organism; the survival potential of the organism is great due to the possibility of continuing contamination of the public water supply.

16a. Snow had identified a problem and made observations concerning the spread of cholera from prior outbreaks of the disease. He then described the 1854 outbreak by place and time. He compared the rates of disease occurring in houses exposed to different water sources. These comparisons are actually the relative risk of cholera. He made logical deductions based upon his observations of the epidemiologic distribution and occurrence of the disease. These deductions led him to reject the prevailing notion that the disease was caused by miasmata.

16b. Of special importance is the conclusion that even though the actual disease agent is not known, the epidemic could have been prevented by eliminating the vehicle of the disease, i.e., by controlling access to the contaminated water! If you can visualize development of the disease as a chain of related events, then breaking the chain at any point would result in prevention or control of the disease.

EXERCISE 9. PRINCIPLES OF CAUSATION

Goals

Upon completion of this exercise you should be able (1) to identify different types of cause and effect relations and (2) to understand the epidemiologic criteria for inferring causal associations.

Methods

In order to achieve these goals you will need to understand

I.   CONCEPT OF CAUSATION
II. HISTORICAL CONCEPTS OF CAUSATION
III. EPIDEMIOLOGIC CRITERIA OF CAUSATION. THE ASSOCIATION BE-
     TWEEN SMOKING AND LUNG CANCER

Terms

Direct and indirect associations, spurious association, web of causation, net of effects, correlation, correlation coefficients, correlation matrix, ecologic fallacy, Koch's postulates, Mill's canons, retrospective studies, prospective studies, cross-sectional studies, case reports.

Suggested readings

Lilienfeld and Lilienfeld, Foundations of Epidemiology, Ch. 12.
Mausner and Bahn, Epidemiology, Ch. 5, pp. 91-111.
MacMahon and Pugh, Epidemiology; Principles and Methods, pp. 17-27, pp. 32-39.
Freidman, Primer of Epidemiology, pp. 3-6, pp. 48-49, pp. 173-191.
Susser, Causal Thinking in the Health Sciences, pp. 48-63, pp. 64-72.
Stewart, Trends in Epidemiology, Ch. 2, pp. 23-100.
Peterson, Epidemiology and Clinical Problems, pp. 32-48.
Li, C.C., Path Analysis: A Primer, Pacific Grove: Boxwood Press, 1975, pp. 135-186.

I. CONCEPT OF CAUSATION

The concept of "cause(s)" is fundamental to epidemiology. A CAUSE of the frequency and distribution of a disease or health problem in a population is defined as a factor or habit whose reduction (or removal) leads to reduction in the incidence of the disease or health problem. This exercise raises some issues involved in judging whether or not a causal explanation can be invoked when an observed relationship exists between variables:

1. What issues are important in drawing valid conclusions about cause?
2. How are judgments about the validity of causal theories and hypothe-
    ses made?

3.   How do we determine whether observed statistical associations are in a cause and effect relationship?

Other questions raised by a discussion of causation have been debated by epidemiologists and public health personnel for many years. Some of these questions are listed to stimulate your thinking, but will not be explicitly answered in this exercise.

4.   Does a causal explanation necessarily permit prediction? Must a causal explanation be rejected if it does not permit prediction?
5.   What is meant by the expression "degree of probability"? Are such concepts as "proof" or "certainty" useful, or even meaningful, in epidemiology?
6.   Are the requirements for evidence to support causal claims in epidemiology subject to standardization?
7.   Is it the role of the epidemiologist to be the "etiologist" for public health research?
8.   What evidence constitutes sufficient grounds for advocating a particular public health policy?

Such questions suggest that even though the search for causes is of central importance to epidemiology there may be doubt about when "cause" has been proven. Epidemiology uses many expressions in speaking and writing in which the notion of "cause" is implicit, such as "influenced by," "would result in," "would tend to reduce," "a factor in producing," "in reaction to," "have an impact on," "accounts for," "yields a difference between," "an effect of," "in consequence of," "explained by." The sense of a causal association connecting events is implicit in all of these expressions, yet <u>the</u> <u>direct</u> <u>statement</u>, <u>x</u> <u>causes</u> <u>y</u>, is rarely used in epidemiologic reports.

If one were to have considered why or how we invoked "causation" prior to the study of epidemiology, one would probably have mentioned <u>direct</u> <u>observation</u>, <u>personal</u> <u>experience</u>, and the <u>sequence</u> <u>of</u> <u>events</u>, i.e., temporal proximity (time) of the factor thought to be the cause of an event, and the outcome (result or endpoint) resulting from that factor. In many daily situations you would be inclined to believe that "chances are pretty good" that A causes X if the sequence of events is very rapid and one's prior experience and direct observation were consistent with that conclusion. However, in epidemiology, direct observation may not be possible, experience may be lacking and the sequence of events either unclear or difficult to determine.

The following problems will demonstrate why direct observation, personal experience, and temporal proximity of exposure and outcome might not be the only ways to search for "causes."

A small village in a developing country is located on the Equator. Every afternoon at 4:55 p.m. the villagers gather in the square. At 5:00 p.m. the church bell strikes and within an hour the sun sets. This sequence of events has occurred without fail as long as the townspeople can remember. Half the villagers believe that their daily gathering causes the sun to set (group A) while the other half believes the ringing of the church bell causes the sun to set (group B). Each group uses observation, personal experience, and the interval of time between an event and a subsequent outcome in judging what caused the sun to set.

Question 1

Identify the fallacy in each group's argument based upon your enlightened understanding of why the sun REALLY sets.

Several persons representing each of the groups decide to conduct an experiment to determine which of their opinions is true. Members of both groups travel to a distant village and there they observe that the sunset precedes the 5 p.m. church bell.

Question 2

How might each group explain this finding and retain belief in their original opinion?

Question 3

Suppose both groups agreed that neither of their earlier opinions was warranted by the facts. What might they do to better understand this curious phenomenon? What alternative explanations might be proposed?

Question 4

Suppose that a causal relation exists between a cause "A" and a disease "B." Why might it be difficult for an epidemiologist to prove that relation if the onset of disease followed the cause by:

a.   1-2 days

b.   1-2 months

c.   1-2 years

d.   10-20 years

e.   What if the disease "B" appeared in the children of those exposed to
     cause "A," as for example, vaginal cancer in female children of mothers
     exposed to the hormone Diethylstilbestrol (DES) during pregnancy?

From the preceding examples, it should be evident that the criteria that we
use for "proving" causation in our daily activities are not always adequate.
When searching for the causes of disease in human populations the problems
are more complex. To understand how epidemiologists prove causation consider
the types of relations thought to occur in the causation of disease. Epidemiologists refer to a relation as an ASSOCIATION. The term association refers
to a statistical and measurable relation observed or existing between two variables. Many associations are of interest when a p value of <0.05 (<0.01,
<0.001, etc.) is observed as a result of statistical analysis. The p values of
these magnitudes are termed STATISTICALLY SIGNIFICANT, and refer to the
probability that the measured or observed differences between two variables
being compared could have occurred by chance if they were derived from the
same universe (population); or that an observed value for one variable differs
from the true mean of the universe (population) from which it may have been
drawn, by the probability or p value observed.

As pointed out earlier, some may be prone to equate statistically significant differences with establishing proof of a biologic association between the factors under investigation. This is not true! Statistical significance establishes associations but this is not the same as proving causation! Biostatistics has a very important and useful role in epidemiology, in that it provides techniques that are helpful in demonstrating whether or not the observations from one study are consistent with results of other studies that have been performed.

Evidence from a single study is seldom sufficient to determine "causal" association because of the difficulties involved in carrying out population-based studies. The conclusion that an association is a causal explanation is usually the result of an extensive body of supporting BIOLOGICAL AND STATISTICAL EVIDENCE derived from several studies. To understand the implications of the use of the term "cause" it is helpful to describe some of the ways in which events may be related, although the statistical associations observed may be spurious, indirect, or causal.

Examples of causal relations can be diagrammed as follows:

1.   A ─────────► B

This model suggests that A causes B. It implies that when the factor A is present, the disease B must result. Conversely, when the disease is present, the factor must also be evident. A relationship in which the cause always produces the disease seldom occurs; however, measles may be one disease in which such a relation exists.

2.   A + C ─────► B

This relation implies that both A and C are required to produce the disease. The relation is probably the correct model for many diseases. For example, although there is little doubt that smoking (A) causes lung cancer (B), not all smokers get cancer. Some other factor (C) may mediate or influence the development of the disease. In most infectious diseases etiologic microorganisms are frequently found in nonill persons. Additional factors such as a susceptible host (low or absent resistance) and proper environmental conditions also must be present for clinical disease to occur.

                                  A ──────┐
3.   ►► B
                                  C ──────┘

This relation implies that either A or C acting alone is capable of causing B. An example is death (B), which may result from oxygen deprivation (A) or electrocution (C); or hepatitis, which may result from viral infection or chemical agents. This model is important because it establishes that a disease may be caused in different ways.

4.

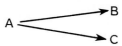

This relation implies that A is a cause of either B or C. An example is asbestos dust exposure (A), which may cause chronic lung disease (B) or cancer of the lung (C). This model also establishes the principle that one cause can produce different outcomes.

5.

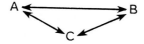

This model implies a chain of events to cause disease C. Both A and B are incidental steps leading to the disease. For example, tooth decay or gum disease (A) may lead to inadequate nutrition (B), which in turn may result in vitamin deficiency disease (C).

6.

This model implies that each factor may be either the cause or the result (outcome) of other factors. This chain of events may begin at any point of the triangle. For example, protein or other dietary deficiency (A) may lead to or be the result of intestinal malabsorption of nutrients (B), which in turn may lead to or be the cause of malnutrition or generalized debilitation (C).

Question 5

Based upon your understanding of the models of "cause" define or give an example of:

a. direct association

b. indirect association

c. spurious association

d.   one additional type of association is termed the <u>ecologic</u> <u>fallacy</u>. In this situation, attributes or characteristics of an ecologic area or group are assumed to be true for individual members. Give an example.

The notion of "causative" agents becomes complex when one attempts to study human diseases:

Cause	Diseases
M. tuberculosis	pulmonary tuberculosis, meningitis
T. pallidum	congenital syphilis, valvular heart disease, neurologic disease
Air pollution	respiratory illness, eye irritation
Smoking	lung cancer, hypertension

or the same disease state may be caused by several different organisms or factors:

Disease	Causes
Pneumonitis	staphylococcus, streptococcus, pneumococcus, tuberculosis, viruses, industrial chemicals or other toxins,
Hepatitis	virus, bacteria, alcohol, cleaning solvents, antibiotics.

Figure 1. Some components of the association between treatment for syphilis and icterus.

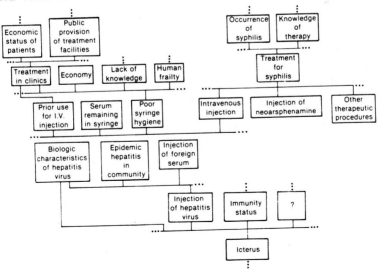

Source: MacMahon and Pugh, <u>Epidemiology</u> <u>Principles</u> <u>and</u> <u>Methods</u>, Little Brown and Co., Boston, 1970, p. 24.

Figure 2. Cause and effect: web of causation in cardiovascular diseases.

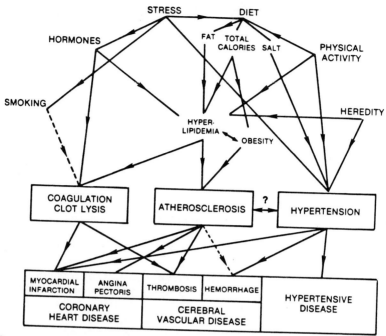

Source: Adapted from Stallones, R.A., Public Health Monograph 76, USDHEW,
           PHS Publication Number 1441.

As more factors or variables are implicated in the disease process the notion of
causation becomes confusing. The number of important variables soon spreads
to include a large, diverse body of information, which is called the WEB OF
CAUSATION. This notion is illustrated in Figures 1 and 2 which show the
components of an association between syphilis and serum hepatitis, and the
complex relationship of causative factors in several cardiovascular diseases.
The web of causation implies that a disease has many causes, while its corol-
lary, the concept of NET OF EFFECTS suggests that a single factor can be a
cause of many different diseases because of its interaction with other factors
that may be important in the disease etiology. The disease results from the
relative importance of and relationship between the different causes.

From the foregoing, you can see the difficulty of defining the term "cause."
Many factors can be regarded as causes of a disease. We must then resort to
thinking about the relative importance of these causes to each other. In practical terms, we observe events and describe relations with the purpose of
controlling and preventing illness. Thus, epidemiologists define the term as
follows: A CAUSE OF AN EVENT IS ANYTHING THAT, IF ALTERED, IS FOL-
LOWED BY AN ALTERATION IN THE EVENT. As the science of epidemiology
has evolved, certain CRITERIA* have evolved to help us decide when an association may be considered a causal association which can explain the etiology of
the disease or account for its pattern.

1.   The STRENGTH OF ASSOCIATION is high; indicated by high relative risk.
2.   The TIME SEQUENCE IS LOGICAL; exposure precedes disease onset.
3.   The ASSOCIATION IS SPECIFIC for the disease, i.e., when few causal factors can produce a disease there will be a stronger association between that disease and the separate factors than will be observed if there are many causal factors.
4.   The ASSOCIATION IS CONSISTENT when studied in different groups and at different times.
5.   The association AGREES WITH KNOWN BIOLOGIC FACTS OR THEORY.

Having invoked a causal association might lead one to theories that predict other associations correctly, or modifications that change the incidence, severity, or prognosis of the disease.

The following example[§] will demonstrate the difficulty of establishing or confirming causal associations. In this example, the association appears statistically strong, consistent in time and place, and biologically feasible. However, the association may still be spurious. We need to sort through the numerous plausible associations with a good deal of care and thought, and decide if the evidence for causality is strong enough to warrant preventive action.

A few years ago, an inverse association between hardness of domestic water supplies and coronary heart disease death rates was reported. This observation was epitomized in the phrase, "Hard water, soft arteries." The meaning of the finding is still somewhat obscure, although the presence of various trace elements might have a role. An analysis was performed from the point of view that if the association between hard water and soft arteries is spurious, then it ought to be possible to demonstrate this by finding stronger associations that appear to be biologically implausible. Before presenting those data a brief introduction to the concept of correlation is necessary.

One method for determining the degree of association between two characteristics is to compute a <u>correlation coefficient</u>. Correlation coefficients measure the linear relationship between variables and are calculated from standard formulas found in any statistical text. The coefficients range from 0 to 1. A correlation coefficient of 0 indicates no linear relationship exists, while a correlation of 1.0 means that the two variables exhibit a perfect linear relationship. Correlation coefficients include a sign that is either positive or negative, so that the actual range of correlation coefficients is from -1.0 to +1.0. A <u>positive correlation</u> is one in which both variables change in the same direction, for example, a rise in illegal drug use and an increase in hepatitis. A

---

*Source: Smoking and Health: Report of the advisory committee to the Surgeon General of the Public Health Service, U.S. Dept. HEW, 1964.

[§]Adapted from Stallones, R.A., and Buechley, R., unpublished.

negative correlation is one in which the variables change in opposite directions, for example, an improvement in surgical skill and a decrease in operative complications.   The degree of association between variables determines
whether the coefficient is closer to 0 or 1.0, while the sign depends upon
whether a change in one variable causes the other variable to change in the
same (positive correlation) or opposite direction (negative correlation).   Correlation coefficients between 0 ± 0.2 are said to exhibit weak correlation, while
coefficients $> \pm 0.7$ reveal strong correlation.   The term strength of association
refers not only to relative risk, but may also refer to a change (either positive or negative) in the correlation coefficient away from zero.

Figure 3 contains correlations of selected variables with coronary heart disease.   Only one of these correlations, lynchings (death by hanging; -.614 for
males and -.681 for females), is much larger than that of hardness of water
(-.419 for males, -.390 for females), and is clearly implausible.   The remaining
correlations are not clearly implausible and because there is a very strong
positive correlation one might study the question, "Why do psychiatrists cause
coronary heart disease?"   However, the method of analysis has shown the
implausibility of the coronary-disease-hard water hypothesis.

Question 6

Rank in order the correlations greater than hardness of water (whether positive or negative) for males and females from Figure 3.   How do these findings
support your opinion about the causes of coronary heart disease?

Exercise 9-11

Figure 3. Coronary, age-adjusted mortality, White males and females, 1950. Correlations with social and geographic variables.

Variable	Males	Females
Geographic trend	.720	.758
Log population	.219	.236
Percent male	-.347	-.376
Log density of population	.508	.650
Percent urban	.742	.721
Percent males divorced	.237	.166
Percent females divorced	.305	.182
Log divorce rate	-.380	-.536
Per capita income	.639	.641
Log percent nonvoters	-.293	-.346
Log percent Negro	.009	-.049
Log no. lynchings	-.614	-.681
Traffic mortality	-.389	-.517
Mental patients/1000 population	.633	.671
Log MDs/1000 population	.745	.745
Log internists/1000 population	.584	.585
Log psychiatrists/1000 population	.766	.808
Log percent MDs/GP	-.478	-.451
Farm owners/1000 population	-.689	-.645
Farm labor/1000 population	-.501	-.603
Percent labor manufacturing	.673	.701
Percent labor agriculture	-.728	-.698
Log hard H_2O	-.419	-.390
Rainfall	.201	.235
Log altitude	-.374	-.398
Percent farms cotton	-.291	-.337
Percent farms wheat	-.169	-.189
Log no. farms	-.348	-.338
Log acres/farms	-.349	-.401
Log value/acre farms	.594	.606

Question 7

What differences are there in correlations observed for males and females? How might some of these be explained?

Rather than looking for causes of disease by searching for variables that correlate highly with the event we wish to explain, one might attempt to explain the etiology of the disease by considering the whole correlation matrix, or as much of it as possible, i.e., trying to tie together many of the "causes" into a coherent and plausible hypothesis.

Mortality records have long been scrutinized for clues to the causes of heart disease to support hypotheses of causation. Generally, in technologically advanced countries, the fact of death is promptly and completely reported. Wide variation in the assignment of cause of death may, however, be attributable to other than true biological forces, so that interpretation of the differences in cause-specific death rates for different geographic areas becomes a matter for dispute. Despite reporting problems and errors due to mistaken diagnoses, death data are readily available and easily related to a defined population base, so that they are useful for epidemiologic study. Certain of the mortality data are included in the correlation matrix shown in Figure 4.

Figure 4 presents a matrix of correlation coefficents of selected variables. To read the table, locate a variable from the vertical list on the left side of the table. For each variable the series of numbers on the corresponding line indicates the correlation coefficient of that variable for all other variables in the table. All variables are also listed horizontally at the top of the table. Thus, to determine the correlation coefficient between a variable selected from the vertical list and a second variable from the horizontal list, merely locate the intersection of the line of numbers for each variable. Those numbers without a sign indicate a positive correlation. A minus sign (-) indicates a negative correlation coefficient.

Figure 4. Correlation coefficients of selected characteristics of the U.S.

VARIABLE	ASHD. MALE	HBP. MALE	STROKE. MALE	DENSITY	PERCENT URBAN	INCOME	PERCENT VOTING	PERCENT NEGRO	TRAFFIC DEATHS	MENTAL PATIENTS	DOCTORS	INTERNISTS	PSYCHIATRISTS	FARM OWNERS	MFG LABOR	HARDNESS OF WATER	RAINFALL	ALTITUDE
AGE-ADJUSTED, MALE DEATHS	.408	.247	-.011	.186	.309	.301	-.093	.110	.302	.192	.187	.205	.203	-.601	.180	-.201	-.057	.140
AGE-ADJUSTED, ASHD, MALE		.130	-.150	.625	.742	.639	.286	-.133	-.389	.509	.754	.642	.786	-.689	.673	-.432	.201	-.294
HYPERTENSION, DEATHS, MALE			.387	.220	-.039	-.250	-.532	.699	.057	.061	-.076	.210	.026	-.088	.367	-.536	.675	-.495
STROKE DEATH, MALE				-.134	-.441	-.429	-.403	.431	.139	-.099	-.433	-.328	-.371	.385	.138	-.195	.372	-.401
POPULATION DENSITY					.662	.400	.194	-.075	-.521	.327	.490	.541	.638	-.527	.673	-.362	.370	-.400
PERCENT URBAN						.744	.381	-.305	-.363	.542	.773	.741	.749	-.816	.570	-.118	.021	-.089
PER CAPITA INCOME							.689	-.581	-.331	.393	.699	.519	.660	-.568	.332	.114	-.349	-.130
PERCENT VOTING								-.888	-.477	.058	.458	.128	.400	-.235	.130	.336	-.523	.304
PERCENT NEGRO									.398	-.013	-.388	-.039	-.322	.223	-.002	-.415	.666	-.433
TRAFFIC DEATHS										-.214	-.462	-.312	-.488	.178	-.499	.222	-.233	.382
MENTAL PATIENTS											.580	.626	.564	-.365	.348	-.136	.165	-.239
DOCTORS/POPULATION												.802	.919	-.640	.466	-.221	-.004	-.070
INTERNISTS/WHITE POPULATION													.772	-.629	.449	-.309	.228	-.252
PSYCHIATRISTS/POPULATION														-.621	.576	-.291	.087	-.192
FARM OWNERS/POPULATION															-.568	.322	-.093	.020
PERCENT MANUFACTURING LABOR																-.509	.538	-.589
HARDNESS OF WATER																	-.639	.449
ANNUAL RAINFALL																		-.844
ALTITUDE																		

Some variables from Figure 4 are presented below, suggesting one of several possible relations between the variables and ASHD in males.

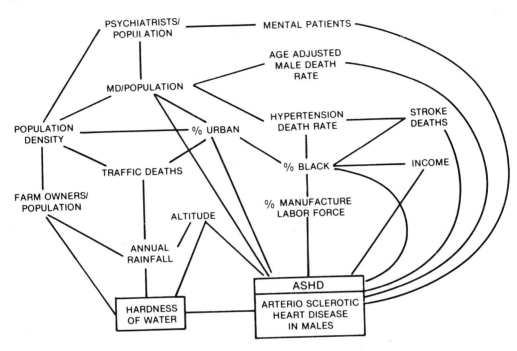

Question 8

a. From the correlation matrix, determine the correlation between pairs of variables and write the value on the line connecting those variables, in the above diagram. Which variables in this model are the best predictors of ASHD in males, i.e., which pairs have the highest correlation coefficients? Choose the best predictors and try to explain why there is such a strong correlation.

b.   From the observed correlations, what is your impression of the possibility that hardness of water plays an important role in causing ASHD?

c.   <u>Optional</u>.   Make a model to illustrate how ASHD or some other disease might be correlated with the variables in Figure 4 (add other variables if you believe them to be important).   Some independent library research ought to enable you to estimate the correlation coefficients for variables of your own choosing.   Examine the coefficients and see if you can explain the cause(s) of the disease in a logical way.   You may wish to apply the analytical technique of path analysis (Li, C.C., 1975).

II. HISTORICAL CONCEPTS OF CAUSATION

The facts that a given characteristic or factor can vary in its ability to produce a particular disease in any particular individual or group and that the characteristic or factor will vary greatly in its relation to different diseases complicates the epidemiologist's task of uncovering "the cause" of a disease as well as explaining the relationship between factors that may play a role. With these problems in mind, let us now examine the ways in which epidemiologists judge whether or not biologic associations are causally related.

Rarely can any individual establish the proof of an association without considerable help from others. The criteria that establish proof have been derived over many years by a host of scientists, scholars, and philosophers. Sir Isaac Newton once remarked,

> If I see farther than others, it is because I stand on the shoulders of giants...the past.

Fracastorius in the sixteenth century arrived at some remarkably accurate conclusions regarding the infectious nature of tuberculosis and its method of transmission, but it was not until 1865 that Villemin transmitted the disease from man to rabbits. Baumgarten may have seen the bacillus in infected tissues in 1878 but credit for the discovery of the cause of tuberculosis goes to Robert Koch, who isolated the tubercle bacillus in 1882. Koch (a) FOUND THE BACILLUS associated constantly with the clinical disease, (b) ISOLATED IT in pure culture, (c) REPRODUCED THE DISEASE in guinea pigs and rabbits with the culture, and (d) RECOVERED THE BACILLUS in pure culture from the experimentally infected animals. Koch stated that these four requirements must be strictly fulfilled before a particular microorganism can be accepted as the cause of a specific infectious disease. The requirements are now known as KOCH'S POSTULATES.

During Koch's era the great majority of human ills both in terms of morbidity and mortality were due to infectious diseases caused by microorganisms. Koch's postulates were intriguing and also supported by fact for many years. However, biology does not always support theory. The etiology of some diseases, including leprosy and certain viral infections cannot be proved strictly adhering to Koch's postulates because the responsible organism CANNOT BE ISOLATED from a diseased host, cannot be CULTURED IN A LABORATORY setting, and/or the DISEASE CANNOT BE PRODUCED IN LABORATORY ANIMALS. Nevertheless, Koch's postulates still stand as a landmark in the history of clinical medicine because of their requirements of objective and rigid criteria in the application of clinical and laboratory skills.

In the 1900s Darwin's ON THE ORIGIN OF SPECIES and Snow's researches ON CHOLERA were important statements of logic in scientific thought and contributed to understanding of biologic causation. Another landmark in the development of the concept of causation occurred in the work of John Stuart Mill, a midnineteenth century English philosopher-scholar. Mill wrote a book entitled

SYSTEM OF LOGIC, which proposed principles that came to be known as MILL'S CANONS. The canons were logical strategies from which the existence of causal relationships might be inferred. Among a number of canons, four are especially noteworthy. Mill named these the METHODS OF "DIFFERENCE," "AGREEMENT," "CONCOMITANT VARIATION," and "RESIDUES."

In the method of difference, the situations compared are alike in all variables but one. This is the case of the classic experiment. In the method of agreement, the situations compared have only one circumstance in common. In the method of concomitant variation, the factors under study vary in the same direction through a range of situations. In the method of residues, known causal factors are removed systematically in order to isolate and measure the contribution of remaining factors. Removal of variation due to known causes leaves a residue due to other causes.

By means of Mill's logic, many hypotheses can be validated or rejected; but Mill's canons DO NOT ALLOW CAUSAL INFERENCES to be drawn in human research. The reason is that Mill's methods require simplifying assumptions, which are not usually possible in the study of human diseases. Mill requires that the situation shall be "alike in all circumstances but one" or shall have "only one circumstance in common." His methods are not strictly applicable to epidemiology because in human populations WE CAN NEVER BE SURE THAT ALL THE RELEVANT FACTORS THAT COULD INFLUENCE THE DISEASE PROCESS UNDER STUDY HAVE BEEN DETERMINED AND TAKEN INTO ACCOUNT.

Mill's canons have been modified over the years to adapt to the difficulties encountered in epidemiologic research. A more appropriate set of criteria for invoking causation was listed earlier (Exercise 9-9). These criteria were cited in Smoking and Health: Report to the Surgeon General of the Public Health Service, 1964, and have been used by epidemiologists for many years.

The Surgeon General's Report states 5 criteria for assessing the importance of epidemiologic and other clinical data on the etiology of disease in human populations, when controlled experimental evidence is not available. These criteria were applied to clinical, pathological, and laboratory evidence of smoking and lung cancer to confirm or refute the hypothesis that a causal association exists. Results from the epidemiologic studies provided the basis upon which the judgment of causality was established.

In carrying out epidemiologic studies, investigations must first determine whether or not an association actually exists between an attribute or agent and a disease. Judgment may be based upon either indirect or direct evidence. If it is shown that an association exists, then the question is asked: "Does the association have a causal significance?" The Surgeon General's Report summarizes epidemiology's position:

> Statistical methods cannot establish proof of a causal relation when an association has been demonstrated. The causal significance of an association is a matter of judgment which goes beyond any statement

of statistical probability. To judge or evaluate the causal significance of the association between the attribute or agent and the disease, or effect upon health, a number of criteria must be utilized, no one of which is an all-sufficient basis for judgment. These criteria include:

1. The strength of the association
2. The temporal relationship of the association
3. The specificity of the association
4. The consistency of the association
5. The coherence of the association

III. EPIDEMIOLOGIC CRITERIA OF CAUSATION. THE ASSOCIATION BETWEEN SMOKING AND LUNG CANCER.

This section will illustrate the epidemiologic criteria for establishing whether or not an observed association plays a causal role in the etiology of a disease. The data are from the Surgeon General's Report on Smoking and Health, 1964. Numbers in parentheses are the references cited in that report.

A. Illustrating the criteria

Before presenting data a brief introduction to terminology is necessary. The report refers to epidemiologic data derived from retrospective, prospective, and cross-sectional studies. These subjects will be considered at greater length in Exercise 10. For the present it will suffice to know that <u>retrospective studies</u> establish the presence of an association between variables, and elicit the strength of the association by estimating relative risks. <u>Prospective studies</u> measure the incidence rate of disease, which follows exposure to variables suspected of having an association with a disease. <u>Cross-sectional studies</u> determine the prevalence of various diseases.

Retrospective studies

Twenty-nine retrospective studies of the association between tobacco smoking and lung cancer are summarized in Figures 5 and 6. As these tables suggest, the studies varied considerably in design and method.

Figure 5. Variables used in the study of smoking and lung cancer.

<u>Subject Selection</u>

1. Males and/or females
2. Occupational groups
3. Hospitalized cases
4. Autopsy series
5. Total lung cancer deaths in an area
6. Samplings of nationwide lung cancer deaths.
7. Sample size: 43-2,356 cases or records

<u>Control Selection</u>

1. Age matched
2. Healthy individuals
3. Patients hospitalized for other cancers
4. Patients hospitalized for causes other than cancer
5. Deaths from cancers of other sites
6. Deaths from other causes than cancer
7. Samplings of the general population.
8. Sample size: 86-34,339 persons or records

Figure 5.   (continued)

Method of Interviewing

1.   Mailed questionnaires
2.   Personal interviewing of
     subjects (or relatives) and
     controls
     (a) by professional personnel
     (b) by nonprofessional personnel

Tobacco-Use Histories

1.   By type of smoking (separately
     and combined)
2.   By amount and type
3.   By amount, type, and duration
4.   By inhalation practices

Other Variables Concurrently Studied

1.   Geographic distribution
     a)   Regional
     b)   Urban-rural
2.   Occupation
3.   Marital Status
4.   Coffee and alcohol consumption
5.   Other nutritional factors

6.   Parity
7.   War gas exposures
8.   Other pathologic condi-
     tions
9.   Hereditary factors
10. Air pollution
11. Previous respiratory
     conditions

Figure 6. Relative risks of lung cancer for smokers from retrospective studies.

Author and Reference	Year	Sex	Relative risk—Smokers: non-smokers
Sadowsky et al. (301)	1953	M	4.6
Doll and Hill (82)	1952	M	13.8
Wynder and Graham (381)	1950 [1]	M	13.6
Breslow et al. (38)	1954	M	7.7 age 50–59 4.6 " 60–69 17.0 " 50–59 25.5 " 60–69 }very heavy smokers
Randig (283)	1954	M-F	5.1 M 2.2 F
Schwartz and Denoix (313)	1957	M	8.0
Lombard and Snegireff (222)	1959	M	2.4 light smokers 34.1 heavy smokers
Haenszel (147)	1962	M	4.1<1 pack/day 16.6>1 pack/day
Haenszel (152)	Unpublished	F	2.5<1 pack/day 10.8>1 pack/day

[1] Calculated by Sadowsky et al. (301) from other authors' data.

The Surgeon General's Report states:

This listing of varying methods is by no means complete, nor does it imply that the individual retrospective studies should be criticized for their choice of study methods and factors for observation. The individual points of criticism have usually applied to one or two studies but not to all. Most striking is the fact that every one of the retrospective studies of male lung cancer cases showed an association between smoking and lung cancer. All have shown that proportionately more heavy smokers are found among the lung cancer patients than in the control populations and proportionately fewer nonsmokers among the cases than among the controls. Furthermore, the disparities in proportions of heavy smokers between "test" groups and controls are statistically significant in all the studies. The differences in proportions of nonsmokers among the two groups are also statistically significant in all studies but one (236); in the latter study, although there were fewer nonsmokers among lung cancer patients, the difference was very small.

In the studies which dealt with female cases of lung cancer, similar findings are noted in all of them with one exception (238). In this latter study, although significantly more heavy smokers were found among the lung cancer cases than among the controls, the proportion of nonsmokers among the cases was distinctly higher than among the controls. This is the only inconsistent finding among all the retrospective studies. Interpretation of this one inconsistent finding is not clear but the authors have indicated that nonresponse among their female cases was 50 percent.

The weight to be attached to the consistency of the findings in the retrospective studies is enhanced when one considers that these studies vary considerably in their methods.

Germane to this concordance is a study (386) of Seventh Day Adventists, a religious group in which smoking and alcohol consumption are uncommon. On the basis of expectancy of male lung cancer incidence derived from the control population, only 10 percent of the cases expected were actually found among Seventh Day Adventists.

2. Prospective studies

Figure 7. Mortality ratios for lung cancer by smoking status, type of smoking, and amount smoked, from seven prospective studies.

Study	Doll and Hill	Hammond and Horn	Dorn	Dunn, Linden and Breslow—Occupational	Dunn, Buell and Breslow—Legion	Best, Josie and Walker	Hammond
MORTALITY RATIOS:							
All Smokers	12.8	10.7	6.0	-	-	•25.2	†8.1
1–14 gm. tobacco	6.7	-	-	-	-	-	-
15–24 gm. tobacco	12.3	-	-	-	-	-	-
25 gm. tobacco	23.7	-	-	-	-	-	-
Current:**							
Cigarettes only	†20.2	†10.0	†12.0	†15.9	†4.9	†11.7	†9.6
<10	4.4	†5.8	†5.2	(5)- 8.3	-	†8.4	-
10–20	10.8	†7.3	†9.4	(10)- 9.0	-	†13.5	-
21–39	} 43.7	†15.9	†18.1	(20)-19.4	-	} †15.1	-
40+		†21.7	†23.3	(30)-25.1	-		
				(40)-28.7			
≤1 pack †	8.1	6.9	8.1	13.6	4.2	11.8	-
>1 pack †	43.8	16.9	18.0	24.1	7.4	15.1	-
Pipes only	5.4 }	2.6 }	1.3 }	-	-	†1.1 }	†1.5 }
Cigars only	} †4.6	1.0 } †1.3	1.5 } †1.6	-	-		
Pipes and cigars		-	-	-	-	†24.4	
Cigarettes, pipes and cigars	9.7	10.7	6.2	-	-		
Occasional	-	1.3	-	-	-	-	-
Ex-Smokers:							
>10 yrs. since stopped	5.0	-	-	-	-	-	-
<20 cigarettes	-	2.4	-	-	-	-	-
>20 cigarettes	-	17.8	-	-	-	-	-
<10 yrs. since stopped	8.4	-	-	-	-	-	-
<20 cigarettes	-	10.4	-	-	-	-	-
>20 cigarettes	-	22.8	-	-	-	-	-

Figure 8. Expected and observed deaths and mortality ratios of current smokers of cigarettes only, for selected cancer sites, all other sites, and all causes of death; each prospective study.

Site of cancer		British doctors	Men in 9 States	United States veterans	California occupational [1]	California Legion [1]	Canadian veterans	Men in 25 States [1]	Total
Lung and bronchus,	Observed	129	233	519	138	98	317	399	1,833
	Expected	6.4	23.4	43.3	8.7	19.9	27.1	41.5	170.3
	Ratio	20.2	10.0	12.0	15.9	4.9	11.7	9.6	10.8
Larynx	Observed	7	17	14	3	6	5	23	75
	Expected	0.0	1.3	2.4	0.0	4.0	0.0	6.3	14.0
	Ratio	--------	13.1	5.8	--------	1.5	--------	3.7	5.4
Oral Cavity	Observed	6	22	54	7	10	20	33	152
	Expected	0.0	7.8	8.1	7.2	5.2	5.1	3.6	37.0
	Ratio	--------	2.8	6.6	1.0	1.9	3.9	9.2	4.1
Esophagus	Observed	7	18	33	4	9	22	20	113
	Expected	3.3	2.7	5.2	5.5	1.8	6.8	8.4	33.7
	Ratio	2.1	6.6	6.4	0.7	5.1	3.3	2.4	3.4
Bladder	Observed	12	41	55	13	7	38	50	216
	Expected	13.9	17.2	31.4	2.2	1.8	22.3	22.8	111.6
	Ratio	0.9	2.4	1.8	6.0	4.0	1.7	2.2	1.9
Kidney	Observed	8	21	34	10	6	13	28	120
	Expected	0.0	14.0	23.1	0.0	8.3	9.5	24.1	79.0
	Ratio	--------	1.5	1.5	--------	0.7	1.4	1.2	1.5
Stomach	Observed	31	76	90	24	25	76	91	413
	Expected	28.3	33.7	61.5	31.4	20.5	41.2	68.6	285.2
	Ratio	1.1	2.3	1.5	0.8	1.2	1.9	1.3	1.4
Prostate	Observed	15	51	106	4	19	48	75	318
	Expected	29.0	32.4	53.7	8.6	22.1	32.3	74.9	253.0
	Ratio	0.5	1.6	2.0	0.5	0.9	1.5	1.0	1.3
All Other Sites	Observed	116	290	671	141	106	237	571	2,132
	Expected	112.0	228.3	505.7	109.4	120.6	192.1	423.8	1,692.0
	Ratio	1.0	1.3	1.3	1.3	0.9	1.2	1.3	1.3
All Causes of Death.	Observed	1,672	3,781	7,236	1,456	1,264	4,001	6,813	26,223
	Expected	1,161.8	2,227.7	4,043.1	818.5	799.4	2,420.1	4,183.3	15,653.9
	Ratio	1.44	1.70	1.79	1.78	1.58	1.65	1.63	1.68

[1] Includes all cigarette smokers (current and ex-smokers).

Question 9

Which of the criteria used to infer causation are illustrated by the data of Figures 6-8?

B.   Reviewing data from Exercise 3 will illustrate another criterion.

Doll and Hill sent questionnaires on smoking habits to all the 59,600 physicians in the United Kingdom in October 1951. Usable replies were received from 40,701 physicians, 34,494 men, and 6,207 women. These were followed for 4 years and 5 months by obtaining notifications of physicians' deaths from the Registrars General, the General Medical Council, and the British Medical Association. For every death certified as due to lung cancer, confirmation was obtained by writing to the physician certifying the death and also, when necessary, to the hospital or consultant to whom the patient had been referred. Part of the results follow:

Figure 9. Standardized death rates per year per 1000 men aged 35 years or more, in relation to the most recent amount smoked.

Cause of death	No. of death	Death rate per 1000 among		
		All men	Non-smokers	All smokers
Lung cancer	84	0.81	0.07	0.90

Source: Doll, R., and Hill, A.B., Lung cancer and other causes of death in relation to smoking. Brit. Med. J. 2:1071, 1956.

Question 10

Compute the relative risk for smokers vs. nonsmokers in Figure 9 and indicate how this can be used to infer causation.

Compare the death rates of lung cancer for the various categories of smoking. Compute the relative risk for each category of smokers vs. nonsmokers using the data from Doll and Hill's study, shown in Figure 10.

Figure 10. Standardized death rates per year per 1000 men aged 35 years or more in relation to the most recent amount smoked.

Cause of death	No. of deaths	Death rate among					
		All men	Non-smokers	All smokers	Men smoking daily average of cigarettes		
					1-14	15-24	25 or more
Lung cancer	84	0.81	0.07	0.90	0.47	0.86	1.66

Source: Doll and Hill, Brit. Med. J. 2:1071, 1956.

Question 11

Which of the criteria used to infer causation is implied?

C.   A third criterion

Cigarette smoking has been implicated in a variety of disorders including coronary heart disease, and other respiratory illness as shown in Figure 11.

Compute the relative risk and attributable risk of smokers and nonsmokers for each of these diseases.

Figure 11. Standardized death rates per year per 1000 men aged 35 years or more, in relation to the most recent amount smoked.

Cause of death	No. of deaths	Death rate per 1000 among			Men smoking - daily average of cigarettes		
		All men	Non-smokers	All smokers	1-14	15-24	25 or more
Lung cancer	84	0.81	0.07	0.90	0.47	0.86	1.66
Other respira-tory diseases	126	1.10	0.81	1.13	1.00	1.11	1.41
Coronary thrombosis	508	4.78	4.22	4.87	4.64	4.60	5.99
Other causes	779	6.79	6.11	6.89	6.82	6.38	7.19
All causes	1714	15.48	13.25	15.78	14.92	14.49	18.84

Source: Doll and Hill, Brit. Med. J. 2:1071, 1956.

Question 12

Which of the criteria used to infer causation is implied?

D.   A fourth criterion.

Figure 12. Death rate from cancer of the lung and rate of consumption of tobacco and cigarettes.

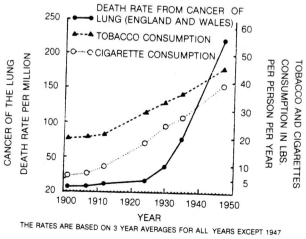

THE RATES ARE BASED ON 3 YEAR AVERAGES FOR ALL YEARS EXCEPT 1947

Source: Doll and Hill, Brit. Med. J. 4682:739, 1950.

Question 13

Which of the criteria used to infer causation is implied in Figure 12? In what type of epidemiologic study can this criterion be better demonstrated?

E. A fifth criterion.

The following information also may help you invoke causation. Data and references are from the Surgeon General's Report, 1964. Numbers in parentheses are cited references.

CARCINOGENICITY OF TOBACCO AND TOBACCO SMOKE IN ANIMALS

There is evidence from numerous laboratories (31,42,92,93,105,132, 139,262,296,338,372,373,382,383) that tobacco smoke condensates and extracts of tobacco are carcinogenic for several animal species. In order for smoking to cause cancer, it implies the presence of a substance (a carcinogen) in the tobacco smoke that is capable of producing cancerous change or that initiates a process mediated through other carcinogens, the end result being cancer.

Skin

Many investigators have shown that the application of tobacco tar to the skin of mice and rabbits induces papillomas and carcinomas (31, 42,92,93,105,132, 139,263,296,297,338,372,373,382,383). Wynder et al. (382) applied a 50 percent solution of cigarette smoke condensate in acetone to the shaved backs of mice so that each received about 10 gm. yearly. More than 5 gm. annually was required for the induction of epidermoid carcinoma and more than 3 gm. for the induction of papillomas (372,373). Since the carcinogenic potency of a smoke condensate can be altered by varying conditions of pyrolysis, the manner of preparation of the tar is of importance (392). Extracts of tobacco usually have weaker carcinogenic activity than do the condensates of cigarette smoke (93,390).

Gellhorn (126) and Roe et al. (290,293) have reported that condensates of cigarette smoke have cocarcinogenic (cancer promoting) properties. It was found that the application of a mixture of benzo-pyrene plus condensate of cigarette smoke to the skin of mice resulted in the production of many neoplasms, whereas the same concentration of benzo-pyrene alone failed to elicit tumors. Gellhorn (126) found that the tobacco smoke condensate appeared to accelerate the transformation of papillomas to carcinomas. Anti-carcinogens have also been reported in condensates of cigarette smoke (107).

Nicotine is not usually considered a carcinogen on the basis of animal experiments (346,391). Removal of nicotine or other alkaloids did not diminish the carcinogenicity of condensates of smoke for the skin of mice. The induction of pulmonary adenomas in mice by urethan (120) and of skin tumors in mice by ultraviolet radiation (121) are not altered by the administration of nicotine or some of its oxidation products.

Subcutaneous Tissue

Druckrey (92) found that cigarette smoke condensates or alcoholic extracts of cigarette tobacco regularly induced sarcomas in rats at the site of subcutaneous injections. Approximately 20 percent of the animals in each experiment developed the neoplasms. Druckrey also carried out similar experiments with benzo-pyrene and found that the amount of this polycyclic aromatic hydrocarbon in smoke condensates or tobacco extracts cannot account for more than a few percent of the activity of the tobacco products. This same discrepancey between the quality of benzo-pyrene in smoke condensates and the carcinogenic potency of the condensates has been reported by several investigators using the mouse skin test (92,93, 126,372,390).

Mechanism of the Carcinogenicity of Tobacco Smoke Condensate

Tobacco smoke contains many carcinogenic polycyclic aromatic hydrocarbons (Table 2, Chapter 6). Benzo-pryrene is present in much larger concentrations than is any other carcinogenic polycyclic hydrocarbon.

SUSCEPTIBILITY OF LUNG OF LABORATORY ANIMALS TO CARCINOGENS

Polycyclic Aromatic Hydrocarbons - Epidermoid carcinoma has been induced in mice by the transfixion of the lungs or bronchi by a thread coated with a carcinogen (5) and by treatment with an aerosol of ozonized gasoline plus mouse-adapted influenza viruses (191).

Kuschner et al. (197,197a) induced epidermoid carcinomas in the lungs of rats by the local application of polycyclic aromatic hydrocarbons, either by thread transfixation or pellet implantation. Distant metastases (spread of the tumor) occurred from some of the carcinomas. The changes in the bronchial tree at different times prior to the appearance of cancer included hyperplasia, metaplasia and anaplasia of the surface epithelium as well as of the subjacent glands. These changes resembled those described in the tracheobronchial tree of human smokers (9).

Epidermoid carcinoma [was induced] in the lungs of rats that had received 3-methylcholanthrene intravenously. The carcinogen was deposited in areas of pulmonary infarction (324).

Saffiotti et al. (302) produced squamous cell bronchogenic carcinomas in hamsters by weekly intubation and insufflation of benzo-pyrene (4%) ground with iron oxide (96%). A proliferative response followed by metaplasia preceded the appearance of the carcinomas, but was not an invariable antecedent.

Viruses - Bronchogenic carcinoma has been induced in animals inoculated with polyoma virus (282). Carcinogens enhance the effect of viruses known to cause cancer in animals (99) and localize the neoplastic lesions at the site of inoculation of the virus (98). [Herpes virus (cervical cancer) and Hepatitis B virus (liver cancer) have been implicated in the etiology of cancer in man.]

Possible Industrial Carcinogens - Vorwald reported that exposure of rats to beryllium sulfate aerosol resulted in carcinomas of the lung; 12 percent were epidermoid but most were adenocarcinomas. The tumors usually arose from the alveolar of bronchiolar epithelium. He also produced bronchogenic carcinomas in two out of ten rhesus monkeys injected with beryllium oxide and in three out of ten exposed to beryllium oxide by inhalation (357).

The production of epidermoid cancer of the lung in rats [was reported following] radioactive cerium. Other investigators have [also] succeeded in producing carcinomas of the lung, predominantly of the epidermoid type, in a high percentage of rats and mice with other radioactive substances [after] exposure [by] inhalation, intratracheal injection, or insufflation and implantation of wire or cylinder.

Hueper exposed rats and guinea pigs to nickel dust and found metaplastic and anaplastic changes in the bronchi (180). Following up earlier work in which squamous metaplasia of the bronchial epithelium was found in rats exposed to nickel carbonyl (341), Sunderman and Sunderman (342) induced bronchogenic carcinoma in rats by exposure to this compound. This group also found 1.59 to 3.07 μg of nickel per cigarette in the ash and in the smoke in several different brands. About three-fourths was contained in the ash. Although Hueper and Payne (182,183) and Payne (270) have demonstrated that pure chromium compounds will produce both sarcomas and carcinoma, in several tissues in rats and mice, bronchogenic carcinomas have not been produced by inhalation of chromium compounds in experimental animals. Experiments designed to test the carcinogenicity of arsenic compounds have been either negative or inconclusive.

Asbestosis can be produced without difficulty in experimental animals by inhalation of asbestos fibers (359), but efforts to produce bronchogenic carcinoma have been unsuccessful (129,181,227,358).

Summary - The lungs of mice, rats, hamsters and primates have been found to be susceptible to the induction of bronochogenic carcinoma by the administration of polycyclic aromatic hydrocarbons, certain metals, radioactive substances and oncogenic viruses. The histopathologic characteristics of the tumors produced are similar to those observed in man and are frequently of the squamous variety.

HISTOPATHOLOGIC ALTERATIONS INDUCED IN THE RESPIRATORY TRACT AND IN PULMONARY PARENCHYMA BY TOBACCO SMOKE

A variety of histopathologic studies from diverse points of view indicate clearly that smoking is associated with abnormal changes in the structure of both the surface epithelium and wall of the airways, including the mouth. Many of the studies are open to criticism because of inadequate numbers, lack of proper controls, and defects of experimental design, but specific criticisms are different for each study, and the sum of the evidence points unmistakably to the reality of deleterious consequences upon the respiratory tract from tobacco smoke.

Several reports implicate smoking, in particular pipe smoking, as an important etiologic agent in the development of a condition of the hard palate, and less often the soft palate, known as stomatitis nicotina (34,70,172,181). This condition is associated with excess proliferation of the surface epithelium and overproduction of keratin; the hyperplasia frequently involves the stomas of the salivary glands, leading to blockage and subsequent dilettation of the ducts. Epithelium lining the ducts commonly shows squamous metaplasia. This condition is believed to be very common in pipe smokers but usually disappears upon cessation of smoking.

A somewhat similar morphologic change has been described in the larynx that correlates closely with the cigarette smoking history (45,170). Epithelial hyperplasia with hyperkeratosis and variable degrees of chronic inflammation and squamous metaplasia are present in the true vocal cords, false cords, and the subglottic area.

The trachea and bronchi show many morphological changes in the cigarette smoker as compared to the nonsmoker (9,10,11,31,33,35,38, 171). Various degrees of hyperplasia, with and without overt atypical change, and metaplasia of the surface epithelium have been described. Deviations from the normal have also been found in the goblet cells, cilia, and mucous glands of smokers. Significant increases in the number of goblet cells and in the degree of mucous distension of the goblet cells were present in whole amounts of bronchial epithelium of smokers (31). Hyperplasia and hypertrophy of mucous glands and a higher proportion of cells with shorter cilia

also were observed more frequently in smokers (33,171). The hypertrophy and hyperplasia of mucous glands from miners correlated
much better with the degree of smoking than with exposure to silica
(35). Even though the number of nonsmokers among the miners was
small, the relation between smoking and mucous gland alteration was
very striking.

Question 14

Which of the criteria used to infer causation is implied?

E.   The following data will illustrate the epidemiologic evidence of causation
     not specific to the above criterion.

Figure 13.   Annual probability of dying for nonsmokers and selected groups of
             cigarette smokers and ex-cigarette smokers who stopped for other
             than doctor's orders, 1954 cohort.

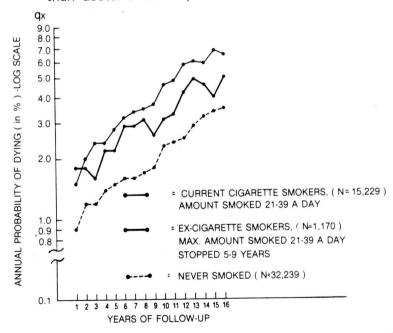

Source: Rogot, E. Smoking and general mortality among U.S. veterans, 1954-
          1969. U.S. DHEW, PHS, NIH, 1974. Publication No. (NIH) 74-544.

Figure 14. Lung cancer mortality ratios of Japanese by age at initiation of cigarette smoking (1966-1970).

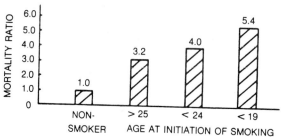

Source: Hirayama, T.   Smoking in relation to the death rates of 265,118 men and women in Japan, American Cancer Society's 14th Science Writer's Seminar, 1972.   City in The Health Consequences of Smoking, U.S. DHEW, PHS, January 1973.

Doll reported that one-third of British physicians who smoked in 1951 were nonsmokers ten years later.   During this period, the average cigarette consumption in Great Britain increased.   Hammond and Horn demonstrated additional evidence of the result of quitting the smoking habit.

Figure 15.   Mortality from lung cancer of physicians in relation to all men, ages 35-84.

Group	Lung cancer deaths per 1000 per year		
	1954-57	1958-61	1962-64
All men, England & Wales	1.49	1.71	1.86
British doctors	1.09	0.83	0.76

Source: Doll, R.   Cancer bronchique et tabac.   Bronches 16:1399-1410, 1966.

Figure 16.   Death rates per 1000 per year for microscopically confirmed cases of bronchogenic carcinoma, excluding adenocarcinoma.

Smoking status	Death rates per 1000 per year by smoking category		
	Never smoked	<1 pack a day	1+ packs a day
Still smoking in 1952		57.6	157.1
Stopped smoking <1 year		56.1	198.0
Stopped smoking 1-10 years		35.5	77.6
Stopped smoking 10+ years		8.3	60.5
Never smoked	3.4		

Source: Hammond, E.C., and Horn, D., Smoking and death rates.   JAMA 166:1294, 1958.   Copyright, 1958, American Medical Association.

Question 15

Why may causation be inferred from the data of Figures 13, 14, 15, and 16?

SUMMARY

While statistical analysis of data is of enormous help in the evaluation of clinical data, the following statement from "Smoking and Health: Report of the Advisory Committee to the Surgeon General of the Public Health Service" (1964) summarizes the epidemiologist's point of view. "Statistical methods cannot establish proof of a causal relation in an association. The causal significance of an association is a matter of judgment which goes beyond any statement of statistical probability. To judge or evaluate the causal significance of the association between cigarette smoking and lung cancer a number of criteria must be utilized no one of which by itself is pathognomonic or a sine qua non for judgment."

Question 16

a. The criteria cited in the preceding paragraph have been illustrated in part III of this exercise. List the criteria useful in establishing proof of causation.

b. Review Snow's work on Cholera (in Exercise 8) and indicate which of the above criteria he used. How does your answer compare to your answer for Question 14 in Exercise 8?

Question 17

Of what value are correlation coefficients in judging possible causal associations?

Question 18

What is the difference between association and causation?

As you may recall from Figure 11, the relative risk for smoking and coronary heart disease was 1.15, the attributable risk 0.65/1000, and the attributable risk percent 13.3. While these are lower than the corresponding figures for smoking and lung cancer, the fact that coronary heart disease is a much more common disease than lung cancer suggests that the result of antismoking programs might have greater overall benefit for the public's health by reducing death from heart disease rather than from reducing deaths due to lung cancer.

An interesting trend in cardiovascular disease has been observed. Between 1965 and 1976, coronary heart disease mortality in the U.S. has decreased by about 20%. A portion of these data, from a study by Kleinman et al., Am. J. Pub. Health 69:795, 1979, is shown below.

Figure 17. Percent distribution of adults aged 35-64 by cigarettes smoked per day according to age, sex, and race: U.S., 1965 and 1976.

	1965				1976			
	Cigarettes smoked per day				Cigarettes smoked per day			
Race, sex age	None [a]	Less than 15 [b]	15-24 [b]	25 or more [b]	None [a]	Less than 15 [b]	15-24 [b]	25 or more [b]
White Male								
35-44 years	43.3	12.1	25.4	19.2	53.5	8.0	18.8	19.7
45-54 years	45.3	11.8	25.3	17.6	57.3	6.5	17.7	18.5
55-64 years	54.9	13.3	19.8	11.9	62.2	6.7	17.3	13.9
White Female								
35-44 years	56.1	15.9	19.9	8.1	61.9	11.3	17.3	9.6
45-54 years	61.8	15.9	16.5	5.7	61.8	11.0	17.6	9.6
55-64 years	74.3	11.3	11.0	3.5	69.3	11.2	13.4	6.1
Black Male								
35-44 years	32.7	28.6	30.6	8.1	41.1	22.6	26.4	9.8
45-54 years	37.6	25.3	30.6	6.6	43.3	19.5	27.4	9.8
55-64 years	48.2	30.0	17.9	3.9	59.5	15.6	22.3	2.5
Black Female								
35-44 years	57.1	27.2	13.0	2.6	58.7	24.9	15.7	0.6
45-54 years	67.8	21.5	9.6	1.2	63.4	16.5	16.5	3.7
55-64 years	83.5	12.8	3.2	0.5	59.9	25.3	10.7	4.2

a) Excludes respondents with current smoking status unknown.
b) Excludes respondents with number of cigarettes smoked unknown.
SOURCE: Health Interview Surveys 1965 and 1976.

Figure 18. Death rates per 10,000 from coronary heart disease by age, sex, and race: U.S., 1965 and 1976.

Race, sex age	1965 [a]	1976 [b]	Per Cent Change
White Male			
35-44 years	8.8	6.4	-27.3
45-54 years	36.1	27.6	-23.5
55-64 years	96.1	75.2	-21.7
White Female			
35-44 years	1.5	1.2	-20.0
45-54 years	7.6	5.8	-23.7
55-64 years	29.9	22.7	-24.1
Black Male			
35-44 years	15.0	9.9	-34.0
45-54 years	44.3	35.5	-20.6
55-64 years	107.9	84.6	-21.6
Black Female			
35-44 years	7.7	3.7	-51.9
45-54 years	24.5	16.7	-31.8
55-64 years	77.9	45.1	-42.1

a) Based on extrapolating 1968 rates for ICDA 410-413 (8th revision) using 1965-67 trend for ICDA 420 (7th revision); see Appendix.

b) CDA 410-413 (8th revision).

SOURCE: Division of Vital Statistics, NCHS

Although most epidemiologists and health professionals in both the private and public health sectors agree that there is a causal association between smoking and lung cancer, that view is not universally accepted. The U.S. tobacco industry and other related organizations maintain an active interest in arguing against the causal association evidence. An article by T.D. Sterling, "A critical reassessment of the evidence bearing on smoking as the cause of lung cancer," Am. J. Pub. Health 65:939, 1975, raises several points at issue with the generally accepted view of the smoking and lung cancer evidence. Among the points raised are the lack of definitive experimental evidence, and a host of methodologic problems in the design of retrospective and prospective studies. The same issue also devotes space to a rebuttal of Sterling's argument, by Weiss, which is reproduced below. The debate continued with a subsequent answer to criticism by Sterling and further criticisms by Ibrahim, Bross, and Higgins, all of which appeared in the Am. J. Pub. Health 66:2, 1976. While you are urged to read the articles, many of the problems discussed may not be understandable to you at this time. However, if you are presently unable to follow the technical arguments reread the articles after you have completed Exercises 10, 11, and 12.

Smoking and Cancer

A Rebuttal

WILLIAM WEISS, MD

The views expressed by Dr. Sterling in the preceding article are rebutted.

In his paper entitled "A Critical Reassessment of the Evidence Bearing on Smoking as the Cause of Lung Cancer," Dr. Theodor D. Sterling has reiterated his stand against a generally accepted hypothesis which is the basis for one of the most important advances in preventive medicine during the past two decades. The evidence underlying the hypothesis has been thoroughly surveyed by the United States Public Health Service in a series of seven published reports from 1964 to 1973 so there is no need to review it in detail. Suffice it to say that the Public Health Service has concluded that cigarette smoking is the major cause of lung cancer in the United States as a result of detailed epidemiological, clinical, autopsy, and experimental data.

While it is true that an association between smoking and lung cancer does not constitute proof that the association is one of cause and effect, the judgment that the association is causal is based on the criteria of consistency, strength, specificity, temporal relationship, and coherence. The data fulfilling these criteria were covered adequately in *Smoking and Health*, the initial report of the Advisory Committee to the Surgeon General of the Public Health Service in 1964 (pp. 179–189). The later reports have summarized newer data which continue to support the validity of the hypothesis.

Dr. Sterling has chosen to ignore most of the clinical, autopsy, and experimental data and concentrate his criticism on the epidemiological evidence. His dissertation is characterized by the sins of omission, misinterpretation, overgeneralization, inconsistency, and innuendo. Without being exhaustive I would like to discuss some examples of these sins in Dr. Sterling's paper.

Dr. Sterling's major contention is that the prospective epidemiological studies are biased by selection of the

populations surveyed and he singles out the American Cancer Society investigation of more than one million people for detailed criticism. He asks us to consider the possibility that the several deficiencies in method operate in such a way that the population was loaded with smokers who developed lung cancer and nonsmokers who did not. This presumes remarkable perspicacity among the volunteer workers who recruited the population. He then generalizes and assumes that the same deficiencies characterize other prospective studies despite the lack of documentation. He omits reference to the several prospective studies, such as the Philadelphia Pulmonary Neoplasm Research Project,[1] which screened populations with periodic chest roentgenograms so that the prevalence cases were readily separated from the incidence cases without altering the strong association between cigarette smoking and lung cancer risk.

While on the one hand it suits Dr. Sterling to invalidate the prospective studies on the grounds of population selection, he uses the immigration studies as an argument against the hypothesis. Certainly immigrants are self-selected.

Dr. Sterling's use of the Japanese study by Hirayama of a quarter million people is a flagrant distortion. He chooses to ignore the 5-year results of this prospective study which duplicate those of all of the other prospective investigations (see *The Health Consequences of Smoking*, pp. 68—69. Public Health Service, U.S. Department of Health, Education, and Welfare, Washington, DC, 1973), in favor of a preliminary 15-month report by Hirayama and contends that the mortality rates of smokers and nonsmokers were "largely the same." The data do not confirm his interpretation. Indeed, the ratio of observed deaths in smokers to deaths expected from the rates in nonsmokers was 1.06 for males and 1.17 for females even in the short period of 15 months. The ratio for lung cancer was 2.92. This was exceeded only by the ratios for cancer of the pancreas and cancer of the bladder but these were based on smaller

Dr. Weiss is Professor of Medicine, Hahnemann Medical College, Philadelphia, Pennsylvania 19102.

numbers of cases and in the 5-year report these ratios were lower than that for lung cancer.

There is an interesting contrast between Dr. Sterling's footnote lament that he must depend on unpublished (in scientific journals) data from Hirayama's study and his glib quotations of erroneous accounts in the lay press of the alleged difficulties Hammond and Auerbach encountered in publishing their studies of lung cancer in smoking beagles. Since I was assistant editor of the *Archives of Environmental Health* at the time, I can testify to the following facts: Dr. Auerbach did make his slides available for independent review; the manuscripts were not rejected by the *Journal of the American Medical Association*, they were returned to the authors for revision; and the editor of the *Archives of Environmental Health* subjected the manuscripts to out-of-office reviewers who recommended publication after certain revisions were made.

The leveling off of lung cancer mortality rates is an exaggeration.[2] It is true that the *rate of increase* has begun to diminish but mortality rates continue to rise except in the younger age groups. But the younger age groups contribute proportionally fewer cases of lung cancer than the older age groups. Undue emphasis is given to the changes in the rates among the younger age groups by plotting the rates on a logarithmic scale. The relative importance of changes in the age-specific curves would be better seen on an arithmetic scale. Furthermore, the few lung cancer cases that occur in the young may have a different etiology from those in older people, a possibility suggested by differences in the distribution of histological types.[3]

Even if the lung cancer incidence were to level off, this would not constitute an argument against the smoking-lung cancer hypothesis. It could be readily explained by invoking a saturation effect. Only the most naive person would deny that chronic diseases like cancer have a multifactorial etiology. Since the occurrence of lung cancer in a particular individual depends not only on a major factor but on other factors as well, there is a ceiling on its incidence in a given population with a given set of conditions. The proportion of susceptibles in the population is limited by the secondary factors. Therefore, after the level of smoking has reached a certain point in the population, further increases in smoking may produce no increase in the incidence of lung cancer.

Dr. Sterling has proposed the process of selection as an explanation for many of the epidemiological observations which favor the smoking-lung cancer hypothesis. It is easier to show that the process of selection has operated in his choice of data to oppose the hypothesis. For example, he states "The constant difference between men and women in the incidence of lung cancer has persisted although the frequency of smoking among women has increased more rapidly than among men" and in 1975 he compares figures in 1965 with those in 1950. In 1972 Burbank[4] showed that in recent years lung cancer death rates have risen proportionately more rapidly in women than in men and his analysis suggested "that the difference between male and female rates is a simple function of the difference in their past cigarette tobacco use, a dose-response effect."

Much of the rest of Dr. Sterling's paper is simple diversionary obfuscation, warranting no further comment. Truth is better served by recognizing that the evidence in favor of the smoking-lung cancer hypothesis is overwhelming. No matter where we look, the association is consistent, strong, and specific (considering the quantitative aspect of the association), smoking precedes the lung cancer, and coherence between the various lines of evidence is of a high order.

The importance of this lies in the fact that the hypothesis provides us with a potent tool of disease prevention and control. The change in the risk of lung cancer among ex-smokers relative to the risk in continuing smokers is a strong point in the evidence favoring the hypothesis. Whether the risk in ex-smokers declines or stabilizes at the rate established at the time smoking is stopped,[5] the change is a salutary one which fits the observation of Auerbach et al.[6] that the prevalence of atypical cells in the bronchial mucosa of ex-smokers decreases with the passage of time after stopping smoking.

As a clinician who treats patients with lung cancer, I find it very disheartening to deal with a disease so rapidly destructive and realize that in most cases the illness would not have developed if the patient had not smoked.

References

1. Boucot, K. R., Cooper, D. A., Weiss, W., Carnahan, W. J., and Seidman, H. The Philadelphia Pulmonary Neoplasma Research Project: Basic Risk Factors of Lung Cancer in Older Men. Am. J. Epidemiol. 95:4—16, 1972.
2. Weiss, W. Predictions of Lung Cancer Mortality: The Dangers of Extrapolation. Arch. Environ. Health 28:114—117, 1974.
3. Kyriakos, M., and Webber, B. Cancer of the Lung in Young Men. J. Thorac. Cardiovasc. Surg. 67:634—648, 1974.
4. Burbank, F. U.S. Lung Cancer Death Rates Begin to Rise Proportionately More Rapidly for Females Than for Males: a Dose-Response Effect? J. Chronic Dis. 25:473—479, 1972.
5. Doll, R. The Age Distribution of Cancer: Implications for Models of Carcinogenesis. J. R. Stat. Soc. 134:133—166, 1971.
6. Auerbach, O., Stout, A. P., Hammond, E. C., and Garfinkel, L. Bronchial Epithelium in Former Smokers. N. Engl. J. Med. 267:119—125, 1962.

SUGGESTED RESPONSES
Exercise 9--Principles of Causation

1. Both groups are using personal experience, observation, and temporal
    sequence of the suspected causal agent and resultant outcome to support
    their conclusions. However, unknown to both groups, these events are
    all merely coexisting in time and space and are not truly cause/effect.
    The problem is that there are no physical laws that might be plausible
    explanations of the observed facts. If this were a health problem, we
    would never find a plausible biologic trigger to explain the outcome.

2. Each group might propose that once having ventured out of this village,
    "all bets are off." Group A might argue that the original group is no
    longer constituted and whatever special effect might be generated by the
    entire group cannot be produced by the smaller sample of persons far
    from home. Group B might claim that the bell does not have the same
    power as their bell at home.

3. They might agree to experiments--alter the number of villagers present,
    the time of the bell ringing, etc., to see whether the sun sets in re-
    sponse to those variables. If they observed many different events lead-
    ing to the same outcome they might eventually decide that the causal
    relationship is more complex than they believed.

4a. Comparison of characteristics and activities of ill and nonill persons ought
    to be fairly easy. Information concerning activities, meals, persons con-
    tacted, etc., for the previous 24-48 hour period should be accurate.
    However, ill persons may recall the preceding events with more complete-
    ness than the nonill, or the ill may emphasize the incorrect facts.

4b. Three problems must be faced. First, the accuracy of recall by ill and
    nonill persons may differ for events that happened some time ago. For
    most individuals, recall of minor details will be inaccurate for events
    occurring more than 7-30 days ago. Try it yourself. Can you remember
    meals? activities? persons contacted for events of the past month?

    Second is memory bias. Ill persons may be more likely than nonill per-
    sons to recall certain events or activities. This may sometimes produce
    an erroneous association between some event and an illness and lead to an
    incorrect conclusion that the event and illness are causally related.

    Third, many intervening factors could have occurred if exposure to the
    disease agent and onset of disease are widely separated in time. What
    could happen? Marriage, pregnancy, other illnesses, changes in diet,
    occupation, socioeconomic status and lifestyle, place of residence, etc.
    Do any of these influence the development of different diseases? Is there
    any effect exerted by several factors acting together?

4c,d. The issues discussed in responses 4a and 4b apply. The problem is increased if the exposure and onset of disease are separated by 10-20 years. People may die from different diseases or leave the area in that interval. Those who survive or who remain may not be an adequate representation of the original group of people who were exposed and were developing the disease before they died or migrated.

4e. The number of intervening variables is further increased when the disease is transmitted by a mother (who is not harmed by the medication) to a developing fetus, which may develop an unusual form of cancer many years later. We now have to consider all of the potential characteristics of the mother and daughter, plus inaccurate memory and survivorship. In this case the search for the causal mechanism involved looking back at pregnancy records to determine medications used at the time the genital organs were developing in utero.

5a. Direct association--a statistical relationship between variables where there are no intervening variables or where the intervening variables are related in a chainlike series of events.

5b. Indirect association--a statistical relationship that occurs between a variable of interest and a disease due to other known or unsuspected factors common to both.

5c. Spurious association--an association resulting from observations obtained in a biased manner. Selection of cases or controls or the manner of collection of data may help to produce an association when none actually existed.

5d. Suppose you wish to compare two communities for some health condition. Community A has a higher rate of illness than B and also uses more electric power. If you concluded that if individuals used electric power they would have a higher risk of developing the disease, you probably fell prey to the ecologic fallacy. In an ecologic relation, many factors can be present and coexist without there actually being any causal association. More knowledge of the community situation might reveal that community A has many more older persons than community B. In fact, a third variable, the age distribution is responsible for the illness rate differences. Accepting ecologically based observations, correlations, or associations and concluding that what is true for the community will also be true for the individual members of that community or group is a failure to recognize that other variables may enter the causal process. In this instance the more important relation is the close association between disease and age. For further discussion of association including the ecologic fallacy, see Susser, M., Causal Thinking in the Health Sciences, Oxford University Press, 1973, pp. 48-63.

6.   <u>Males</u>   <u>Females</u>

Psychiatrists/1000 (+)   Psychiatrists/1000 (+)
MDS/1000 (+)   Geographic Trend (+)
% Urban (+)   M.D.s/1000 (+)
% Labor Agriculture (-)   % Urban (+)
Geographic Trend (+)   % Labor Manufacturing (+)
Farm Owners/1000 (-)   % Labor Agriculture (-)
% Labor Manufacturing (+)   No. Lynchings (-)
Per Capita Income (+)   Mental Patients/1000(+)
Mental Patients/1000 (+)   Density (+)
No. Lynchings (-)   Farm Owners/1000 (-)
Value/Acre Farms (+)   Per Capita Income (+)
Density (+)   Value/Acre Farms (+)
Farm Labor/1000 (-)   Farm Labor/1000 (-)
% M.D.'s/G.P. (-)   Internists/1000 (+)
Hard H_2O (-)   Divorce Rate (-)
                                           Traffic Mortality (-)
                                           % M.D./G.P (-)
                                           Acre/Farm (-)
                                           Altitude (-)
                                           Hard H_2O (-)

7.   The order of items is different and more factors have stronger correlation
for women than men. Many factors denote urbanization and available
medical care. Perhaps the more physicians there are, the more use of
services and consequently more diagnosed CHD. Women are known to
make more visits to a physician a year than men. Perhaps marriage and
low-altitude living are less "protective" of women than of men. The
negative correlations with farming might be due to lower degree of stress
or other factors relating to the quality of life in urban societies. Some
research suggests that many traffic deaths are actually due to heart
attacks. Add your own ideas.

8a. Figure for 8a is shown on the next page. Psychiatrists/population; phy-
sicians/population; % urban; farm owners/population; % manufacturing
labor.

Physicians and particularly psychiatrists are concentrated in urban areas.
Manufacturing is also an urban activity. ASHD may be "caused" by
urban lifestyle or it may occur because the types of individuals who may
be susceptible to the disease live in urban centers.

8b. The possibility of a causal association is not terribly impressive based on
this type of analysis. Trying to pick out a common thread seems to
diminish the importance of the proposed association. Many other factors
would seem to be involved more directly than water hardness, although
that does not preclude the possibility that water hardness is somehow
involved, e.g., the presence of certain trace metals may play a role.
However, the correlation is not striking.

Figure for 8a.

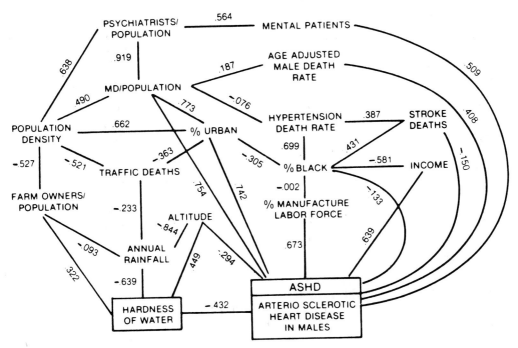

9.   The criteria illustrated are that consistency of observations is evident despite widely varying study methods, and the relative risks of these different methods are consistently and greatly in excess of 1.0.

10. Relative risk illustrates the criterion of the strength of association. The relative risk of 12 is extremely high. Relative risks are rarely observed to be this high.

11. The criterion illustrated is another aspect of the strength of association as demonstrated by the dose-response to smoking. As dose increases, death rates increase. The relative risk increases from 6.7 for light smokers to 23.7 for heavy smokers.

12. The criterion illustrated is the specificity of the association between agent and the disease. Although smoking plays a role in many diseases, the greatest effect is seen with lung cancer. Thus, it is more likely to play a more direct and causal role in lung cancer than in other diseases.

13. The graph provides indirect evidence to illustrate the temporal relation between exposure to the agent and onset of disease. Exposure must precede onset of the disease. This criterion can also be illustrated by prospective studies but not by retrospective studies.

14.   A causal association is supported by the coherence of the available data. A plausible physiologic mechanism is suggested by the laboratory data.

15.   These are other illustrations of a dose-response relation.   Figure 13 shows that removal of the presumed cause, smoking, results in lower probability of death for exsmokers compared to current smokers.   The probability for exsmokers seems to be approaching that for nonsmokers. Figure 14 shows the increased risk of death among men who began smoking at younger age.   Figure 15 shows that among all men, the risk of lung cancer death has increased by 24.8% (1.86/1.49 x 100) but doctors have shown a decrease of 30.3% (1 - .076/1.09 x 100) during the same period.   Figure 16 also shows an overall decrease in lung cancer death rates among exsmokers, particularly for light smokers who quit over 10 years prior to the study.

All these data help confirm the hypothesis linking smoking to lung cancer by showing that groups at high risk of the disease can reduce their risk when not exposed to the presumed causal agent.

16a. 1.   Temporal association
      2.   Strength of association
      3.   Specificity of the association
      4.   Coherence of the observation (plausibility)
      5.   Consistency of the observation to other observations.

16b. Snow's research was consistent with criteria 1 and 2.   At the time of his work, the cholera organism had not been discovered, and there was little evidence to support the hypothesis that water was the vehicle of the disease.   Thus it was difficult for other scientists to accept Snow's data. While Snow's study supported his own findings, his data differed with the accepted facts of his day (criteria 3-5).

17.   Correlation indicates the amount of association between variables.   However, it cannot be used to invoke causation because the sequence of exposure preceding disease cannot be assumed to have occurred.   Knowledge that the correct temporal sequence of exposure to the suspected cause precedes onset of disease is necessary.   Second, correlation does not measure risk.   Correlation measures the degree or amount of linear relationship between two variables.   It may be said that causation implies correlation but correlation does not imply causation.   Causation in epidemiology is based upon the criteria illustrated in the text.

18.   Association is a statistical relationship between variables.   Causation is a judgmental assessment of the meaning of observed associations.   Causal relationships also imply that some action might be taken to reduce, eliminate, or modify the dependent variables through knowledge of independent or antecedent variables.

PART IV. STUDY DESIGN AND INTERPRETATION OF DATA

Epidemiologists are concerned with several aspects of disease processes in their efforts to control and prevent illness in a community. These include identifying and describing the health problem, determining contributing or causative factors, developing, implementing, and managing a program to control or prevent the problem, and finally evaluating the effectiveness of the program. There is an important need for systematic methods of data collection for all of these activities. Epidemiologists therefore have a major role in the critical activities of the design, conduct, analysis, and interpretation of research studies. Part IV of the guide consists of Exercises 10-14, which will examine issues concerning study design and data collection.

EXERCISE 10. STUDY DESIGN IN EPIDEMIOLOGIC INVESTIGATION

Goals

Upon completion of this exercise you should be able (1) to recognize an epidemiologic problem, (2) to formulate a research question, (3) to recognize the objectives and features of different types of epidemiologic studies, and (4) to select an appropriate study design with regard to the research objectives.

Methods

In order to achieve these goals you will need to understand

I. IDENTIFICATION OF AN EPIDEMIOLOGIC PROBLEM AND FORMULATION OF A RESEARCH QUESTION.
II. OBJECTIVES OF EPIDEMIOLOGIC STUDIES
    A. Type A--The Prevalence Study or Cross-Sectional Survey
    B. Type B--The Retrospective or Case-Control Study
    C. Type C--The Prospective or Cohort Study
III. DESIGN OF A STUDY: IDENTIFYING ADVANTAGES AND LIMITATIONS
IV. CONSIDERATIONS IN THE DESIGN OF EPIDEMIOLOGIC INVESTIGATIONS: SELECTING ALTERNATIVES

Terms

Descriptive and analytic design, case report, cross-sectional study, retrospective, case-control, case-comparison, trohoc, prospective, longitudinal, cohort, follow-up, intervention, experimental, historical prospective studies, odds ratio.

Suggested Readings

White, C., and Bailar, J.C.   Retrospective and prospective methods of study-
    ing association in medicine. Am. J. Public Health 46:35, 1956.
Cornfield, J., and Haenszel, W.   Some aspects of retrospective studies. J.
    Chronic Disease 11:523, 1960.
Mantel, N., and Haenszel, W.   Statistical aspects of the analysis of data from
    retrospective studies of disease. J. Nat. Cancer Inst. 22:719, 1959.
Dorn, H.F.   Some application of biometry in the collection and evaluation of
    medical data. J. Chronic Disease 1:638, 1955.
Cochran, W.   Observational studies (Chapter 6) in Statistical Papers in Honor
    of George W. Snedecor.   T.A. Bancroft, ed., Iowa State University
    Press, 1972.
Mausner and Bahn, Epidemiology, pp. 112-125; 307-340.
Friedman, Primer of Epidemiology, pp. 48-56; 58-166.
MacMahon and Pugh, Epidemiology, Principles and Methods, pp. 207-300.
Lilienfeld, Research Methods in Cancer, pp. 69-84.
Lilienfeld and Lilienfeld, Foundations of Epidemiology, pp. 191-288.
Fleiss, J.L. (ed.) Statistical methods for rates and proportions John Wiley
    and Sons, N.Y., 1981, pp. 53-66.
Kerlinger, F. N., Foundations of Behavioral Research, Holt, Rinehart and
    Winston, 1967, pp. 411-462.
Abramson, J.H., and Livingstone, C., Survey Methods in Community Medicine,
    Willmer Bros. Ltd., Birkenhead, Great Britain, 1974.

I.   IDENTIFICATION OF AN EPIDEMIOLOGIC PROBLEM AND FORMULATION OF A RESEARCH QUESTION

FORMULATION OF THE QUESTION TO BE ANSWERED IS AN IMPORTANT INITIAL STEP in an epidemiological study. Although this appears to be easy, not infrequently this step may require a good deal of time and effort; and if not performed well the study may prove to be a wasted effort.   The formulation of the question requires that we carefully determine what is known, pertinent to the disease, including literature review of current general knowledge, and theories and facts specific to the problem.   These facts are helpful to understand the variables likely to influence the distribution of the health problem.   They also suggest the type of study to be performed and how the results of any particular study stands relative to a general epidemiological strategy.

Epidemiologists face several problems when formulating a study question.   The variables to be included and their use as independent or dependent variables must be decided, the means by which each variable will be ascertained must be specified, and an appropriate reference or study population from which observations are made and to which conclusions will be referable must be selected.

Question 1

For each of the following statements (1) formulate the study question, (2) specify additional information you need to determine if a health problem exists, and (3) identify whether or not the study questions are epidemiological issues.

a. The missed appointment rate for the health clinic is 15/100/month.

b. This is the second angiosarcoma of the liver reported among workers in plant X in the past three years.

c. The birthrate for the age group less than 15 years was 3/1000 in 1960.

d. The incidence rates for tuberculosis by socioeconomic status in 1973 were: UPPER 12/100,000; MIDDLE 22/100,000; LOWER 56/100,000.

e. The survey of female textile workers showed 8% had bacteria in their urine.

f. Twenty percent of the navy recruits had a positive heterophile reaction, suggesting an outbreak of infectious mononucleosis.

Question 2

Formulate questions to investigate each of the following problems:

a. In reviewing the neonatal mortality, a health official states that the problem is too many "grannies" (midwives) are delivering babies.

b. Following an assessment of the completion-of-therapy rate for tuberculosis relapse cases, it was concluded that there were not enough home nursing visits.

c. While comparing community mortality rate reports, the conclusion reached was that the problem was a lack of coronary care units.

d. The problem is that many restaurants and food markets are sources of contaminated food.

e. A positive heterophile reaction is usually observed with infectious mono-nucleosis, but, eighty-seven percent of navy recruits with a positive heterophile reaction had a recent history of glandular fever while seven-teen percent of navy recruits with a negative heterophile reaction had a recent history of glandular fever.

f. Residents in the vicinity of an industrial-wastes disposal site claim to have a high rate of spontaneous abortion (miscarriage) during pregnancy.

g. Community leaders wish to close down the nuclear reactor because they fear that radioactive material leaking into the atmosphere will cause cancer.

h.   Volcanic eruptions in Washington state left 10 cm deposits of ash over a wide area of Washington and Oregon. The air was so thick with dust that residents were forced to wear a mask over their nose and mouth.

II. OBJECTIVES OF EPIDEMIOLOGIC STUDIES

Epidemiologists use data derived from three sources--vital statistics (mortality and natality), morbidity, and surveys. The purpose, design, and value of a particular study vary greatly and depend upon the skills and intelligence of the investigator, the time, money, and personnel available to accomplish the study, the suitability of the problem for investigation, the adequacy and availability of existing data, or the feasibility of collecting new information. Appropriate analysis and appropriate interpretation of the research findings also depend on the type of study design chosen, and the validity and reliability of the measurements made. Figure 1 indicates some of the different approaches that were used to investigate the association between smoking and lung cancer. Note the variety of sources for obtaining case and comparison groups, and the different methods of data collection.

Figure 1. Outline of methods used in studies of smoking in relation to lung cancer.

Investigator, year, and reference	Country	Sex of cases	Number of persons and method of selection		Collection of data
			Cases	Controls	
Müller 1939 (250)	Germany	M	86 Lung cancer decedents, Bürger Hospital, Cologne.	86 Healthy men of the same age	Cases: Questionnaire sent to relatives of deceased. Controls: Not stated.
Schairer and Schoeniger 1943 (309).	Germany	M	93 Cancer decedents autopsied at Jena Pathological Institute, 1930-1941.	270 Men of the city of Jena aged 53 and 54 (average age of lung cancer victims= 53.9).	Cases: Questionnaire sent to next of kin (195 for lung cancer). Controls: Questionnaire sent to 700.
Potter and Tully 1945 (280)	U.S.A.	M	43 Male patients aged over 40 in Massachusetts cancer clinics with cancer of respiratory tract.	1,847 Patients of same group with diagnoses other than cancer.	Cases and controls interviewed in clinics
Wassink 1948 (363)	Netherlands	M	134 Male clinic patients with lung cancer.	100 Normal men of same age groups as cases.	Cases: Interviewed in clinic. Controls: Not stated.
Schrek et al., 1950 (311)	U.S.A.	M	82 Male lung cancer cases among 5,003 patients recorded, 1941-48.	522 Miscellaneous tumors other than lung, larynx and pharynx.	Smoking habits recorded during routine hospital interview.
Mills and Porter 1950 (237)	U.S.A.	M	444 Respiratory cancer decedents in Cincinnati, 1940-45 and in Detroit, 1942-46.	430 Sample of residents matched by age in Columbus, Ohio, from census tracts stratified by degree of air pollution.	Cases: Relatives queried by mail questionnaire or personal visit. Controls: House-to-house interviews.
Levin et al., 1950 (207)	U.S.A.	M	236 Cancer hospital patients diagnosed lung cancer.	481 Patients in same hospital with non-cancer diagnoses.	Cases and controls: Routine clinical history taken before diagnosis.
Wynder & Graham 1950 (381).	U.S.A.	M-F	605 Hospital and private lung cancer patients in many cities.	780 Patients of several hospitals with diagnoses other than lung cancer.	Nearly all data by personal interview; a few cases by questionnaire; a few from intimate acquaintances. Some interviews with knowledge or presumption of diagnosis, some with none.
McConnell et al., 1952 (236)	England	M-F	100 Lung cancer patients, unselected, in 3 hospitals in Liverpool area, 1946-49.	200 Inpatients of same hospitals, matched by age and sex, without cancer, 1948-50.	Personal interviews by the authors of both cases and controls, with few exceptions.
Doll and Hill 1952 (82)	Great Britain.	M-F	1,465 Patients with lung cancer in hospitals of several cities.	1,465 Patients in same hospitals, matched by sex and age group; some with cancer of other sites, some without cancer.	Personal interviews of cases and controls by almoners.
Sadowsky et al., 1953 (301)	U.S.A.	M	477 Patients with lung cancer in hospitals in 4 states.	615 Patients in same hospitals with illnesses other than cancer.	Personal questioning by trained interviewers.
Wynder and Cornfield 1953 (379).	U.S.A.	M	63 Physicians reported in A.M.A. Journal as dying of cancer of the lung.	133 Physicians of same group dying of cancer of certain other sites.	Mail questionnaire to estates of decedents

Figure 1. (continued)

Koulumies 1953 (192)	Finland	M–F	812 Lung cancer patients diagnosed at one hospital in 16 years.	300 Outpatients of same hospital aged over 40, living in similar circumstances, and without cancer, February and March 1952.	Cases and controls questioned about smoking habits when taking case histories.
Lickint 1953 (211)	Germany	M–F	246 Lung cancer patients in a number of hospitals and clinics.	2.002 Sample of persons without cancer living in the same area and of same sex and age range as cases.	Personal interviews by staff members of cooperating hospitals and clinics, corresponding in time to interviews of cases.
Breslow et al., 1954 (38)	U.S.A.	M–F	518 Lung cancer patients in 11 California hospitals, 1949–52	518 Patients admitted to same hospitals about the same time, for conditions other than cancer or chest disease, matched by race, sex, and age group.	Cases and controls questioned by trained interviewers, each matched pair by the same person.
Watson and Conte 1954 (365).	U.S.A.	M–F	301 All patients of Thoracic Clinic at Memorial Hospital who were diagnosed lung cancer, 1950–52.	468 All patients of same clinic during same period with diagnoses other than lung cancer.	The 769 consecutive patients of case and control groups were questioned by the same trained interviewer.
Gsell 1954 (138)	Switzerland	M	135 Men with diagnosis of bronchial carcinoma.	135 Similar hospital patients with diagnoses other than lung cancer, and of the same age.	Personal interviews, all by the same person.
Randig 1954 (283)	Germany	M–F	448 Lung cancer patients in a number of West Berlin hospitals, 1952–1954.	512 Patients with other diagnoses, matched for age.	Controls were interviewed at about the same time as the cases, each case-control pair by the same physician.
Stocks and Campbell 1955 (337).	(Preliminary; see 1957 report below.)				
Wynder et al., 1956 (375)	U.S.A.	F	105 Patients with lung cancer in several New York City hospitals, 1953–55.	1,304 Patients at Memorial Center with tumors of sites other than respiratory or upper alimentary, 1953–1955.	Cases: Personal interview or questionnaire mailed to close relatives or friends Controls: Personal interview.
Segi et al., 1957 (316)	Japan	M–F	207 Patients with lung cancer in 33 hospitals in all parts of the country, 1953–55.	5,636 Patients free of cancer in 420 local health centers, selected to approximate the sex and age distributions of cases.	Cases and controls by personal interview using long questionnaire on occupational and medical history and living habits.
Mills and Porter 1957 (238)	U.S.A.	M–F	578 Residents of defined areas dying of respiratory cancer, 1947–55.	3,310 Population sample approximately proportional to cases as regards areas of residence, and 10 years or more in the area.	Cases: From death certificates, hospital records, and close relatives or friends. Controls: Personal home visits or telephone calls, usually interviewing housewife.
Stocks 1957 (335)	England	M–F	2,356 Patients suffering from or dying with lung cancer within certain areas.	9,362 Unselected patients of the same area admitted for conditions other than cancer.	Cases: Histories taken at the hospital or from relatives by health visitors. Controls: Personal interview in hospital.

There are two general classes of epidemiologic investigation: Descriptive studies characterize the occurrence of disease in terms of person, place, and time; or characterize factors related to host, agent, and environment; or characterize exposure and susceptibility status. Descriptive studies characterize a disease distribution and enable us to develop hypotheses about that disease pattern. Analytic studies go beyond simply describing the distribution of, or pattern of occurrence of disease, and attempt to analyze the reasons for them. Hypotheses derived from descriptive studies may be tested using analytic study methods.

Much confusion arises from the variety of names given to the different types of study design used in epidemiology. Studies have been designated with the names descriptive, analytic, observational, case report, retrospective, trohoc, case-control, case-comparison, cross-sectional, prevalence, incidence, prospective, longitudinal, cohort, follow-up, intervention, experimental, and historical prospective. Frequently, the distinctions between these designs are unclear and in some situations an incorrect or inappropriate name has been assigned to a study, adding to the confusion. Much of the confusion can and ought to be eliminated. The following explanation should clarify the issues involved; however, you will still need to be familiar with the above list of names because they are commonly used, a fact not likely to change in the near future.

The basis of all clinical and epidemiologic research is the CASE REPORT. The objectives of case reports are to describe clinical observations, interesting or unusual variations of disease, results of new treatment modalities, and to call attention to unexpected findings. A CASE SERIES refers to a group of similar cases, which may enable us to discern a clinical pattern to identify character-istics common to the cases, or to describe a noteworthy aspect of a disease. Case reports and case series may refer to illness observed in private clinical practice or in the public health sector, or in an occupational setting, or they may refer to health problems other than disease. While their primary purpose is to describe something, the observer usually proposes an explanation of the phenomenon or suggests an hypothesis to account for the observation. A great many varieties of case reports may be encountered, but essentially they are still case reports, which DESCRIBE SOMETHING occurring in an individual or group. Of particular importance is that they are NOT POPULATION BASED. Therefore, estimates of risk cannot be derived from them.

Epidemiologic data from studies designed to determine whether or not statistical associations exist or to examine the incidence of a disease following exposure to a presumed cause are frequently presented in the form of the 2 x 2 (four-fold or contingency) table:

Disease

		Present	Absent		
	Present	a	b	a+b	type C
Factor	Absent	c	d	c+d	
		a+c	b+d	N	
		type B		type A	

Two variables are included, namely, "factor" and "disease." Factor refers to one or more attributes or characteristics that a host either has (present) or does not have (absent); or factor can be something to which the host is ex-posed or not exposed; or factor can be the presumed or suspected cause of a disease. In some tables the terms "exposed" and "not exposed" replace the terms present and absent, respectively. Disease refers to any disease of interest to the investigator. In some tables, an outcome of a disease, a stage in the natural history of a disease process, or a health problem other than disease may be substituted. In any event, the host will be recognized to either have (present) or not have (absent) the condition. Depending upon how the research question was formulated, factor could either be an indepen-dent variable or a dependent variable, and the disease would be the dependent or independent variable, accordingly.

Suppose we have a population of N individuals, all of whom could be categor-ized with respect to a factor, e.g., red hair, and a disease, e.g., Tinea infection (ringworm) of the scalp. Some individuals would have both red hair and Tinea, others would have neither, and some would have one but not the other. If all individuals in these categories were designated as a, b, c, or d depending upon which CELL of the table they occupied, the total of N persons would equal the total of a+b+c+d. If we added the horizontal rows and vertical columns, we would obtain the MARGINAL TOTALS, a+b, c+d, a+c, and b+d.

A.   Type A--THE PREVALENCE STUDY OR CROSS-SECTIONAL SURVEY

If one had no knowledge prior to the start of a study, regarding how individual members of the population would be distributed in each of the cells, the investigator would have to study the entire population N (or a sample or a particular subgroup of it).   After examination of the hair color, and presence or absence of Tinea had been determined, individuals would be categorized in the appropriate cells.   Ratios

$$\frac{a}{a+b}, \quad \frac{b}{a+b}, \quad \frac{c}{c+d}, \quad \frac{d}{c+d}, \quad \frac{a}{a+c}, \quad \frac{c}{a+c}, \quad \frac{b}{b+d}, \quad \frac{d}{b+d}, \quad \frac{a...d}{N}$$

could be calculated depending upon how the investigator phrased his question, i.e., whether the factor or the disease was to be considered the independent variable.   Studies based upon N or a sample of N are termed PREVALENCE or CROSS-SECTIONAL STUDIES.   These studies describe or identify health problems at a point in time or over a short period of time.   They are like a photograph or snapshot of the population or community at a given time.

B.   Type B--THE RETROSPECTIVE OR CASE-CONTROL STUDY

Studies whose purpose it is to investigate PERSONS KNOWN TO HAVE A DISEASE AND OTHERS WHO ARE FREE OF DISEASE will, by definition, compare all diseased persons (a+c) and compare them to nondiseased persons (b+d) for the presence or absence of the factor red hair.

If all persons who would be categorized as cases (a+c) or controls (b+d) cannot be studied, then it may be appropriate to substitute a sample of each group.   Studies that compare the groups (a+c) and (b+d) for the presence or absence of a factor are called RETROSPECTIVE, CASE-CONTROL, CASE-COMPARISON, or TROHOC studies.   (The term trohoc is cohort spelled backwards, and has been proposed by Feinstein.)   The purpose of this class of studies is TO ESTABLISH WHETHER OR NOT AN ASSOCIATION EXISTS BETWEEN THE FACTOR AND THE DISEASE.   However, in most situations it is not possible to clearly determine if the host had the factor or was exposed to it BEFORE the disease process began.   When there is uncertainty about whether the factor preceded the onset of disease, it is not possible to establish that an observed association is causal when only this type of study design has been used.   For example, if an association between alcoholism and tuberculosis was observed we could not be sure if alcoholism led to tuberculosis or if tuberculosis cases became alcoholics after their disease began.   A second problem with this class of studies is that relative risk cannot be calculated because incidence rates cannot be determined in these studies.   The cross-products ratio, often called the ODDS RATIO (calculated as ad/bc) is an approximation of the relative risk, IF THE DISEASE IS RARE.   Thus, like relative risk, it expresses the strength of association between the variables measured.

C.   Type C--THE PROSPECTIVE OR COHORT STUDY

Studies of PERSONS FREE OF DISEASE AT THE START OF THE OBSERVA-TION PERIOD, SOME OF WHOM HAVE BEEN EXPOSED AND OTHERS NOT EX-POSED TO A FACTOR, are called PROSPECTIVE, LONGITUDINAL, COHORT, HISTORICAL PROSPECTIVE, INCIDENCE, or EXPERIMENTAL STUDIES. The essential feature is that disease-free persons exposed to or having the factor red hair (a+b) are compared to persons not exposed to and not having the factor (c+d), to determine the proportion of each group that develops the disease tinea. Because the participants are free of disease at the beginning of the observation period, it is clear that any suspected cause precedes the onset of disease. Therefore, these studies are very useful in "proving" that a causal association exists. <u>Relative</u> <u>risk</u> <u>can</u> <u>be</u> <u>calculated</u> because the ratios a/a+b and c/c+d actually represent the rates of disease (incidence or attack rates) of exposed and unexposed groups.

SUMMARY

Although many names are used, there really are only 3 possible approaches to defining the study groups. Selection of the study type depends upon how the populations are selected. The study populations must be defined in terms of "denominators." Those using denominators that are:

Type A.   based upon the distribution of the total or a sample of the population N.

Type B.   selects and compares persons with and without a disease (cases and noncases).

Type C.   selects and compares persons free of disease at the start of the period of observation, some of whom are exposed and others not exposed to a suspected disease agent.

Figure 2. Schematic outline of the types of epidemiologic studies.

		Disease			
		Present	Absent		
	Present	a	b	a+b	} type C
Factor	Absent	c	d	c+d	
		a+c	b+d	N	
		type B		type A	

When reviewing data of epidemiologic studies one can avoid the confusion arising from the incorrect use of the terms retrospective and prospective by some authors, if the readers focus attention on which of the three types of denominators is being used.

Each of the categories that present epidemiologic information (case reports, cross-sectional studies, retrospective, and prospective designs) have a distinct role to play in the epidemiologic strategy for discovering the cause(s) of the disease and developing measures for the control or prevention of a disease or health problem. Generally speaking, the purpose of each may be summarized:

Case reports and case series call attention to the problem.

Cross-sectional studies indicate the extent of the problem.

Retrospective studies test hypotheses of association or identify factors that may be related to the disease or health problem in ill and nonill persons.

Prospective studies of exposed and nonexposed persons test hypotheses of "causal" association that have been derived from case reports, cross-sectional studies, or retrospective studies.

Obviously, an investigator's choice of which study design to select depends upon what information is being studied and how the question is stated. At any point in time, a review of the scientific literature will disclose that large numbers of studies of each type are in progress simultaneously.

III. DESIGN OF A STUDY: IDENTIFYING ADVANTAGES AND LIMITATIONS

Ability to distinguish the types of studies is helpful because it will enable you to identify the inherent limitations of the study and some of the methodologic problems the investigator faced. You will also be able to judge the quality of the study by examination of the ways that the investigator attempted to overcome problems in the design of the study or collection of data.

Each of the following eight abstracts describes a health problem to be investigated. Identify the type, major variables, useful features, and limitations of the study design decribed.

Question 3

You wish to study the effect of suspended particulates (the stuff that pollutes air) on mucous membranes and respiratory apparatus. Fifty members of a single strain of white mice of similar ages are selected and divided into two groups. One group is placed in cages whose atmosphere is drawn from the outside air by a large intake fan. The second group also has its air piped in from the outside except that a sophisticated set of filters screen out solid particulates before they enter the cages. Cage temperature, humidity, and diet of both groups are identical. After two weeks, both sets of animals are sacrificed and respiratory organs are examined using an electron microscope.

a.   Identify the study design and independent and dependent variables of this method.

b.   Identify useful features of this study technique.

c.   identify limitations of this study technique.

Question 4

A physician observes an unusual 45-year-old male patient having orange skin associated with gastrointestinal abnormality, including changes in bowel habits. Never having seen an orange man before he feels obligated to report this case in his favorite medical journal. He describes the pertinent medical history, physical examination, laboratory tests, and clinical course of the patient, and speculates about the etiology or pathologic process of this unusual phenomenon.

a.   Identify the method of study used.

b.   Identify useful features of this study technique.

c.   Identify limitations of this study technique.

Question 5

You would like to study the occurrence of prematurity among women who have experienced an induced abortion. You obtain a list of all households in your area from the postal system and select a 2 percent sample at random. Following this, you send interviewers to each household and inquire about the occurrence of previous pregnancy including abortion. You separate women into those with and without a history of abortion and compute prematurity rates for the appropriate pregnancies in women in each group.

a.   Identify the study design and independent and dependent variables.

b.   Identify useful features of this study technique.

c.   Identify limitations of this study technique.

Question 6

The relation between mild hypertension and the use of antihypertensive agents
is of interest.   A study is organized that involves several medical centers
across the nation.   A large number of patients is screened for the presence of
hypertension.   After identification of a group of individuals with hypertension,
the patients are divided into three groups using a random process of allocation.
Group 1 is treated with mild tranquilizers; group 2 is treated with a combination of antihypertensive and diuretic agents; group 3 receives no particular
treatment.   All groups are followed for three years to determine whether the
incidence of stroke or death differs with respect to mode of therapy.

a.   Identify the study design and independent and dependent variables.

b.   Identify useful features of this study technique.

c.   Identify limitations of this study technique.

Question 7

Information concerning the frequency of hepatitis antibody among prostitutes
may be helpful for understanding the mode of transmission of the virus.   A
roster of women known to be so employed is identified from police records.
With difficulty, you are able to locate the women, convince them of the usefulness of their participation, and obtain suitable blood specimens from each.
Laboratory tests on the blood measures the presence and quantity of hepatitis
antibody.

a.   Identify the study design and independent and dependent variables.

b.   Identify useful features of this study technique.

c.   Identify limitations of this study technique.

Question 8

You would like to improve the effectiveness and efficiency in delivering health services through your clinic.   After selecting a 10 percent sample of all patient visits during the past six months you are able to characterize the patient population utilizing your clinic in terms of age, race, sex, method of referral, diagnostic category, therapy provided, method of payment, daily patient load, and clinic staff work schedules.

a.   Identify the study design.

b.   Identify useful features of this study technique.

c.   Identify limitations of this study technique.

Question 9

It has been suggested that users of oral contraceptives are at greater risk of thromboembolic (blood clots) disease than those who do not use the drugs. Through the ICDA Code used by Medical Records, you are able to identify 100 women diagnosed as having thromboembolic disease during the past two years and a comparison group of 100 women who are similar to the cases with respect to age, race, and parity (pregnancy history) but who do not have thrombo-embolic disease. A careful review of each woman's medical chart reveals that a higher proportion of women with thromboembolism reported using oral contra-ceptives than did the comparison group.

a.   Identify the study design and independent and dependent variables.

b.   Identify useful features of this study technique.

c.   Identify limitations of this study technique.

Question 10

You are interested in finding out whether middle aged-men who have premature heartbeats are at greater risk of developing a myocardial infarction (heart attack) than men whose heartbeat is regular. Electrocardiogram (ECG) exam-inations are performed on all male office employees 35 years of age or older who work for oil companies in Houston. The ECG tracings are classified into those with irregular heartbeats (arhythmias) and those with regular heart rhythm. Repeat examinations are performed each year for five years to ob-serve potential changes in the ECG. Employee medical and health insurance records are collected over the five-year period. At the conclusion of the study, myocardial infarction rates are calculated according to the electrocar-diogram status at the beginning of the study.

a.   Identify the study design and independent and dependent variables.

b.   Identify useful features of this study technique.

c.   Identify limitations of this study technique.

Question 11

In order to understand both useful and limiting features of epidemiologic study designs, consider the factors, listed in Figure 3, that concern epidemiologists. Indicate which of the epidemiologic study designs would be advantageous to use for each item by writing an A in the appropriate column of Figure 3. For those studies that are at a disadvantage with respect to the item, write a D in the appropriate column. It is not necessary to write either A or D for all study types, only those which are made appreciably better or worse with regard to each item.

Figure 3. Advantages and disadvantages of epidemiologic study designs.

Items to be considered	Case reports	Prevalence or cross sectional	Retro-spective	Pros-pective
Many hypotheses to test				
Rare diseases				
Baseline data				
Selective recall of important events				
Attrition (death, migration, loss of participation)				
Nonresponse				
Time needed to complete study				
Cost				
Control of confounding variables				
Temporal relation of etiologic factor and disease onset				
Quantitation of risk				
Inference to population				
Source of data collection specific to investigators need				
Establishing directness of association				
Selection of controls leading to bias				
Interpretation fallacy (spurious association)				
Health hazard to participants				
Placebo effect				
Establishing strength of association				

IV. CONSIDERATIONS IN THE DESIGN OF EPIDEMIOLOGIC INVESTIGATIONS: SELECTING ALTERNATIVES

The following section considers the important features of good epidemiologic research. These features are not unique to epidemiology and are sometimes used in other fields of investigation. The term "epidemiologic method" really implies that the investigator is attempting to use sound scientific principles; i.e., CAREFUL OBSERVATION OF THE PHENOMENA (OF HEALTH AND DISEASE) LEADING TO LOGICAL INFERENCES AND DEDUCTION OF CONCLUSIONS DERIVED FROM THOSE OBSERVATIONS.

Features that distinguish good from bad research should be clearly understood by public health professionals since intelligent decision making ought to reflect both knowledge of scientific data and understanding of the ways in which data are obtained.

In the following eight examples, a research problem will be posed, and two alternative methods of study (A and B) briefly described. With respect to the alternative methods, try to determine the major differences between A and B; identify the major problems or disadvantage (if any) introduced by each research method; identify the special attributes and advantages (if any) introduced by each research method; and designate which alternative design is more likely to yield useful results.

In some cases it may be difficult to decide which alternative is better because the methods may have both good and bad features. Such is the nature of research!

Question 12

You wish to study the effect of an oral hypoglycemic drug on the clinical course of diabetes mellitus.

Method A

From medical records of patients in your large practice you identify those patients who are taking the medication and those who are using either no medication or a different medication. The group using the oral hypoglycemic agent is designated as <u>cases</u> and all other patients comprise the control or <u>comparison group</u>. You determine the rate of a variety of signs and symptoms and monitor health changes in each group over a two-year period.

Method B

You identify diabetic patients from your medical records and assign a study number to each record and a treatment code number to each therapy you wish to evaluate. You place all the patient study numbers in one bag and treatment code numbers in a second bag. After shaking both bags, you close your eyes and select a number from each bag until all patients are assigned to one of the

therapy groups.   Having assigned cases and comparison groups you determine
the rate of signs and symptoms and monitor changes in the health status of
each group over a two-year period.

a.   Identify major differences between A and B.

b.   Identify major problems of the methods.

c.   Identify special advantages of the methods.

d.   Which is the better method?

Question 13

You wish to study the effectiveness of a new vaccine against pneumococcal
pneumonia.

Method A

You assign people to be vaccinated or not vaccinated by randomly selecting
colored tags placed in your favorite black bag.   The medical record of each
patient is tagged in red (vaccinated) or blue (not vaccinated).   During the
next month you treat your patients as necessary.   At the end of the month
you calculate attack rates of infection for vaccinated and nonvaccinated groups.

Method B

A nurse assigns patients to be vaccinated or not vaccinated by selecting the
colored tags from the black bag.   She writes the method of treatment on a
piece of paper and places it in a sealed envelope.   The patients receive the
assigned therapy, but the nurse does not reveal to you which category of
treatment the patient has received.   At the end of one month attack rates for
each therapy are calculated.   The sealed envelopes are opened and the nurse
then tells you which data represent the vaccinated and nonvaccinated patients.

a.   Identify major differences between A and B.

b.   Identify major problems of the methods.

c.   Identify special advantages of the methods.

d.   Which is the better method?

Question 14

You wish to determine the pulmonary status of heroin users.

Method A

You carefully monitor the roster of patients seen in the emergency room of the
city hospital. All patients seen for drug-related problems receive a chest
X-ray and respiratory function tests. They are carefully interviewed about
drug use and those with a history of heroin use are referred to the respiratory function laboratory for additional pulmonary function studies. You express your findings as a percentage of abnormal tests among heroin users
examined.

Method B

You canvass the local halfway houses and methadone treatment programs and
offer free chest X-ray and pulmonary function studies to any individuals who
wish to receive them. You compare the abnormal lung findings of those with
to those without a history of heroin abuse, making appropriate comparisons for
age and gender.

a.   Identify major differences between A and B.

b.   Identify major problems of the methods.

c.   Identify special advantages of the methods.

d.   Which is the better method?

Question 15

You wish to measure the distribution of blood pressure among military recruits on four separate bases.

Method A

Recruits are requested to report to the base dispensary or hospital during their free time. Upon reporting, recruits are instructed to sit down and relax for a few minutes in the waiting room or treatment room (depending upon the presence of other patients). After a few minutes they are requested to roll up a shirtsleeve, whereupon a blood pressure reading is performed and results recorded.

Method B

Recruits are requested to report to the base dispensary or hospital between 7:00 and 8:00 a.m., and instructed not to eat, drink, smoke, or use any medication between midnight and the time they appear for the examination. Upon reporting they are taken to a quiet area of the facility reserved for the examination. They are requested to remove their shirts and lie down on an examination table. After 5 minutes, a blood pressure is taken using the patient's left arm, which is raised slightly to the approximate level of the heart. Pressures are measured using a standardized procedure. After another 10 minutes, a second pressure is recorded, following the previous procedure. The average pressure of the two readings is recorded on a standard form, which includes demographic information about the patient, as well as the date and time of examination and identity of the person performing the procedure. The equipment type and format of examination are the same on all four military posts.

a.   Identify major differences between A and B.

b.   Identify major problems of the methods.

c.   Identify special advantages of the methods.

d.   Which is the better method?

Question 16

You wish to determine the prevalence of rheumatoid factor in the blood of arthritis patients.

Method A

Patients attending the medical and surgical outpatient clinics are given a brief questionnaire asking whether or not they ever had or now have arthritis or painful joints. Those responding "yes" receive a blood test for rheumatoid factor as part of their physical examination.

Method B

Correspondence with the Arthritis Society of America reveals that there are several diagnostic criteria of arthritis including pain, tenderness and swelling of the joints, limitation of motion; changes in the appearance of the skin over the affected joint; and possible deformity of the joint. Symptoms recur periodically with a gradual progression and deterioration of function.

Patients attending the medical and surgical outpatient clinics are given a questionnaire that inquires about the above criteria. Patients meeting these criteria are designated as active or inactive (in remission) cases. Bloods are drawn and analyzed according to current disease status.

a.   Identify major differences between A and B.

b.   Identify major problems of the methods.

c.   Identify special advantages of the methods.

d.   Which is the better method?

Question 17

You wish to test the allergic potential of a new antibiotic by giving a small challenge dose injected subcutaneously into the skin of the forearm.

Method A

Subjects are volunteers from among the inmates of the city prison system. Skin reactions are observed and recorded according to standardized dermatologic practices 24 and 48 hours later.

Method B

You select the name of every fifth child currently on your roster of 1500 pediatric patients at your large public hospital and inject the challenge dose at the time of their next check-up. Patients are requested to return at 24 and

48 hours to have the skin reaction observed and recorded according to standardized dermatologic practices.

a.   Identify major differences between A and B.

b.   Identify major problems of the methods.

c.   Identify special advantages of the methods.

d.   Which is the better method?

Question 18

You wish to determine whether physicians on your hospital staff are correctly
diagnosing and treating those serious conditions that lead to patient deaths.

Method A

Without identifying patients by name, an abstract of the medical history,
preliminary diagnosis, laboratory results, treatment, clinical progress and any
other pertinent information of patients dying in the hospital is prepared by the
chief of the hospital staff.   A panel of five senior attending physicians is
selected and asked to review these records.   Each physician scores the abstract for each of the above factors on a scale of 1 to 5.   The same record is
submitted to each physician a second time six weeks later.

You score the results in two ways: First, you determine the mean score of
the five physicians for each category of the disease.   Second, you compare the
results of the physician's first determination against his second determination.

Method B

An autopsy is performed on all deceased patients and results are entered by the pathologist on a score sheet, that uses a graded scoring system from 0 to 4 indicating the diagnosis and severity of pathology present in each body organ.   Clinical findings and therapy are then evaluated against the patho- logical evidence to determine accuracy of the attending doctor's diagnosis and his choice of therapy.

a.   Identify major differences between A and B.

b.   Identify major problems of the methods.

c.   Identify special advantages of the methods.

d.   Which is the better method?

Question 19

You wish to discover the etiology of the Sudden Infant Death Syndrome.

Method A

Using a variety of sources including hospital and clinic records and interviews with the infant's family and family friends, you collect as much information about each of the 114 cases that occurred in your hospital's area as you can. After putting all the information on computer cards you determine the fre- quency distributions of all variables and perform cross tabulations of all com- binations of variables to determine those which are statistically significant.

Method B

After reviewing the scientific literature you determine that the etiology of
Sudden Infant Death Syndrome is unknown, although many factors have already been investigated. You further learn that some investigators believe
that abnormal rhythms of the heart beat may be produced by irregular breath-
ing patterns and chronic hypoxia in infants, and these abnormal cardiac
rhythms may be a precipitating factor in the occurrence of sudden infant
deaths. You propose to perform electrocardiogram (ECG) examinations of all
newborn infants on your hospital's obstetrical service to determine the nature
of the cardiac rhythms. In the event of an infant death attributed to Sudden
Infant Death Syndrome, the electrocardiograms would be reviewed. Findings
would support or refute the hypothesis that cardiac arhythmias were related to
the mechanism of death.

a.   Identify major differences between A and B.

b.   Identify major problems of the methods.

c.   Identify special advantages of the methods.

d.   Which is the better method?

SUGGESTED RESPONSES
Exercise 10--Study Design in Epidemiologic Investigation

1a.   (1) What is the monthly incidence rate of missed appointments for our clinics?   (2) The desired or acceptable rate of missed appointments is needed for comparison.   (3) This is primarily an administrative problem, not an epidemiological one.

1b.   (1) What is the number of cases reported from plant X for the past three years?   (2) For the population of plant X how many cases of angiosarcoma might be expected during three years?   The expected rate of this tumor would also be useful.   (3) This is an epidemiologic problem.

1c.   (1) What is the age-specific birth rate for our population in the age group less than 15 years during 1960?   (2) The expected or estimated age-specific birth rate for our population in the less than 15 years age group during 1960 would be needed.   This is usually based on the data observed for similar age groups in prior years.   (3) It is an epidemio-logical problem if there is an underlying health problem, otherwise it is a demographic problem.

1d.   (1) What is the socioeconomic-specific tuberculosis incidence rates for our population during 1973?   (2) The estimated or expected incidence rates by socioeconomic status are needed.   (3) It is an epidemiological issue.

1e.   (1) What is the prevalence rate of bacteriuria in female textile workers?   (2) The expected prevalence rate for a comparable group of women is needed.   (3) It is an epidemiological problem.

1f.   (1) What is the prevalence rate of positive heterophile reactions in our Navy recruits?   (2) The expected prevalence rate of positive heterophile reactions in a similar group of persons is needed.   (3) This is an epide-miological problem.

2a.   (1) Is there a correlation between the neonatal mortality rate of counties and the number of "grannies" delivering babies?   (2) Do neonates deliv-ered by "grannies" have a higher mortality rate than those delivered by other health professionals, e.g., doctors?

2b.   Is the completion-of-therapy rate causally related to home nursing visit coverage?

2c.   Are the mortality rates from specific diseases and number of coronary care units causally related?

2d.   What is the incidence (or prevalence) of diarrheal episodes (or epidemics) in the community related to the use of restaurants and food markets?   Are cases of reported food-borne illness located in proximity of restaurants or food markets?

2e. What is the sensitivity and specificity of a heterophile reaction test for glandular fever?

2f. Are the spontaneous abortion rates similar for women living in the vicinity of the dump site compared to those residing farther from the site? Can we demonstrate a gradient (dose-response) of abortion--high rates proximal to the site, and low rates distant from the site?

2g. What is the observed/expected ratio of cancer incidence in this community? What is the rate of contaminated discharges into the atmosphere? What is the per capita exposure of residents to contaminated discharges?

2h. What is the pattern of cardiovascular and pulmonary mortality and morbidity preceding, during, and after the eruptions?

3a. This is an animal laboratory experiment that is a <u>prospective study</u> of type C. The independent variable is suspended particulates. The dependent variable is respiratory tissue pathology.

3b. Exposed and unexposed mice are similar with respect to genetic background, age, and living conditions except for the experimental variable air.

3c. If animals and humans differ in their response to the variables being studied, results from animal studies would not be ascribable to humans.

4a. This is a <u>case report</u> that describes an unusual finding.

4b. It calls attention to an unusual finding or variation in a disease process and alerts the health community to potentially new diseases or clinical situations. It generates hypotheses to be tested.

4c. Common things happen commonly, rare things happen rarely! Rare diseases may not generate hypotheses that are testable. Conclusions concerning etiology based on samples of 1 or 2 cases usually (but not always) are proved to be incorrect. It is difficult to generalize findings to the community or a population at risk from a single observation or report.

5a. This is a <u>cross-sectional survey</u> of type A, which has both descriptive and analytic features. For analytic purposes, induced abortion is the independent variable, prematurity (low birth weight) is the dependent variable.

5b. Community-based probability samples allow the study results to be generalized to the community or a population at risk. Incidence rates can be directly calculated. Information not readily available in existing medical records may be obtained directly from the participants.

5c.   Nonresponse or nonparticipation may be a problem. Interviewers' skill in obtaining information may vary. Subjects recall of important events may vary. The sequence of events and their time of occurrence may be incorrectly given. Subjects may not admit the truth when questioned about sensitive subjects. Data are not easily reproducible or validated.

6a.   This is a human experiment (clinical trial) with a <u>prospective</u> (type C) or <u>longitudinal</u> design. It is an analytic study; the independent variable is method of treatment. The dependent variables are stroke and/or death.

6b.   Incidence rates can be calculated from each treatment group. A specific set of questions may be answered, particularly in establishing risk among different populations. Common protocol and procedures help to produce a successful study.

6c.   Length of time to complete the study, cost, and possibility of patient loss to follow-up may be problems. Patient loss may occur because of death, migration or lack of desire to continue in the study. Also, patients or health professionals may break the code and destroy the "double blind" aspect of the study (if it is used). Participants may not comply with instructions concerning diet or therapy. Randomization might not produce similar case and comparison groups since <u>randomization</u> <u>is</u> <u>a</u> <u>process</u> <u>not</u> <u>an</u> <u>outcome</u>.

7a.   This is a <u>prevalence study (type A) or cross-sectional survey</u> whose purpose is to describe a factor in a particular population. Occupation is the independent variable, antibody to hepatitis is the dependent variable.

7b.   A specific population is chosen for study. Characteristics of occupational exposures are well suited to the study of transmission of microorganisms.

7c.   Findings are not necessarily generalizable to the entire community. <u>Incidence</u> rates (new cases per year or risk of acquiring a disease) cannot be calculated. <u>Temporal</u> relationship of exposure and development of disease may be difficult to discover. Interpretation of the prevalence ratio is difficult because there is no comparison group.

8a.   This is a <u>cross-sectional (type A) descriptive study</u> of a population of clinic patients.

8b.   It attempts to make administrative decisions based on facts. The probability sample allows the investigator to generalize findings to the entire population of clinic patients.

8c.   Records that are used are not specific to the investigation being attempted. Incomplete data (missing or poor quality information) from the records may make it difficult to use general medical records.

9a.   This is a <u>retrospective</u> (type B), case-comparison study using matched comparison subjects. It is an analytic study in which thromboembolism is the independent variable and use of oral contraception is the dependent variable. We don't know whether or not use of oral contraception preceded the onset of the disease process. In retrospective studies the disease is the independent variable and the "factor" is the dependent variable. In prospective studies, the opposite is true.

9b. Retrospective studies are the most powerful design to uncover an association between variables IF an association exists. Cost and time to complete these studies are less than prospective studies. There is no loss to follow up.

9c. The temporal relation between the agent and disease onset may be difficult to discover. Patient recall may affect the determination of whether events occurred. A suitable comparison group may be difficult to locate if hospital subjects are used as cases. Incidence rates cannot be calculated for retrospective studies. Hospital records may have missing or imprecise observations.

10a. This is a prospective study (type C), in which the heart rhythm at the start of the study is the independent variable, and the dependent variable is development of myocardial infarction.

10b. Incidence of disease following exposure/nonexposure to the factor in question is a powerful technique in proving causation because exposure preceding disease onset can be documented. A large population of diverse subjects is used which will give a more representative sample of middle aged males. Incidence rates can be calculated.

10c. Loss to follow up, time to complete study, cost, etc., are limitations of prospective designs.

11. Figure 3 shows a general classification of advantages and disadvantages. Exceptions to this schema may occur in some instances.

Figure 3. Advantages and disadvantages of epidemiologic study designs.

Items to be considered	Type of study			
	Case reports	Prevalence or cross sectional	Retro-spective	Pros-pective
Many hypotheses to test			A	D
Rare diseases	A	D	A	D
Baseline data	A	A	A	
Selective recall of important events			D	A
Attrition (death, migration, loss of participation)		A	A	D

Figure 3. (continued)

Items to be considered	Case reports	Prevalence or cross sectional	Retro-spective	Pros-pective
Nonresponse		D	A	D
Time needed to complete study	A	A	A	D
Cost	A		A	D
Control of confounding variables			D	A
Temporal relation of etiologic factor and disease onset		D	D	A
Quantitation of risk	D	A	D	A
Inference to population	D	A	D	A
Source of data collection specific to investigators need		A	D	A
Establishing directness of association		D	D	A
Selection of controls leading to bias			D	A
Interpretation fallacy (spurious association)	D		D	A
Health hazard to participants			A	occasional D
Placebo effect				D
Establishing strength of association		A	A	A

12a. Method A uses a de facto definition of treated and untreated patients. Treated patients may be more seriously ill than the untreated; hence the study may be biased from the outset. The physician may let personal feelings or other factors influence his judgment in deciding who should be treated or left untreated.

Method B removes the physicians influence over who is treated and who is untreated. Patients have an equal probability of being in either group. Random allocation attempts but does not guarantee that cases and comparison groups will be similar.

12b. By knowing which patients are treated and which are not treated the observer may consciously or subconsciously be more attuned to symptoms and illnesses in one group compared to the other. This would influence the rate of diseases calculated at the end of the study.

12c. Randomization equalizes the probability of a subject being assigned to the case or the comparison group and removes that decision from potential bias of the investigator.

12d. Method B is preferable.

13a. Both methods use randomization but method B also uses the "blind" technique in which the person making judgment about the disease outcome is uninformed of the treatment group to which the patient is assigned. A "double blind" technique would mean that patients also are not aware of the treatment groups to which they are assigned.

13b. The investigator might not exercise the same degree of objectivity in trying to determine illness rates for the case and comparison groups. It would be relatively easy to bias the study according to the investigator's preconceived prejudices as to which group <u>ought</u> to do better.

13c. "Blinding" prevents investigators from knowing which is the treated and which the nontreated group. This helps to eliminate observer bias. Double blinding would help to minimize patients' subjective bias in evaluating how they feel when they are aware of being treated/not treated.

13d. Method B is preferable.

14a. Method A uses no comparison group. Method B uses a comparison group but it consists of volunteers.

14b. Absence of a comparison group does not allow a standard of comparison to be introduced. One might express rates of disease among subjects but you would not know if this were more than, less than, or equal to the amount of disease expected in the population at risk. Volunteers are a self-selected group who might differ from nonvolunteers with respect to factors related to the disease.

14c. Halfway houses and methadone programs probably give a better cross section of drug users (representative sample) than a hospital, which might attract the sicker drug users. Use of comparison groups offers a standard of comparison.

14d. Method B is better particularly if the investigator can assure that volunteers do not introduce any serious bias into the study. Conclusions would be more generalizable to the entire population of drug users.

15a. Method A does not use a standard protocol.

15b. Observations made in study A are not made in a systematic manner. Each base may use different procedures for measuring blood pressure. Any differences observed between bases may arise from the variety of ways in which measurements are made.

15c. Observations made when a strict and rigid protocol is used allow comparison of data collected at different places. Differences between bases would not be explained by the manner in which observations are made.

15d. Method B is preferable.

16a. The methods differ with respect to how cases are defined. In both methods patients "self report" their illness. In method B, clear criteria are established to evaluate the medical history.

16b. Vague criteria used to define method A cases may result in misclassification of the diagnosis, i.e., subjects may be categorized incorrectly. Conclusions are of less value than studies in which this bias does not exist. Both studies use self-administered questionnaires that may be difficult for arthritis patients to fill out.

16c. In method B, careful delineation of the criteria used for defining what a case is removes ambiguity. Your peers may disagree with your definitions/criteria, but they will certainly understand whom and to what your findings refer. Careful definition of cases (as well as methods) will also permit others to attempt to reproduce your findings.

16d. Method B is preferable.

17a. The methods differ with respect to how subjects are selected, i.e., volunteers versus a probability sample.

17b. Volunteers are a self-selected group in all instances. When they come from a prison, they do not represent all segments of society and so the subjects may not be representative of any particular population at risk. It is difficult to generalize findings among prison inmates to the community at large.

Hospital-based studies also may not be representative of the community at large. Hospitals tend to attract the more severely ill persons and the most interesting diseases. Furthermore, hospitals are selective for patients who can afford to pay for treatment. All community residents do not have an equal probability of being hospitalized or treated at the hospital even if they suffer from the same diseases.

Some children may not come back after 24 or 48 hours and a portion of the study will be lost. Prison inmates will not be lost to follow-up.

Allergic response may differ in adults and children.

17c. Observations are made and recorded in a systematic way at similar times.

17d. If the allergen is specific for adults rather than children, method A is preferable even though volunteers are used. If children are more responsive to the allergen, then method B is preferable. Generally, studies using probability samples are preferable to those using volunteers because volunteers are not necessarily representative of the general population or a population subgroup that may be at increased risk.

18a. The methods differ with respect to the ways in which reproducibility and accuracy of observations are determined.

18b. Measurements made in A may be reproducible, but this does not establish that the diagnosis is valid or accurate; they may be difficult to interpret.

Diagnoses determined in B are probably valid but might not be completely reproducible if the graded scoring system requires subjective judgment. It would be useful to know if the pathologist was consistent in his scoring at different times.

18c. Method A attempted to discern the reproducibility (precision) of its measurements. Method B gave valid results but several pathologists might disagree with the diagnosis made from the surgical specimens. Both precision and validity are desirable.

18d. Both methods have desirable elements of study design as well as limitations. The best epidemiologic studies are designed to achieve both precision and validity!

19a. The methods differ with respect to the analysis of your data and consideration of legitimate hypotheses.

19b. The shotgun approach of method A may produce many statistically significant results but few will be realistic in terms of the biological features of the disease. Many wild goose chases might result from a shotgun approach. Further, many important but unsuspected factors about which you have no information might be overlooked in this approach to determine etiology. Method B proposes to relate an ECG result to the occurrence of death at a future time. Many things could happen between the ECG and time of death that could confound the association.

19c. Studies designed to test specific hypotheses may be somewhat easier to perform. Pertinent data specific to the investigator's needs can be collected, offering the economy of time, energy, and money.

If one is lucky, a shotgun approach may yield some interesting information and generate testable hypotheses. Use of a computer allows us to sift through a large amount of data very quickly.

19d. Method B is preferable. It uses what is already known in the literature and attempts to add to it.

EXERCISE 11. PROBLEMS IN THE DESIGN OR PRESENTATION OF DATA OF EPIDEMIOLOGIC STUDIES

Goals

Upon completion of this exercise you should be able to identify commonly encountered problems in the design or in the interpretation of data from epidemiologic studies.

Methods

In order to achieve this goal you need to understand the problems related to

I.   COMPARABILITY OF CASE AND COMPARISON (CONTROL) GROUPS
II. PERIOD OF EXPOSURE TO RISK
III. VOLUNTEERS
IV. ASSOCIATIONS, CORRELATIONS, AND TRENDS
V.   INFERENCES DERIVED IN THE ABSENCE OF A POPULATION AT RISK

Terms

Proportionate mortality

Suggested Readings

Readings suggested for Exercise 10 will also be useful for Exercise 11.

This exercise will consider some of the major problems in design of a study or presentation of the data.

The following illustrations refer to studies using comparison (control) groups. Data refer to a hypothetical disease, Sasquatch fever. Each illustration reveals a problem or error that the unsuspecting investigator or student may encounter. However, the investigator learns from the mistake of the previous example and tries to improve the study design by correcting that mistake in the subsequent problem.

I.   COMPARABILITY OF CASE AND COMPARISON (CONTROL) GROUPS.

Perhaps the most serious problem is in not using comparison (or control) groups. Lack of an appropriate standard of comparison can prevent an investigator from drawing valid conclusions, although uncontrolled studies on occasion may yield valid observations.

In any study involving comparisons of two or more study groups, or comparison of the characteristics of cases to an available population or existing data set (the standard of comparison), the investigator must strive to assure that the GROUPS ARE COMPARABLE. Lack of comparability will frequently invalidate the study results. The ways in which groups may lack comparability can vary greatly, as illustrated in the following series of problems:

A. You wish to study the effectiveness of a new surgical technique (the independent variable) for patients with Sasquatch fever. Patients are age-
matched with untreated controls. The dependent (outcome) variable is
death.

Figure 1. Survival of Sasquatch fever by method of treatment.

Therapy	Outcome			
	Survived	Died	Total	Percent died
Treated	88	32	120	26.7
Untreated	60	30	90	33.3

Statistical analysis of this 2 × 2 contingency table reveals that the results of
therapy are not statistically significant (χ^2 = 1.10; 0.30 > p > 0.20), although
there is a substantial and intriguing difference in survival between the groups.

Question 1

a. What variables other than age should the investigator present in order to
establish that treated and untreated subjects are comparable?

b. If treated and untreated groups were comparable might it be reasonable
to conclude that therapy caused the lower death rate?

Question 2

Suppose the medical literature indicated that Sasquatch fever was a sex
(gender)-linked disease and more detailed analyses of the previous data revealed the associations shown in Figure 2.

a. Compare the sex-specific death rates for treated and untreated cases.
How can you explain the difference in the total death rates?

Figure 2.   Death rate per 100 by sex and treatment, Sasquatch fever.

Mode of therapy	Males		Females		Total	
	Cases	Deaths	Cases	Deaths	Cases	Deaths
Treated	40	16	80	16	120	32
Death rate		40		20		26.7
Untreated	60	24	30	6	90	30
Death rate		40		20		33.3

Question 2 (continued)

b.   Identify one option the investigator has in design and one option in the analysis of the data that will eliminate noncomparability of treated and untreated groups.

design:

analysis:

B.   <u>You wish to compare the 5-year survival of Sasquatch fever patients treated at two different hospitals.</u>

A series of 800 consecutive patients admitted with Sasquatch fever were selected from each hospital.   The results:

Hospital	Cases	Deaths	Rate per 1000
A	800	40	50
B	800	81	100

The investigators argued that hospital A had better medical care because equal numbers of cases should assure comparability between the hospitals.

Question 3

a.   To test the validity of the conclusion, and to avoid the sex bias encountered in "A," consider the more detailed data in Figure 3.   Calculate the death rates by age, sex, and severity of disease for each hospital. Compare the age-sex-severity specific rates in both hospitals.

Exercise 11-4

Figure 3. Death rates per 100 by sex, age, severity and hospital, Sasquatch fever.

Sex	Age	Severity of disease	Hospital A			Hospital B		
			Cases	Deaths	Rate per 100	Cases	Deaths	Rate per 100
male	>60	more	40	10		160	40	
	>60	less	100	5		200	10	
	≦59	more	60	6		100	10	
	≦59	less	200	4		50	1	
		TOTAL	400	25		510	61	
female	>60	more	40	6		100	15	
	>60	less	100	4		50	2	
	≦59	more	60	3		40	2	
	≦59	less	200	2		100	1	
		TOTAL	400	15		290	20	

b. What differences exist between patients from Hospital A and B?

c. Given the more detailed analyses, is the conclusion justified?

d. Is the error likely to be in study design or in presentation of the data, or in both?

e.   The issue of the degree to which cases and controls must be comparable
     is difficult to resolve.   Obviously no two people are exactly alike in all
     respects when we consider genetic inheritance, personal habits and cus-
     toms.   For how many or for what type of variables is it necessary to
     establish comparability?

II.   PERIOD OF EXPOSURE TO RISK.

A second frequently encountered problem occurs when one does not consider
changes that might have occurred during the period of time that one is exposed to the risk of contracting a disease.   In a sense this is another example
of noncomparability, but it does not involve the inherent or acquired characteristics of the host.

A.   A vaccine for Sasquatch fever was tested on 600 individuals over a
     2-year period.

Several comparison groups were selected, totaling 1600 persons.   The case and
comparison groups were balanced for such major demographic characteristics as
age, sex, race, and socioeconomic status, and for medical history including
allergy, thereby avoiding the comparability problems of Part I.   The results
were:

	Number	ill	Percent ill
Inoculated	600	15	2.5
Not Inoculated	1600	106	6.6

Question 4

a.   Calculate the vaccine effectiveness (i.e., the percent reduction in illness).

b.   Give reasons for concluding that the vaccine is effective.

c.   How might insufficient consideration of the period of exposure to risk re-
     sult in failure to detect that the vaccine might be ineffective?

To see how the period of exposure can affect the disease rate in cases and controls you must remember that the relationship between illness and vaccination status is a function of the relationship between

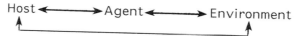

Although they exist in a steady state, this does not imply that the relationship is static. Change often occurs in one or more members of the triad. Therefore, the investigators ought to consider the role of TIME more explicitly. Reassess the vaccination data to determine the role of the period of exposure to risk. Note that the total ill, nonill, treated, and untreated remains the same as before.

d. Calculate the percent ill by year and enter it in Figure 4.

Figure 4. Percent ill by treatment status and year of vaccination, Sasquatch fever vaccine trial.

Study Year	Inoculation Status	Number	ill	Percent ill
1	Yes	100	10	
1	No	1000	100	
2	Yes	500	5	
2	No	600	6	

e. Restate the conclusions of the study.

f. How does the period of exposure affect the findings?

g. Was an error committed in the study design or presentation of data?

B. A community screening program was implemented to determine if vaccination of women of reproductive ages might be effective in reducing Sasquatch fever. If contracted during pregnancy, the disease causes congenital illness of the baby.

The investigator, having learned to avoid the errors noted in the previous examples, decided to match his inoculation and comparison groups by major demographic characteristics. He also employed a laboratory technician to run serial in vitro cultures to determine any changes in the virulence of the organism (which, you may be happy to learn, did not vary over the study period). The results:

Figure 5. Attack rate per 100 pregnant women by inoculation status, Sasquatch fever vaccine trial.

Inoculation status	Persons exposed	Number ill	Attack rate/100
Yes	1000	110	11.0
No	4000	890	22.3

Question 5

a. Can you suggest how the results shown in Figure 5 could occur if the vaccine was totally ineffective?

If you cannot answer Question 5a, reexamine the above data using person-years of exposure as the denominator of the attack rate as shown in Figure 6. We will assume that the attack rate for Sasquatch fever (cases/no. exposed per unit time $\times$ 100) is 5% per calendar quarter but that people become vaccinated at varying times during the year depending upon availability of the vaccine, their awareness of the vaccine program, and their willingness to be vaccinated. Recalculating the attack rate using person-years of exposure more accurately reflects the way vaccination occurred during the year.

b. Examine Figure 6 to determine how person-years exposed and persons ill are derived. Then complete the table for both groups.

c. Review the conclusions of the study by comparing the attack rates observed when person-years rather than persons exposed is used as the denominator of the rate. Can you explain the different results shown in Figures 5 and 6?

MORAL. One of the most useful and often repeated questions raised by epidemiologists is, WHAT IS THE DENOMINATOR? This question refers to the quality (the intensity or severity of exposure to risk including the way in which exposure occurs) and also to the quantity (the number and/or period of exposure to risk) of persons participating in the study.

Figure 6. Attack rate per 100 person-years by immunization status, Sasquatch fever vaccine program.

Date of calendar quarter beginning	Persons not inoculated					Persons inoculated				
	Persons exposed to disease in this quarter	Years exposed	Person-years exposed	Persons ill at 5% per quarter	Attack rate/ 100 person-years exposed	Persons exposed to disease in this quarter	Years exposed	Person-years exposed	Persons ill at 5% per quarter	Attack rate/ 100 person-years exposed
	a	b	axb	.05xa		a	b	axb	.05xa	
1 January	5000	¼	1250	250		0	¼			
1 April	4700	¼	1175	235		300	¼			
1 July	4100	¼	1025	205		900	¼			
1 October	4000	¼	1000	200		1000	¼			
End of year	4000	-	4450	890		1000	-			

Question 6

a. Explain why person-years is often an appropriate denominator for epidemiologic studies.

b. In what situations would it be particularly useful?

c. What property inherent to the notion of person-years might complicate interpretation of rates calculated using person-years of exposure?

C.   Period of Observation when Assessing Survivorship

Following treatment, survival without illness or death can be analyzed in different ways. Consider the following example:

You wish to compare the survival time of Sasquatch fever patients treated with two methods of therapy. Method 1 was used between 1969 and 1980 and method 2 was used between 1975 and 1980.

Question 7

a. Calculate the death rates per 100 and per 100 person-years, and the average years survived, and enter them in the appropriate places in Figure 7.

Figure 7. Death rates by treatment method, Sasquatch fever, 1969-1980.

Method	Year	Number treated	Number dead	Death rate per 100	Number person-years survived	Death rate per 100 person-years	Average years survived
1	1969-1980	400	200		3400		
2	1975-1980	400	40		1200		

b.   Compare the rates of the two treatments.   Compare the rates for the same treatment.   From these data, which method seems to be better?

c.   How can you explain the different impressions of effectiveness derived from the above calculations?

Question 7 raises two issues in evaluating survivorship of therapies of different durations; when do you start the period of observation? and how long should you continue follow-up?

When comparing the efficacy of two treatments RxA and RxB you might evaluate patient deaths, remissions, side effects, or other outcomes occurring to each therapy.   For the following example we use deaths as the outcome measure and assume that deaths occur both during and after treatment.   Deaths reflect the severity of the disease in question, relative efficacy and safety of the therapy, and the possibility of death occurring from causes other than the disease being investigated.

Figure 8. Evaluation of treatments after completion of therapy.

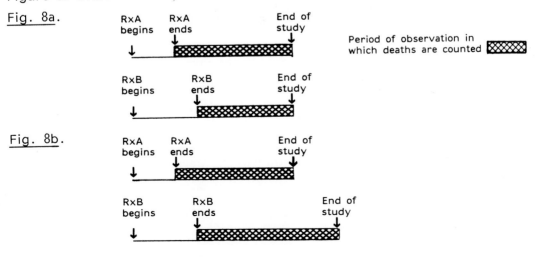

Question 8

a. Contrast Figures 8a and 8b in terms of (1) the period of observation after completing the therapy and (2) the overall length of the study.

b. If the treatments RxA and RxB differ in their effectiveness, what effect does that have on a study whose period of observation begins at the completion of therapy?

Figure 9. Evaluation of treatments from start of therapy.

Fig. 9a.

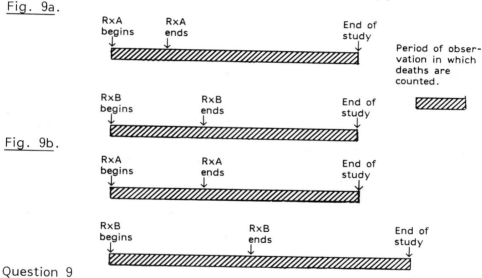

Fig. 9b.

Question 9

a. Contrast Figures 9a and 9b in terms of the period of observation and in terms of overall length of the study.

b. If the treatments RxA and RxB differ in their effectiveness, how might you plan the data analysis of a study whose period of observation begins at the start of therapy?

Is the method used in Figures 8a and 8b better or worse than the method of Figures 9a and 9b? Judgment as to which approach is better depends upon the purpose of the study. If the investigator seeks to learn about efficacy on all members of the treatment cohort then the overall length of the study should be equal for RxA and RxB. If, on the other hand, the investigator is interested to learn what happens to patients who survive treatment, then each treatment group should have similar periods of observation after completion of therapy.

Evaluating the efficacy of two treatments can be further complicated by other considerations, especially whether or not the natural history of the disease is affected. The natural history of most diseases consists of 3 periods. The first is the interval between exposure to the disease agent and onset of disease (incubation period), the second interval occurs between disease onset and diagnosis, and the third period follows diagnosis, during which therapy occurs.

The diseased individual may recover completely, may die from the illness, or may continue to be ill (intermittently or continuously) over a long period of time but not die from the disease. Much of modern medical practice is predicated on the hypothesis that early detection and treatment of disease is effective in controlling the disease's course. While true for some diseases (tuberculosis, bacterial infections) the hypothesis has not been proven for many diseases and in fact may not be true for some diseases.

For example, suppose a disease process begins at age 45 and has an expected duration of 20 years. If diagnosed at age 55, the average survival after diagnosis is 10 years and age at death is 65. If a new screening or diagnostic technique lowered the age at diagnosis to 50, the average survival after diagnosis would increase to 15 years even if the average age of death was unchanged. Moreover, if a new therapy were available and initiated after early detection of the disease or at a less severe stage of illness, there would be an apparent improvement in average survival after treatment, compared to more traditional modes of therapy. This could occur even though the average age at death remained at 65, and the total duration of the disease remained 20 years.

In treating cancer, earlier diagnosis and therapy are desirable. The choice of therapy may be a difficult decision because of problems in accurately assessing the safest and most effective treatment. Treatment of breast cancer may require the doctor and patient to choose between two surgical techniques over which there is considerable debate. For more complete discussion of these issues, the student is referred to the American Cancer Society monograph, Cancer of the Breast, Statistical and Epidemiologic Data, by Herbert Seidman (72-2R-15M-9/73-No 3017-PE).

III. VOLUNTEERS

An investigator places an advertisement requesting volunteers to test a new vaccine for Sasquatch fever.

Question 10

a.   What problems related to data validity might arise by using volunteers?

b.   How might the investigator overcome these problems?

c.   Historically, closed populations such as prisons, mental institutions, and military installations have been the source of volunteers for clinical and epidemiologic study.   What ethical issues are raised?

d.   What effect might these types of volunteers have on the conclusions of the study?

IV.   ASSOCIATIONS, CORRELATIONS AND TRENDS

Figure 10.   Changes in rates over time, selected variables, U.S.

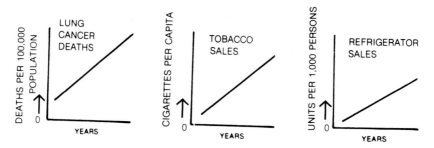

Question 11

a.   Describe the relation suggested by the curves shown in Figure 10.

b.   Are you justified in concluding that a causal relation exists?   Explain. What kind of relation does exist?

c.   How might an epidemiologist validate whether or not these correlations have biologic importance?

Figure 11. Maternal mortality ratio compared to selected health services indices.

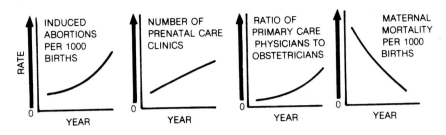

Question 12

Compare the trend of maternal mortality shown in Figure 11 in relation to the trends for the 3 other variables shown above. How would you justify financial support for your program assuming you are

a. Director of a statewide abortion service?

b. Director of the Health Department Maternal/Child Health program?

c. President of the American College of Family Practice Physicians?

A. INTERPRETING TRENDS

Changes over time may occur in the characteristics of a host (exposure or susceptibility), a disease agent, or the environment and these may affect the disease incidence or prevalence. Disease trends that vary over time may, therefore, reflect actual changes in pathogenicity of the disease agent or the host's response to a given exposure as discussed in earlier exercises. Epidemiologists constantly try to differentiate these "real" changes from spurious, artifactual, or random fluctuations, which may mistakenly be interpreted as due to biologic change in the disease. Distinguishing real from spurious variation has great importance in health planning and evaluation of health care services.

Disease rates usually fluctuate over time. A rate may vary if there is a change in either the numerator or denominator (or both). It is therefore possible to explain changing trends in a variety of ways. The change may be "real," or may occur because of nonbiologic factors, such as changes in diagnostic criteria for disease classification, alteration of geographic boundaries of the reference population at risk, change in population characteristics due to migration (in or out) of the area, or change in case finding or reporting procedures by the health agency responsible for data collection.

Question 13

With the above possibilities in mind, list alternative possibilities to explain a change in the Sasquatch fever mortality in the U.S. from 350 to 403 per 100,000 between 1973 and 1980, consistent with the following:

a.   Increase in numerator, denominator remains constant.

b.   Decrease in denominator, numerator remains constant.

c.   Both numerator and denominator increase.

d.   Both numerator and denominator decrease.

Question 14

Suppose the mortality rate had decreased from 403 to 350 during the same period.   List explanations consistent with the following:

a.   Numerator decrease, denominator remains constant.

b.   Numerator constant, denominator increases.

c.   Both numerator and denominator decrease.

d.   Both numerator and denominator increase.

Question 15

What is an appropriate use of trend data in epidemiology?

Question 16

Suggest reasons to explain the following observations. Indicate whether or not the trend is due to change in risk.

a.　An increase in lung cancer deaths among women.

b.　An increase in rape.

c.　An increase in deaths and serious injury involving automobiles.

V.　INFERENCES DERIVED IN THE ABSENCE OF A POPULATION AT RISK

Question 17

a.　Compare the risk of death from Sasquatch fever by age groups, as shown in Figure 12.

Figure 12. Mortality rates by age and cause in a one-year period, U.S., 1980.

Age group	Population	Deaths		Death rate per 100,000	
		All causes	Sasquatch fever	All causes	Sasquatch fever
5-9	3,181,900	6,601	774	207.5	24.3
10-14	3,349,100	4,603	827	138.6	24.7

b.　Calculate the PROPORTIONATE MORTALITY RATIO of Sasquatch fever by age, i.e., the percent of deaths from Sasquatch fever among deaths from all causes.

Ages　5-9　　　　　774/6601　　　=　　＿＿＿＿＿＿

Ages　10-14　　　　827/4603　　　=　　＿＿＿＿＿＿

c.   How would your decision regarding the need for a Sasquatch fever control program among children ages 10-14 change if you assessed the death rate rather than the proportionate mortality?

d.   In assessing risk of death, what is the preferable denominator representing the population at risk?

e.   What does the denominator of the proportionate mortality of deaths from all causes represent?   Is it a suitable denominator for assessing risk?

f.   Why are proportionate ratios of less value than rates in determining risk? When might proportionate mortality ratios be used?

g.   Do you see the value for determining both the quality and quantity of the denominator?

Consider the following data, which contrast infant mortality rates and proportionate mortality.   Both tables are derived from the same data.

Figure 13a. Infant mortality from Sasquatch fever per 1000 births by age, 1980.

	Age at death				
Area	<1 Month	1-2 Months	3-5 Months	6-12 Months	Total
Urban	29.7	20.8	22.8	22.1	95.4
Rural	23.8	12.6	11.0	11.3	58.7

Figure 13b. Percentage of infant deaths from Sasquatch fever by age, 1980.

Area	<1 Month	1-2 Months	3-5 Months	6-12 Months	Total
Urban	31.1	21.8	23.9	23.2	100.0
Rural	40.6	21.5	18.7	19.2	100.0

(column header group spanning: Age at death)

CONCLUSIONS: Because rural areas have higher PERCENTAGE mortality than urban areas for newborn infants (<1 month), a neonatal health program should be implemented in rural areas.

Question 18

a. Comment on this conclusion.

b. Which are more useful for assessing risk, conclusions based upon proportional data when the denominator is not a population at risk or conclusions derived from age-specific rates?

Question 19

A newspaper article stated that 75% of automobile accidents involve drunk drivers. They concluded that drivers who drink are more dangerous than drivers who are nondrinkers.

a. Write the rate or ratio used to calculate this statistic.

b. What is the unit of "exposure" for this statistic? Is this actually a population at risk?

c. Is the conclusion justified? Explain.

SUGGESTED RESPONSES
Exercise 11--Problems in the Design or Presentation
of Data of Epidemiologic Studies

1a. Other variables that might be presented are sex, severity of disease, presence of other medical illnesses that might influence survival, or any specific factors known to affect Sasquatch fever mortality and that might differ between the treated and untreated groups.

1b. It would be tempting, but this is insufficient evidence to invoke a causal association. The statistical association is not significant.

2a. Sex-specific death rates are equal for treated and untreated cases. The total death rates differ because the untreated group contains a larger proportion of males. Males have a higher death rate than females.

2b. An investigator may attempt to design his study such that treated/untreated subjects are comparable in terms of important disease-related factors such as age, sex, and severity of disease. A second option is to adjust or standardize the data for differences between treated/untreated groups during the analysis--age adjust, sex adjust (no pun intended), etc. One may adjust single variables or several variables at the same time. Multiple regression techniques may be necessary if attempting to adjust for more than 3 or 4 variables simultaneously.

3a. <u>Figure 3</u>

			Rate Hospital A	Rate Hospital B
Male rates:	>60	more	25.0	25.0
	>60	less	5.0	5.0
	≤59	more	10.0	10.0
	≤59	less	2.0	2.0
	Total		6.3	12.0
Female rates:	>60	more	15.0	15.0
	>60	less	4.0	4.0
	≤59	more	5.0	5.0
	≤59	less	1.0	1.0
	Total		3.8	6.9

3b. Age-sex-severity-specific rates for both hospitals are identical. Differences in total death rates occur because a greater proportion of hospital B's admissions were older and more severely ill than hospital A's admissions.

3c. There is no evidence to suggest that A had better care than B. The crude unadjusted rates show A to be superior because A had a younger and less severely ill patient population. These data reflect the differences among hospital patients in communities. Thus, crude data from different hospitals should not be compared until specifying appropriate categories or performing suitable "adjustment."

3d. The investigators might not have been aware of the differences in patients' characteristics between their hospitals. If this were true and they
neglected to subject their data to careful analysis, they made a serious
error. If on the other hand they were aware of potential differences and
neglected to present the detailed analysis merely to prove their hypothesis, they were unethical.

3e. Cases and comparison subjects should be similar with respect to important
variables known or suspected of having an association with the disease
process or outcome under study. The most common variables are age,
sex, race, and socioeconomic status. However, any disease may have
specific factors such as smoking history, dietary habits, or occupational
exposure to toxins that are relevant to the disease in question. In some
diseases only a few factors will be necessary, while in other diseases
many variables must be considered. A knowledge of the literature concerning the research area will help to identify the most important variables. Your available time and money may influence the number of variables that can realistically be considered.

4a. Effectiveness (reduction of disease by therapy)

$$= \frac{\text{Percent ill among untreated - Percent ill among treated}}{\text{Percent ill among untreated}} \times 100$$

$$= (6.6 - 2.5) / 6.6 \times 100 = 4.1 / 6.6 \times 100 = 62.1\%$$

4b. Treated and untreated persons are comparable for major demographic and
medical variables that are known to affect the rate of disease. The
variables presented suggest that treated and untreated should be similar
with regard to susceptibility and exposure to the disease.

4c. While demographic and medical characteristics IMPLY treated and untreated
persons are similar, other factors associated with the disease process but
unknown to the investigator might differ between treated and untreated
groups. Each group might have had different periods of exposure
(person-years) to infection, or the risk of infection might vary during
the period of the investigation. To establish that all participants are
similar the investigator must show that both susceptibility and exposure
to infection are similar in qualitative and quantitative terms, thereby
making the vaccine the only important difference between groups. The
requirement is difficult to meet outside a laboratory setting. In this
study neither have been shown, and so it would be premature to accept
the study results as correct.

4d. Figure 4

Study year	Percent ill	
	Treated	Untreated
1	10	10
2	1	1

4e. There is no difference in attack rate when period of exposure is con-
     sidered. The vaccine is not effective.

4f. Considering the period of exposure changes the findings. Differing pro-
     portions of treated and untreated persons entered the study at different
     times during the two years this study was conducted. Something had
     altered the pathogenicity of the disease agent between years 1 and 2.

4g. Perhaps both. It depends upon whether the potential for differing expo-
     sure was considered. In this example the exposure differed from years 1
     to 2. Either susceptibles were not exposed or the pathogenicity of the
     organism may have changed during year 2.

5a. Again, some consideration must be given to the period of exposure. We
     are certain that the cases-controls are likely to have equal susceptibility
     and the organism has not changed over time.

5b. Figure 6.

| | Not inoculated | Inoculated | | |
Date of quarter beginning	Attack rate/100 person-years exposed	Person-years exposed	Persons ill at 5% per quarter	Attack rate/100 person-years exposed
1 January	20	0	0	0
1 April	20	75	15	20
1 July	20	225	45	20
1 October	20	250	50	20
End of year	20	550	110	20

5c. The attack rate in both groups is similar for each quarter (except the
     first) and the attack rate for the full year is identical. The vaccine is
     not effective. The apparent differences between Figures 5 and 6 are due
     to the all-or-none aspect of Figure 5. Figure 6 reflects the rate at which
     illness occurred during the year in relation to the vaccination status of
     the women studied.

     A refinement in the person-years exposed calculation would be to assume
     that the distribution of entry/withdrawal is at the midpoint of each inter-
     val rather than the end of the period as shown in this example. Both
     may be used correctly; it depends on the quality and availability of data
     on hand. Finally, the most accurate denominator would be calculated from
     the actual number of days each person contributed to the inoculated and
     noninoculated groups.

6a. Person-years is appropriate when people may enter or withdraw from the
     study at different points during the period of observation. It may not be
     appropriate to calculate rates in terms of presence/absence of disease
     without regard to the period at which they are at risk and the availability

of observations--i.e., not everyone becomes infected at the same time during the year. Also if some persons leave the study you would still like to be able to process their usable data. Thus, person-years is quite useful in prospective studies.

6b. Person-years of exposure can be used in many situations. In occupational health studies it is important to relate the disease outcome to the exposure dose, and so person-years is useful. In diseases where a person can switch between ill and nonill status during the observation period and for diseases such as cancer, which have long latency periods, rates based on person-years of exposure are suitable and appropriate.

6c. The quality of rates that use person-years frequently is overlooked. For example, 100 person-years may represent 100 persons for 1 year, 1 person for 100 years or any intermediate mixture between these extremes. In addition to presenting the total person-years, an investigator ought to indicate the average contribution (the mean or median number of years exposed) of participants.

7a.

Figure 7

Method	Death rate per 100	Death rate per 100 person-years	Years average survival
1	50	5.88	8.5
2	10	3.33	3.0

7b. Method 1 has higher mortality for each rate. Comparison of the ratio of the rates per 100 suggests method 1 has five-fold increase in mortality (50/10) while the same comparison for 100 person-years shows method 1 mortality excess to be only 1.77 times that of method 2. Selection of denominators can influence the magnitude of difference in effectiveness.

Although death rates per 100 and per 100 person-years reveals method 2 to be superior, the average years-survived reveals method 1 to be superior. The average years survived is 8.5 vs. 3.0, an excess of over 5 years per person.

7c. The problem is that patients treated by method 1 have been observed from 1969 to 1980, an 11-year period. Those treated by method 2 have been observed for only 5 years. Due to the differing periods of observation, survivors of method 1 may contribute an inordinately large number of person-years survived. Their contribution is so large that in this example it is able to reverse the interpretation as to which treatment is more effective.

8a. In Figure 8a the period of observation is longer for RxA than RxB even though the overall length of study is the same. In Figure 8b the periods of observation are similar but study B is of longer duration than A.

8b. Some deaths might occur during the period when therapy is being given and some after the completion of treatment. In Figure 8a there is a longer period after therapy during which deaths would be counted against RxA. Because the periods of observation are not similar for both treatments, there is a possibility that the study's results might favor RxB.

In Figure 8b there is an attempt to resolve this problem by making the counting periods similar. This introduces a problem in that recipients of RxB will be observed for part of the study when they are older than study A participants. Since the risk of death is greater with older age, some patients who receive RxB and who die near the end of the counting period may cause RxB to have a higher death rate than RxA.

9a. In Figures 9a and 9b deaths are counted from the start of therapy. In the former the overall length of study is similar for RxA and RxB; in the latter example RxB is studied for a longer period of time in order to equalize the period of time after completing the therapy.

9b. The investigator might wish to distinguish between those who survive from the outset of treatment as contrasted with those who survive after the completion of the treatment. Figures 8a and 8b are the preferred approaches if the former question is being investigated, while Figures 9a and 9b might be indicated if the latter question is investigated. The effect of age and period of observation must be considered when interpreting results.

10a. Volunteers may be useful to an investigator who needs subjects for study. However, one should have some skepticism about them. Why did they volunteer? What do they gain from participation?

Volunteers may participate for financial reward or to receive extensive health examinations. Some volunteers may come from families or have occupations that have above average risk of developing a disease and thus may be interested in diagnostic services.

Volunteers are not necessarily representative of the general population from which they come. They may be more aware of good health practices than nonvolunteers. They could have certain customs or habits (e.g., they may be joggers and have a diet low in cholesterol and saturated fats), which afford them lower risk for some diseases (e.g., myocardial infarction) compared to the general population. Thus, disease risk for a group of volunteers may either underestimate or overestimate the actual risk compared to the general population.

10b. Careful selection of volunteers according to criteria that exclude persons with known history of disease or exposure to suspected causal factors or factors thought to play a role in the disease etiology should occur. Exceptions to this principle would be necessary if the investigator was trying to evaluate the effect of prior exposure and was using volunteers to minimize the expense of the study.

Randomization of volunteers to either the treatment (test) or comparison groups is an important technique used in study design, when prospective follow-up is necessary. Randomization is expected to yield similar test and comparison groups for variables of interest, but randomization is a PROCESS to achieve similarity and NOT A RESULT. Thus, an investigator must still demonstrate that the randomization process had, in fact, resulted in test and comparison groups that were similar.

An investigator should consider using several comparison groups, including some from the community. Selection of persons from nonhospital populations will help to avoid many potential problems of bias, and also provides information concerning the nonill population in general.

10c. Prisoners may have been forced to participate against their will, or they may not have been informed of potential risks to their health.

Persons from mental institutions may not be capable of evaluating potential risks to their health.

Military personnel may be forced or unsuspecting participants in experiments for the purpose of evaluating some military measure with health consequences.

The principle of INFORMED CONSENT has not always been used in clinical and epidemiologic studies. In recent years, the legal responsibility of investigators to obtain informed consent from research participants has been established and enforced. In many university and hospital settings, it is no longer possible to conduct human research without approval of committees for protection of human subjects. All U.S. government research funds require this type of review.

10d. Data may not be representative of the general community, and therefore the conclusions may not be generalized to the entire community or population.

The biological effect of the factor under study may be over- or underestimates of the actual risk in the general population, depending upon the characteristics and composition of the volunteer population.

11a. All three curves show an increase over time. There would be a positive correlation between these variables.

11b. Review the criteria for invoking causal associations (Exercise 9). These data suggest a correlation between the pairs of variables. Correlation implies that an association exists but we cannot determine that it is causal. From other evidence there is a known direct association between lung cancer and tobacco sales. The correlation between refrigerator sales and cancer deaths is coincidental (spurious).

11c. Perform specific studies of lung cancer vs. non-lung cancer deaths to determine whether these groups used tobacco or purchased refrigerators prior to their disease onset. Also, attempt laboratory experiments on animals to determine if a biologic mechanism exists between the suspected disease agent and clinical illness.

12. Each director has selectively assembled facts of interest to him, which cast his program in the most favorable light. Obviously, there is a correlation between the desired result of decreased maternal mortality and each of the three variables. These variables contribute something to the overall effect of reducing the mortality but it is difficult to know what the particular role of each variable might be. To the unwary each of the arguments might seem strong, but obviously are only a portion of the total picture. Other evidence might be presented by <u>other directors</u> to show the virtues of other programs. Whose data would <u>you</u> believe if <u>you</u> were responsible for allocating health funds to the three programs?

13a. Better case finding; more complete reporting, improved care for other diseases might result in less death from those diseases, and therefore more people are alive who might contract Sasquatch fever.

13b. Outmigration or a large number of deaths due to a severe epidemic reduces the size of the population when the epidemic is over.

13c. Both numerator and denominator increase, but numerator increase must be larger. Better reporting of disease, immigration of susceptible persons, or decline in death rate from other diseases may result in a larger population at risk of Sasquatch fever.

13d. Both numerator and denominator decrease, but denominator decline must be greater. Fewer deaths would occur if many persons who were susceptible to Sasquatch fever migrate out of the population.

In all of the above it is important to recognize that a changing trend may be due either to real or artifactual fluctuation. Changes in reporting practices or population size can produce artifactual fluctuation, even if the biologic factors for developing disease do not truly change. When there is a change over time in the biologic factors known to be causal (e.g., environmental risks or dietary habits), there will be a real change in risk.

14a. A change in reporting practices, e.g., the requirement for mandatory reporting is suspended; or diagnostic criteria may have changed, or a new preventive measure may have become available.

14b. A new treatment method for an unrelated disease enables a larger number of persons to survive. These survivors have zero risk of developing Sasquatch fever. Immigration of nonsusceptible persons would also explain this condition.

14c. Both may decrease for the reasons given above, but the relative decrease of the numerator is less than for the denominator.

14d. The relative increase in the denominator is greater than the relative increase in numerator. This might occur with a large influx of migrants having a lower risk of disease than native residents.

15. Trend data alone are not sufficient to invoke causation. They can be helpful in identifying the emergence or decline of a public health problem. They can provide indirect evidence to support or refute associations or hypotheses of causation. A major limitation is that trends are the resultant of many factors and an investigator may not be knowledgable about these factors or the possible interplay between them.

16a. There was an increase in cigarette smoking among women. Smoking habits of women also changed (more inhalation, smoking the cigarettes down to the tip). Exposure (risk) has increased.

16b. There is an increase in the proportion of victims who report rape and seek treatment. This probably accounts for a large proportion of the observed increase. Some of the increase may also be attributed to increased risk, i.e., an actual increase in violent crime.

16c. There has been a large increase in the number of automobiles and younger drivers. There are many more smaller automobiles and imported cars being driven, to conserve energy. Death and injury rates are higher for young male drivers and for small cars. The trend represents an increase in risk.

17a. There is no significant difference in the age-specific death rates (the actual risk of death) from Sasquatch fever.

17b. Proportionate mortality, ages 5-9 = 11.7%
ages 10-14 = 18.0%

17c. Proportionate mortality shows that Sasquatch fever is a more important cause of death in ages 10-14 than it is in younger children. One might be tempted to consider the 10-14 age group as a target population for a health program if the actual death rates were not considered.

17d. The denominator should be the midyear population estimate for each age group. Death RATES are the best indicator of risk.

17e. It is the number that permits us to assess the relative importance of any cause of death to all other causes. It is not suitable as a measure of risk because it is not directly measured against the size of the midyear populations. It is a problem because it does not measure risk directly but rather in relation to other causes of death whose FREQUENCY may vary each year.

17f. Proportionate data may fluctuate because of the importance of relative changes in the frequency of deaths (up or down) even if the population at risk does not vary. This is shown by the different conclusions derived from using age-specific rather than proportionate mortality. Be suspicious when percentages are used in reporting data! PMRs are sometimes useful when midyear populations or other populations at risk cannot be determined. In developing nations where no census data (or recent reliable data) are available, PMRs may be useful, but keep in mind that these statistics are not the most appropriate indicators of risk.

17g. When asking, "What is the denominator?" one should be careful to assess both the quality and quantity of the denominator. Is the denominator truly a population at risk? Is the number of observations in the denominator sufficiently large to avoid fluctuation produced by small numbers?

18a. The findings are not justified by the age-specific rates. On the contrary, rural areas appear to have better survival of their infants. The percentage for < 1 month in Figure 15b occurs because of the markedly reduced mortality in rural area infants after age 1 month.

18b. Again, rates derived when a population at risk is considered are likely to be superior to proportions as given in the examples.

19a. $\dfrac{\text{Auto accidents with drunken driver}}{\text{Total auto accidents}} = 75\%$

19b. The unit of exposure is not a population at risk. The unit of exposure or population at risk might be "drivers" or "miles driven" while sober or drunk. This problem is another example of the use of two numbers that are outcomes or events usually counted in the numerator. The correct analysis would be to compare the rate of accidents among drivers who drink and the rate of accidents among drivers who don't drink. This would give a ratio (the relative risk) of accidents in both groups of drivers.

19c. If the relative risk of accidents among drunk/sober drivers is greater than unity then the conclusion that alcohol may be a dangerous drug to use if one plans to drive a car may be justified. The difficulty is that it is virtually impossible to know how many persons constitute the population at risk for each category of drinking status. Therefore, the newspaper conclusion is not justified.

EXERCISE 12. BIAS IN EPIDEMIOLOGIC INVESTIGATIONS

Goals

Upon completion of this exercise you should be able to (1) define the term bias and (2) identify the major sources of bias in epidemiologic studies.

Methods

In order to achieve these goals you will need to understand

I.   DEFINITION OF BIAS
II.   BERKSON'S BIAS
III. ATTRITION BIAS
IV.   SOURCES OF BIAS
V.   AVOIDING BIAS
VI.   EXAMPLES OF BIASED DATA

Suggested Readings

Mainland, D., The risk of fallacious conclusions from autopsy data on the incidence of diseases with applications to heart disease, Am. Heart J. 45:644, 1953.
Berkson, J. Limitations of the application of fourfold table analysis to hospital data, Biometrics Bull. 2:47, 1946.
Sackett, D.L. Bias in analytic research, J. Chronic Dis. 32:51, 1979.
Dalenius, T. Bibliography of nonsampling errors in surveys, Int. Statist. Rev. 45:71, 1977; also 45:181, 1977.
Levy, P.S., and Lemeshow, S. Sampling for Health Professionals, Belmont, Calif.: Lifetime Learning Publ., 1980.
Additional readings listed in Exercise 10.

I.   DEFINITION OF BIAS

The introduction of any factor or information in the design or execution of a study that leads to a spurious association between variables being studied, or that masks an association that truly exists, constitutes bias. Bias is a sys-tematic distortion (rather than randomly occurring error) of the relation be-tween variables. It may be introduced because of some characteristic of the study population or because of the way the data are collected, e.g., hospital records or personal interviews. Bias may be blatantly obvious or surprisingly subtle. Investigators and readers of scientific reports must always be alert to its occurrence.

It is rarely possible to conduct epidemiologic research without some bias. The resourceful investigator should attempt to anticipate potential sources of bias in advance of the study to control it as much as possible. An investigator's good intentions do not necessarily prevent bias. Careful planning and scrupu-lous attention to detail are often required to prevent bias from unduly influ-encing a study's data.

II.   BERKSON'S BIAS

A special category of bias is selection bias, which may occur in relation to studies of hospital data.   Known as <u>Berkson's bias</u>, it was first described by Dr. Joseph Berkson in 1946.   The following illustrates the concept of selection bias.

Suppose that we wish to determine the association of disease X with either of two other diseases A and B, by studying hospital records.   The presence or absence of an association between X and A or B will depend upon the biologic characteristics of the diseases, but it may also be affected by nonbiologic factors such as hospital admission rates (selection rates) for these diseases, i.e., who is in the hospital, that we may study.

Suppose that a community has 6000 persons with disease A and 6000 with B, and that disease X affects 20% of each group.   Then the community prevalence is

A with X =   1200 persons; B with X = 1200 persons
A not X   =   4800 persons; B not X   = 4800 persons

If the admission rates for the three diseases [A = 60%, B=25%, X=40%] are applied to the prevalence, then an epidemiologic study of the three diseases from hospital data would reveal:

	X	not X	Total
A	912	2880	3792
B	660	1200	1860
Total	1572	4080	5652

Note:

A not X = .60 x 4800 = 2880;   B not X = .25 x 4800 = 1200
AX = [.60 x 1200 hospitalized for A] + [.40 x (1200-720) hospitalized for X]
AX =   720   +   192   = 912

BX = [.25 x 1200 hospitalized for B] + [.40 x (1200-300) hospitalized for X]
BX =   300   +   360   = 660

Question 1

What percentage of As and Bs are associated with X?

AX / A =   912 / 3792   =

BX / B =   660 / 1860   =

$\chi^2 = 81.3$, $p < 0.001$ (a statistically significant result).

Differences in admission rates (selection rates) have created a spurious association from hospital records when there was no difference in the relationship between disease X and diseases A or B in the community! Because A has a higher admission rate than B, A will provide more subjects for hospital study than does B. That leaves more Bs to be admitted who also have disease X. The result is that an association is observed between X and B that does not exist in the general community. The bias could be avoided if the actual admission rates were available, but for most diseases they are not known!

Berkson's bias may potentially occur when attempting "retrospective," case-control studies (see type B study, Exercise 10) that use hospital patients as the comparison group. The bias arises because

a. A person with two diseases is more likely to be hospitalized than a person with only one disease.

b. Some diseases are more likely to be hospitalized than others. Hospitalized patients are not representative of the distribution of diseases that occurs in the community.

Question 2

Can you suggest ways in which an investigator might avoid Berkson's bias?

III. ATTRITION BIAS

An illustration using incidence and prevalence data shows another way that a spurious association can occur.

Suppose two populations, 1000 Ps and 1000 Qs, are free of a disease or characteristic S. During a period of time Ps have an incidence rate of disease S of 200 per 1000 and Qs have a rate of 100 per 1000. If the populations were surveyed for disease S at the conclusion of the period of observation we would expect:

P with S	= 200	Q with S	= 100
P not S	= 800	Q not S	= 900

How will the study results be affected if PS and QS have differential attrition, i.e., if S has a higher case-fatality rate in population P than in Q; or if PS persons drop out of the study or migrate out of the area to a greater extent than do QS individuals? Suppose that 80% of PS (160 cases) but only 5% of QS (5) individuals are lost to death, follow-up, or migration. Then those present and surveyed at the end of the observation period reveal:

Exercise 12-4

	S	Not S	Total
P	40	800	840
Q	95	900	995

The prevalence of S among Ps = 40/840 = 47.6 per 1000.
The prevalence of S among Qs = 95/995 = 95.5 per 1000.

From these data QS has a prevalence twice that of PS, even though PS had a higher incidence rate! (x^2 = 14.6; p < 0.001.)

IV. SOURCES OF BIAS

The following categories may be sources of error or bias that might occur in epidemiologic studies. While some errors might occur in any study, they are especially important when the case and comparison groups, or the respondents and nonrespondents, are affected to different degrees. This results in the differences between the study groups being increased or decreased from the "true" values for those populations. A second effect of bias is to limit the study data's usefulness for extrapolating results to the general population. A third effect of bias is that there may be actual misclassification of study subjects. In these ways, bias may produce a spurious association, mask a real association, or diminish or increase the magnitude of real associations by reducing our ability to correctly measure the "true" value of the factors under study.

Question 3.

List potential sources of error or bias that might occur for the following:

   a.   Composition or selection of study groups.

   b.   Collection of data.

   c.   Factors relating to the respondent.

   d.   Precision of measurement and classification.

   e.   Conclusions.

V.   AVOIDING BIAS*

A.   In sampling plan

1.   The ideal sample provides each individual in the population an equal opportunity or a known probability for inclusion in the sample(s), and selects groups exactly alike in all respects except for the factor under study.

2.   Some basic rules:
   a.   The sampling frame, i.e., population sampled, must be well defined and include all persons in the population.
   b.   Each individual must have known probability of inclusion in the sample, but the probability must not be zero or one.
   c.   The sampling plan must be precisely described and strictly followed.

3.   Confirm comparability of cases and comparison subjects by checking samples for characteristics other than those used for selecting the study population.

4.   Special considerations in retrospective and prospective studies include:
   a.   Use of internal comparisons between case and comparison groups to establish equivalence.
   b.   Methods of selecting the comparison group should permit control of confounding variables.
   c.   It may be necessary to have several comparison groups, including some selected from the community.
   d.   The term "controls" implies a situation that an investigator seldom has in the study of human disease and health.   Comparison groups is a more suitable term.

5.   When in doubt, consult a sampling expert!

B.   Nonrespondents and dropouts

1.   Avoid nonrespondents and dropouts when possible by obtaining data from several independent sets of records or by attempting additional follow-up efforts.

2.   Substitutes do not overcome the loss of data from nonresponse or dropouts.

3.   Investigate a subsample of, or have another basis for estimating, the known characteristics of nonrespondents or dropouts. If you can demonstrate that the known characteristics of respondents and nonrespondents are similar, you can have more confidence that the nonresponse has not introduced a bias. These measures are only a partial replacement for nonresponse and cannot prove that the data are not biased.

---

*Source: Adapted from White, C., Yale University Dept. of Epidemiology and Biostatistics.

C. Self-selection

    1. Volunteers usually are better-educated, more strongly motivated, and more consistent in following instructions. They may be more likely to show a beneficial effect from treatment. Study results may not be replicable in the general population.

    2. Use of volunteers may be unavoidable when medical procedures or measurements are to be performed or evaluated , especially when multiple examinations are required over a long period of time.

    3. Identify the characteristics and attempt to estimate the effect of using subjects who are self-selected.

    4. Randomization of volunteers to treatment may be a necessary and useful research tool in many situations.

    5. Be aware that the effect of some types of self-selection may tend to either diminish or increase with time.

D. Subjectivity

    1. In experimental studies, subjectivity may be avoided by "double-blind" techniques.

    2. Subjectivity can be avoided or minimized by use of objective tests, independent observers unaware of background information, or certain types of written records that do not rely upon subjective opinions for interpretation.

    3. Extreme efforts are often necessary to establish standard and uniform procedures to assure precise data collection.

E. Interobserver variation

    1. Use the same observers for case and comparison groups.

    2. Record and adjust for interobserver differences.

    3. Subsample independently or interchange observers.

    4. As a last resort, discard data from incompetent observers.

F. Misclassification

    1. Minimize by use of objective criteria whenever possible.

    2. When dealing with historical information minimize errors by training interviewers and data collectors, using precise definitions, and exercising scrupulous care.

VI. EXAMPLES OF BIASED DATA

Bias often cannot be eliminated. Therefore, it is important to detect its presence, its direction, and its magnitude. Bias may act in two directions: the observed value may be either closer to or further from the "true" population value of the variable being investigated. A major reason to try to eliminate bias is because we cannot always know whether our observed result is an under- or an overestimate of "reality."

In designing a study, epidemiologists attempt to eliminate as many potential sources of bias as possible. However, many situations will not permit elimination of all bias. In these cases, the investigator should attempt to measure the bias and assess its direction, i.e., does it lead to an over- or underestimation of the true value. For example, one may discover that the laboratory consistently reports results 10% in excess of results obtained using a known standard; or, in a second case, the results from one technician or interviewer may be substantially different from those of other workers.

In other situations, the bias may not be measureable; the epidemiologist cannot determine either the magnitude or direction of the bias. In these cases, the likelihood of the bias being present should be mentioned so that persons who read the study can speculate about the significance of the bias upon the study results.

Finally, all studies may be subject to unsuspected bias because of gaps in the present state of knowledge. Unsuspected factors may be directly associated with a disease, while others may influence disease occurrence indirectly through a complex interaction with other known or unknown factors. All of the above cause much anxiety in epidemiologic research.

In summary, one may conclude that good epidemiologic research is difficult to perform and, regrettably, there is no perfect study. Each investigation suffers from certain limitations inherent to study design, availability and/or accuracy of data, etc. Because of this, careful investigators devote much effort to eliminate, limit, or control those aspects of their research likely to result in bias. While the limitations of research studies directly concern the investigator, they are also important to administrators or decision makers in health agencies, who are responsible for making logical decisions based on sound scientific evidence. For these reasons it is important for all persons engaged in public health work to be familiar with the techniques and limitations of epidemiologic research and to be sensitive to the possibility of error or bias affecting a study's results.

The following problems contain some error or bias.* See if you can detect how or where the potential for bias or error may occur. Keep in mind that some of the conclusions that may be drawn are highly speculative. Further, the findings may be valid (i.e., indicating the true nature of the relationship between variables) even though bias or error occurs. Bias or error in itself does not mean that the study is not valid.

Question 4

Consider the average length of stay of patients discharged from a mental hospital in a year. Suggest how an improvement in the treatment of previously

---

*Source: Questions 4-16, Dr. Colin White, Yale University Dept. of Epidemiology and Biostatistics.

intractable conditions might lead to an increase in the average length of stay of discharged patients.

Question 5

A WHO survey of the ages of children in Morocco who had been given a complete tuberculin test provided the following frequency distribution:

Age	Number of children (in thousands)
8	63
9	38
10	57
11	26
12	44

Question 6

Judging by the death rates of 1950 in the U.S., the safest occupation for males is that of messenger boy.

Question 7

In a study of malignant melanoma among women, the survival rate among women who became pregnant and completed pregnancy after diagnosis was found to be higher than the rate among nonpregnant women of the same age.

Question 8

A study was made of the interval between operation and recurrence in a series of patients with recurrent breast cancer. If operation and recurrence both occurred before the menopause, the mean disease-free interval was shorter than if the operation preceded and the recurrence followed menopause. Can you conclude that the occurrence of menopause has a beneficial effect in post-poning recurrence of breast cancer?

Question 9

Immediately following the 1918 influenza pandemic there was a sharp drop in the tuberculosis mortality rate of the U.S. This proves that an attack of influenza protects against tuberculosis.

Question 10

In Vermont in 1953 divorces were tabulated by length of marriage:

Length of Marriage	No. of Divorces
0 - 4 years	137
5 - 9	117
10 - 14	86
15 - 19	49
20+	90

This table shows that the longer people are married the less apt they are to be divorced, except for a somewhat higher risk after 20 years. Do you agree?

Question 11

The Pearl pregnancy rate is the number of pregnancies per 100 person-years of exposure. It has been used to study the effectiveness of different methods of contraception; it is defined as

$$1200 \; n/m = \text{pregnancy rate per 100 person-years.}$$

$$\text{where } n = \text{total number of accidental pregnancies}$$
$$m = \text{total months of contraceptive exposure.}$$
$$1200 = \text{12 months per year} \times \text{100 women exposed}$$
$$= \text{1200 person-months or 100 person-years.}$$

The longer a group of women is followed, the lower in general is the Pearl pregnancy rate. Why is this?

Question 12

The death rate from rheumatic fever per 100,000 population in the U.S. increased an alarming 133% (from 0.6 to 1.4) between 1948 and 1950. On the other hand, that from nephritis has shown a 68% decline (from 52.5 to 16.6) in the same period. Serious consideration should be given to changing the allocation of health expenditures for those diseases. Do you agree?

Question 13

Hospital data show that the fatality rate from many infectious diseases is lower in epidemic than in sporadic cases.

Question 14

Estimates from burial inscriptions place the average length of life in Roman times at somewhere from 20 to 30 years. These are biased data. Would you justify their use on the grounds that they are the best we have on the length of life at the time of the Roman Empire?

Question 15

Common biases are often given distinctive names. Explain the terms "non-response bias," "memory bias," "selection bias," "interviewer bias," "digit preference," in terms of the questions or problems that each type of bias presents to an investigator.

Question 16

A study by the American Tobacco Institute shows that not all smokers get lung cancer and that not all lung cancer patients have a history of smoking.   They conclude that smoking does not cause lung cancer.

Question 17

A study of cancer deaths in New Mexico in 1966 revealed that the cancer-death rate was remarkably lower than that of the remainder of the U.S.   The authors could not explain this finding.

Question 18

During the implementation of an epidemiologic study, errors in classification of data or selection of study subjects may occur.   The following observations were made during epidemiologic studies.   Specify the type of problem that may occur by indicating MC for misclassification of a variable and NR for non-representative study population.   What would you do if your own study was affected?

a.   You observed a 15% turnover of residents in census tract 37 each year.

b.   One of the blood pressure takers was found to have a hearing deficiency.

c.   The reference serum titer dropped eight-fold in the last 4 weeks.

d.   You found a 20% dropout rate in your study during the year.

e.   The malaria microscopist is color blind.

f.   The refrigeration was off all weekend in your laboratory.

g.   The overall mortality rate for the study has been 6% per year.

h.   You have not been able to standardize a laboratory procedure.

Question 19.

Investigators studied animal-hospital employees who permitted their blood to be tested for serologic evidence of infection (antibody) to Toxocara canis, a microorganism associated with household pets. They concluded that there was a high risk of infection among these employees. Do you think the findings are valid?

Question 20.

A study was made of 120 male employees newly arrived at an overseas branch of a company to determine the incidence of travelers' diarrhea. Nine men developed diarrhea during the first 4 weeks of observation. At the end of the 4-week period 70 of the 120 men were asked whether or not they had been ill; the remainder were not contacted. In order to obtain a sufficient number of persons with diarrheal disease, 50 males who had arrived about the same time as, but were not part of, the original group of 120 were included. All of them had experienced diarrhea. The investigators concluded that the incidence of illness was 59/170 and described the frequency of symptoms and types of organisms cultured from the feces of cases. Are these findings valid?

SUGGESTED RESPONSES
Exercise 12--Bias in Epidemiologic Investigations

1. $AX/A = 912/3792 = 24.1\%$ $BX/B = 660/1860 = 35.5\%$

2. Alternatives available to avoid Berkson's bias:

    Select comparison subjects very carefully. Be aware of differential rates of disease among hospitalized and discharged patients; also between persons who die and those who are autopsied for specified diseases.

    Select comparison subjects from a wide variety of sources--use several different types of hospitals or clinics. This may help to reduce the biased nature (self selection) of patients admitted to a single hospital.

    Use community-based comparison groups.

    Attempt to avoid bias by making the comparison subjects more "representative" of the community or the disease process under study.

3a. Composition or selection of study groups

    1. Incomplete or incorrect sampling frame
    2. Self-selection: volunteers, hospital admissions
    3. Nonresponse, nonparticipation; dropouts
    4. Attrition; loss to follow-up--death, migration
    5. Inadequate sample size or sampling methods
    6. Use of comparison groups that are not comparable to cases

3b. Collection of data

    1. Poorly designed questionnaires or data collection instrument
    2. Inadequate training of interviewers or data collectors
    3. Nonstandard techniques and procedures for data collection and data recording
    4. Variation in interview techniques: depth of probing, leading questions, subjective interpretation of respondents' answers
    5. Insufficient or incorrect period for observation

3c. Respondents

    1. Poor memory or inadequate knowledge or selective recall or incorrect responses
    2. Subjective interpretation of questions
    3. Changing disease status, change of opinion
    4. Reexposure or onset of disease
    5. Placebo effects
    6. Ancillary information not available for all study subjects

3d. Classification

1. Diagnostic criteria incorrect, subjective, inadequate, or imprecise
2. Inconsistent criteria
3. Laboratory or equipment errors: inadequate accuracy and precision

3e. Conclusions

1. Study results are limited only to the study population and similar groups. Extrapolation of the results to the general population or to other subgroups of a population are valid when the investigator demonstrates that the study population is a representative sample of the general population or comparable to other population subgroups.
2. Unsuspected associations, physiologic mechanisms or other sources of error may exist that the investigator did not consider.

Examples of bias

4. It might require a longer duration of hospitalization in order to complete the therapy.

5. There is an excess number of children of ages 8, 10, and 12 compared to the odd numbered ages 9 and 11. This may reflect digit preference unless some unusual occurrence such as epidemic, war, or outmigration reduced the number of children 9 and 11 years of age.

6. Messenger boys are very young. They would be expected to have low mortality. These data need to be age-adjusted to allow meaningful interpretation.

7. Disease may be severe enough to prevent some women from becoming pregnant. Those who completed pregnancy have an additional 9 months of survival by definition. Malignant melanoma is usually a disease of short duration. Nine months additional survival would bias the rate in favor of pregnant women.

8. First, breast cancer pre- and postmenopause may have different causal mechanisms, as shown by the different characteristics of women with these diseases. (Recall the bimodal curve for incidence and mortality by age.) The investigators may be analyzing different disease situations, which should not be considered as equivalent disease states. Second, disease of premenopausal women must have a shorter disease-free interval. Suppose that the average age of diagnosis is age 35 and age at menopause is 40. Recurrent disease before menopause must be disease-free less than 5 years, while postmenopausal recurrence must be greater than 5 years.

   Finally, by definition, recurrent cases indicate that the original therapy was not completely successful. Perhaps those with recurrent illness were more severely ill than those whose recurrence was postponed, or perhaps the former group did not have as good surgery as the latter.

9. Since both diseases have a respiratory component, it may be that influenza killed those persons who might also be at higher risk of dying from tuberculosis.

10. The conclusion is not based upon divorce rates. There is no denominator. All we know are numerators so we cannot calculate rates (the appropriate statistic of risk) of divorce by duration of marriage.

11. The Pearl pregnancy rate was popular for many years until it was shown that it tends to be biased in favor of the less fertile women and/or more successful contraceptors. Those who are less fertile or who are more successful contraceptors contribute a disproportionate amount to the denominator. Fertile women drop out of the study earlier. Therefore, long term follow-up of any contraceptive method may give a better impression of the effectiveness of the method than is warranted.

12. This poses a problem of magnitude. Uncommon diseases may have rates that fluctuate widely due to the presence or absence of only a few cases from one year to another. If one got excited over this "alarming" increase, one might not concentrate necessary efforts on a disease (nephritis) that is 12 times more common. Keep in mind that the actual rate of disease needs to be considered as well as the relative change over time. Perhaps more money should be allocated to nephritis because a major impact has been made upon the disease mortality in a short time.

13. Criteria for admission to a hospital may vary between epidemic and nonepidemic periods. Accuracy of diagnosis may also change in these periods. Health care might be improved because of "more practice."

14. Almost all data may be biased in some way. If we reject any or all biased data then few studies would merit publication. The investigator should, of course, strive to eliminate as much of the bias as possible. In the event that it cannot be eliminated, the investigator should attempt to define and measure the bias, indicating its direction and size and effect on the reported data (over- or underestimate of the true population value). If it cannot be measured then the bias should at least be described so that others will be aware of its presence and can make up their own minds as to the usefulness of the reported data.

15. Nonresponse bias--suppose 60% of the sample respond to your questionnaire. Are the 40% nonrespondents similar or dissimilar to respondents? What effect does nonresponse have on your data? If nonrespondents are similar to respondents then your data will still be representative of the original sample. If not, your data will either be an over- or an underestimate of the variable you are attempting to measure.

Memory-bias--how long will persons remember events? Will cases and comparison subjects be likely to remember events with equal accuracy? Will events subsequent to diagnosis or treatment of a disease distort the subject's recollection of disease-related events or factors occurring prior to onset of the disease?

Selection bias--are volunteers likely to be representative of all persons with a disease? Are hospital records representative of either the type or extent of disease in the community? Are certain factors more likely to result in one person or group of persons being selected for participation in a study than others?

Interviewer bias--do the interviewers record the subjects' responses accurately or do interviewers introduce their own view or opinions about how the question was or should have been answered? How much distortion of the facts is introduced by the interviewer?

Digit preference--there is a tendency for the data to cluster around even digits (0, 2, 4, 6, 8) or 0s and 5s in measurement of certain variables. Do the ages of respondents get rounded off to convenient numbers such as 18, 20, 21, 25, 30, 35, 40?

16. Few things in biology satisfy an all-or-none rule. For example, in the laboratory we speak of the LD-50, or the amount of chemical that constitutes a <u>lethal dose</u> for 50% of a laboratory strain of animals under controlled conditions. If there can be that much variation in laboratory animals, human beings might be expected to show much more variation. Therefore, expectation of an all-or-none phenomena in humans in unrealistic and unlikely to occur because of differences in age, sex, general background, nutritional state, and medical history. The epidemiologic criteria for proving causation (Exercise 9) provides overwhelming evidence of the existence of the association.

17. The population of New Mexico is much younger than the U.S. These data must be age-adjusted at the start of analysis.

18a. N.R. You might have to make great efforts to locate census tract residents to avoid error introduced by dropouts. Denominators may require person-years of observation.

18b. M.C. Get a hearing aid for or replace the observer. Exclude data for which the amount of error cannot be determined.

18c. M.C. Recalibrate lab equipment to a known standard. If equipment is good, get new reference sera that are well standardized. Contact the company that sells it or the person to whom it belongs to get a new supply.

18d. N.R.   Determine reasons for dropout if possible.   Compare characteristics of continuing and drop out persons to estimate the effect of dropouts. Analyze data including all dropouts or excluding them from the denominator.   This will place low and high limits on the observations for the entire study group.

18e. M.C.   Reexamine the slides if available.   If not available compare the color-blind microscopists future results against those of a competent technician to estimate the amount of error.   Apply the error estimates to the color-blind person's earlier work.

18f. M.C.   Laboratory specimens may be ruined.   Plan to initiate a quality assessment of these specimens over the next few days, comparing them to known and useful specimens if available.   Data for damaged specimens may be irretrievably lost.

18g. N.R.   The effect of any loss to follow-up may be minimal or great depending upon whether or not the survivors and decedents differ appreciably with regard to variables causally associated with the disease.

18h. M.C.   If you cannot eliminate the error, then try to measure the amount and its direction.   If the lab test gives hopelessly confusing data you may have to discard the test completely.

19.   Three points would invalidate the findings.   First, the study subjects were actually volunteers.   We have no idea whether or not these persons are a representative sample of the hospital employees, of pet owners, or of the general population.   Thus, we cannot evaluate the exposure experience.   Second, presence of antibody is a measure of prevalence, i.e., infection at some time in the past, rather than incidence.   Thus, we cannot realistically assess the risk of infection.   Third, we are not informed of the expected prevalence (or incidence) of infection among animal-hospital employees, pet owners or the general population.   This would make it difficult to interpret the findings observed for the study group.

20.   Findings are not valid.   We do not know the incidence in the original group.   Substituting 50 cases for persons about whom we have no information is not appropriate.   We do not know whether the 50 added cases were derived from 50 or from a larger number of persons constituting the second cohort which arrived at the location.   We do not know if the 50 added persons were comparable to the original 120 individuals with regard to exposure or susceptibility variables.

EXERCISE 13. EVALUATION OF EPIDEMIOLOGIC REPORTS

Goals

Upon completion of this exercise you should be able to evaluate an epidemiologic or other scientific report in a systematic way.

Methods

I.   OUTLINE FOR EVALUATING AN EPIDEMIOLOGIC REPORT
II. REPORTS TO BE EVALUATED

    A.   Second trimester abortion after vaginal termination of pregnancy.
    B.   The effect of music on pulse-rate, blood pressure, and final exam scores of university students.

Suggested Readings

Sartwell, P., et al. Thromboembolism and oral contraceptives: an epidemiologic case-control study. Am. J. Epidemiol. 90:365-380, 1969.
Blot, W., et al. Frequency of marriage and live birth among survivors prenatally exposed to the atomic bomb. Am. J. Epidemiol. 102:128-135, 1975.
Merson, M., et al. Shigellosis at sea: an outbreak aboard a passenger cruise ship. Am. J. Epidemiol. 101:165-174, 1975.
Patel, C.H. Yoga, and biofeedback in the management of hypertension. The Lancet: 1053-1055, Nov. 10, 1973.

This exercise will provide you with an approach for evaluating scientific reports. It raises questions RELEVANT FOR PLANNING research, FOR PREPARING OR READING a research report, or FOR EVALUATING data or facts upon which some policy decision may be based. These skills are essential to those who participate in research as well as those who "administrate."

It should be kept in mind that NO RESEARCH IS PERFECT. Every study may be constructively criticized. The investigator should attempt to avoid as many sources of error as possible, and to obtain the most precise and valid data that can be collected given the circumstances of the investigation. Because scientific studies are not perfect, we usually reach conclusions and make decisions in THE FACE OF UNCERTAINTY. It is necessary, therefore, to achieve considerable skill in judging the accuracy and validity of scientific observations. The important point is whether or not bias or error in the study design, or the data analysis could have produced the observed finding.

When evaluating a report a single and rigid approach may not be useful for all epidemiologic reports. The questions used in the critique outline are general and some of them may not be applicable to every report. For a particular report, some questions in the outline will be more relevant than others. Also, other important and relevant questions that are not in the outline may occur to you. Use of the outline will guide you through a systematic and logical appraisal of any report.

After studying the outline, read and criticize the two research studies provided. Compare your critical observations with the suggested responses. If your time and interest permit, read and criticize the articles listed in the suggested readings.

A complete and systematic evaluation of a report should include the following:

1. Determination of the objectives, purposes, and rationale of the study.
2. Careful and thorough examination of the methods.
3. Consideration of the data and their method of presentation.
4. Judgment of the conclusions and relevance to the study objectives.
5. Consideration of the sources of error and bias, and ways in which the study could have been improved.

You may also find the outline useful in planning or developing a proposal for a research study! The outline is formulated to stimulate you to think about WHAT WAS DONE and also OTHER WAYS THE STUDY COULD HAVE BEEN DONE.

I. OUTLINE FOR EVALUATING AN EPIDEMIOLOGIC REPORT

A. WHAT IS THE QUESTION BEING ASKED? WHAT IS THE PURPOSE OR OBJECTIVE OF THE REPORT OR STUDY?

1. Is it clearly stated, vague, or unstated?
2. Is the background and magnitude of the problem addressed?
3. What is known about the problem?
4. Is this question or problem a significant health issue?
5. Is the intent to describe a situation or problem, or to test an hypothesis?

B. HOW IS THE STUDY DESIGNED?

1. What information is needed to answer the study question?

   a. Can it be obtained from existing records or is a population survey or experiment needed to obtain new data?
   b. Can the most appropriate information be obtained from a study of mortality or morbidity data, or from surveys?
   c. What variables should be measured? Are they clearly defined and appropriate to the study objectives?
   d. Can exposure to risk or severity of exposure be defined and measured?

2. What is an appropriate format or study design to answer the study question?

   Description of cases (case report or case series)
   Description of surveillance data

Type A (prevalence) study (cross-sectional survey data)
Type C (incidence) study (cohort or prospective study)
Type B (retrospective) study (so called case-comparison or case-control study)
Type C study--experimental study or clinical trial

a.   If sampling is necessary or if it was used, have the following been addressed?

Is the sampling frame described or defined?
Is the sampling frame complete?
Is the sampling method described?
How is the sample size determined?

b.   Is a comparison group(s) necessary or was it used?

Could conclusions be drawn without comparison to a disease-free or unexposed population?
How is the comparison group determined? How is it defined? How are subjects selected? Is the sampling frame complete?
Are comparison group subjects and cases comparable for important study variables? Is matching used (or necessary) for important variables such as age, race, sex, and smoking history?

c.   Are ethical issues such as undue risks to study participants or need for informed consent likely to occur?
d.   Are potential sources of bias or error considered?

What provisions are made to deal with it?
Are special steps taken to assure precision and validity of the needed information or measurements?

3.   Collection of the needed information

a.   How will the information be collected?

(1)   Are existing records from the following sources appropriate for this study? Hospital or clinic records, health agency or health insurance records, illness or disease registries, census data, membership lists or rosters, directories.
(2)   What are appropriate groups from which ill vs. nonill subjects, or exposed (or treated) vs. unexposed (or untreated) subjects can be identified and selected for study?
(3)   How complete is the data source?

b.   Which of the multitude of collection methods is used:

Self-administered questionnaire; interviewers; medical/hospital records abstractors; computer programmers; laboratory technicians; physicians, nurses, midwives, health auxiliaries, paramedics, etc. Are these adequate to obtain accurate information suitable to the study's objective?

c.   Are data collection techniques, questionnaire, and written records described? standardized? validated?

d.   Are diagnostic procedures and laboratory tests described? standardized? validated?

e.   Is there adequate description of the equipment or instruments used? Is the equipment standardized?

f.   Are data collectors or observers "blinded" during data collection or is blinding not necessary or not feasible?

4.   How are the data analyzed?

a.   Are definitions of terms and diagnostic criteria clear and appropriate?

b.   Are outcome measures specified?

c.   Are measurements and criteria consistent for all subjects? Are they relevant to the study objectives?

d.   Are categories/groupings/classification of variables appropriate for and relevant to the study objectives?

5.   Are findings clearly presented and readily understandable?

a.   Are the findings presented consistently? Are there discrepancies between different tables or graphs? Have all relevant observations been made for each table or graph?

b.   Are there errors in the tables? Do the data for different tables refer to the same number of individuals? If some data are left out, are reasons given?

c.   Are the appropriate statistical tests performed? Are the results correctly interpreted?

d.   Are confounding variables considered? Have case-comparison subjects been demonstrated to be comparable for important variables?

e.   Is "adjustment" (for age, sex, smoking, etc.) necessary to compensate for important differences between cases and comparison group subjects?

C.   WHAT WERE THE CONCLUSIONS?

1.   Do the data justify the conclusions?

2.   Are conclusions appropriate to the study objectives and the population selected for study?

3. Can the conclusions be extrapolated from the study population to the general population? Are these justified or reasonable? Is the population chosen for study representative of the disease or the population at risk?

D. WHAT INSIGHT OR ADDITIONAL INFORMATION IS PROVIDED BY THE DISCUSSION?

1. Is there a discussion of the limitations, errors, bias, or problems encountered in the course of the study? Are the findings discussed in relation to these problems?
2. Are alternative explanations of the findings considered?
3. Is the effect of missing data or confounding variables considered?

E. HOW COULD THIS STUDY HAVE BEEN IMPROVED?

II. REPORTS TO BE EVALUATED

In order to gain some experience in evaluating scientific reports two articles are reproduced from the scientific literature. Read and discuss the articles in the space provided at the conclusion of each paper.

A. Second Trimester Abortion after Vaginal Termination of Pregnancy.

Introduction

The Abortion Act (1967) has resulted in a twentyfold increase in the number of legal terminations of pregnancy in the United Kingdom. Attention has been drawn to the hazards associated with termination in the second trimester, and termination by the vaginal route in the first trimester is usually recommended because of its low maternal mortality and morbidity rates. However, two papers have suggested that vaginal terminations, as performed in the United Kingdom, are not as free from morbidity as had been claimed, and that haemorrhage, cervical laceration, perforation of the uterus, infection, and paralytic ileus are not infrequent complications.

We have investigated our clinical impression that a further complication of vaginal termination is an increased risk of second-trimester abortion or premature labour in a subsequent pregnancy.

Method

All patients who attended Queen Charlotte's Hospital antenatally and who delivered during 1971 were asked at their booking visit for a full obstetric history. Specific questions were asked about all previous miscarriages and abortions to ascertain whether they were spontaneous or had been artificially induced. As much detail as possible concerning any therapeutic abortion was obtained, with emphasis

Source: Wright, C.S.W., et al., The Lancet 1:1278, 1972.

on the length of gestation, method of termination, and the hospital in which termination was performed.

We defined a second-trimester abortion as one occurring spontaneously from the fifteenth to the twenty-seventh week inclusive, in which there was no evidence of maceration or abnormality of the fetus. A premature labour was any labour that occurred spontaneously before the thirty-seventh week of pregnancy.

To assess the effects of vaginal termination on subsequent obstetric-performance, the patients were divided into three groups:

Group A includes only those patients booking for confinement whose preceding pregnancy had been terminated vaginally. To reduce the number of factors which might influence the incidence of complications after termination, we have excluded from group A all patients who gave a history of pregnancy (other than the current one) after termination.

Group B consists of age-matched control patients who had had one spontaneous miscarriage before the present pregnancy.

Group C contains all the deliveries or abortions occurring within the period of study, except group-A patients.

Results

During 1971, a total of 3314 patients delivered or aborted at this hospital. There were 91 patients in groups A and B and 3223 patients in group C.

Group A

Of the 91 patients, 83 (91%) had had no previous pregnancy other than the one which had been terminated (Table 1). Of the 8

Table 1. Group A: obstetric history.

	No. of patients
No. of pregnancies before termination of pregnancy:	
0	83 (91%)
1	4 (4%)
2	2
3	2
No. of terminations before booking:	
1	84 (91%)
2	5 (6%)
3	1
4	1

remaining patients all had been delivered of normal full-term babies before a pregnancy termination. Eighty-four (91%) of the patients in group A had only one previous termination of pregnancy, while 1 patient had had as many as four successive terminations.

Only 19 patients (21%) were aborted in National Health Service hospitals; the remainder were terminated privately (64 patients) or abroad (8 patients).

Table 2. Clinical details of abnormal cases in group A.

Case no.	Age (yr.)	Parity	Termination of pregnancy (wk.)	Time of labour or abortion (wk.)	Comment[ψ]
Intrauterine death:					
1	23	0^{+1}	10 (private 1968)	*	
Premature labour:					
2	16	0^{+1}	12 (private 1968)	35	Live infant, b.w. 2.5 kg.
3	21	0^{+1}	12 (private 1969)	35	Live infant, b.w. 2.3 kb.
4	27	0^{+2}	12 (private 1970)	35	Live infant, b.w. 1.9 kg.
5	25	0^{+1}	10 (private 1968)	34	Live infant,
Cervical incompetence:					
6	22	0^{+1}	13 (private 1970)	†	---
Second-trimester abortion:					
7	26	0^{+3}	10 (private 1964) / 10 (private 1965)	23	---
8	21	0^{+1}	18 (private 1970)	26	Infant lived 2 days
9	30	0^{+2}	8 (abroad 1958)	16	---
10	26	0^{+1}	10 (abroad 1966)	20	---
11	24	1^{+1}	12 (private 1970)	17	---
12	20	0^{+1}	12 (N.H.S. 1969)	18	---
13	37	3^{+1}	11 (N.H.S. 1968)	24	---
14	22	0^{+1}	12 (private 1968)	18	---

*Case 1. Rhesus antibodies at booking. Induction of labour intended at 36 weeks. Intrauterine death on day of induction.
†Case 6. Cervix 2 cm. dilated at booking at 13 weeks' gestation. Cervical suture inserted at 15 weeks; removed at 38 weeks. Spontaneous delivery.
ψb.w. = birth-weight.

From group A, 8 (9%) had a spontaneous second-trimester abortion and 1 had a clinically incompetent cervix that required a suture. There were no first-trimester abortions. Four patients went into premature labour, and there was 1 intrauterine death caused by rhesus incompatibility. Clinical details of the abnormal cases are given in Table 2.

Group B

Of the 91 control patients, 1 had a spontaneous second-trimester abortion and 4 had a first-trimester abortion; 1 patient went into premature labour and there were no stillbirths.

There was a statistically significant increase in the number of second-trimester abortions in group A compared with group B ($\chi^2=4.21$ [Yates' correction], $p<0.05$).

Group C

Out of the 3223 confinements in this group, there were 32 first-trimester abortions (1%) and 42 second-trimester abortions. After excluding 12 pregnancies ending in the second trimester because of missed abortion, abruptio placentae, or intrauterine death, there were 30 spontaneous second-trimester abortions--an incidence of 0.9%. 8 of these 30 patients had already had a previous second-trimester abortion; of the remaining 22, 3 had had a vaginal termination of pregnancy, though not immediately before the aborted pregnancy (thus not qualifying for group A).

215 patients (6.7%) went into premature labour and there were 36 stillbirths (1.1%).

Discussion

During 1971 in Queen Charlotte's Hospital there was a tenfold increase in the number of second-trimester abortions in pregnancies which followed a vaginal termination of pregnancy, compared with all patients who delivered in the same year. This increase strongly indicates that temporary or permanent cervical incompetence is induced by the procedure of dilatation of the cervix during termination. This is further suggested by the fact that a control group had significantly fewer second-trimester abortions. The only important difference between the two groups was that the previous-termination patients had had forcible dilatation of the cervix. This result agrees with the finding of Stallworthy et al. that 4-8% of patients had cervical lacerations after vaginal termination of pregnancy. Our abortion-rate of 9% after this procedure is considerably below the 30-40% rate reported by Kotasek, who did not give details of how his figure was determined. The numbers in group A are small because

we did not make a retrospective study of this subject. In our experience a significant number of patients do not admit to previous
terminations, or refer to them as miscarriages unless specifically
questioned about this aspect of their obstetric history. If the 9%
incidence of second-trimester abortion in our study is correct, then
an additional 10,000 second-trimester abortions may take place annually in the U.K. over the next few years.

We found no difference between the number of subsequent abortions
in patients terminated privately and under the National Health Service. Of the 8 patients in group A who aborted, only 1 had previously been terminated before 10 weeks' menstrual age. Perhaps
earlier termination using the Karman catheter will reduce the risk of
cervical damage. In our study previous termination was not associated with an increased incidence of premature labour or other complications of pregnancy.

We believe that all patients who have had a vaginal termination of
pregnancy should be judged as being at risk of having a second-
trimester abortion in their subsequent pregnancy. Digital assessment of the cervix should be performed every two weeks in the subsequent pregnancy for signs of cervical incompetence. This assessment resulted in the early diagnosis and successful treatment of cervical incompetence in case 6 (Table 2).

Summary

A tenfold increase in the incidence of second-trimester abortion has
been demonstrated in pregnancies which followed vaginal termination
of pregnancy. There was no increase in the incidence of other obstetric abnormalities. Vaginal termination of pregnancy by present
techniques seems to induce cervical incompetence in a succeeding
pregnancy.

Question 1

Evaluate the article.

B.   The effect of music on pulse-rate, blood pressure, and final exam scores of university students.

Introduction

Many people are familiar with the tensions, nervousness, and apprehensive uneasiness which students experience in the process of taking a final academic examination. Even prior to taking a written examination, many students will stay up half the night studying and preparing for the ordeal. Hence, sleep, proper relaxation, and diet may suffer to some extent.

It is well-known that music plays an important role in physical education activities where proper cadence and rhythmic patterns are necessary. Some medical clinics and hospitals also use music as a therapeutic device in aiding the mentally handicapped, especially those who may display symptoms of anxiety, depression, irritability, and other emotional instabilities.

Purpose of Study

The basic purpose of this study was to ascertain the effect that music might have on pulse-rate, blood-pressure, and final academic scores of a group of university students.

The Sampling Population

A total of 254 university students, 124 being males and 130 being females, between the ages of 20 and 31 volunteered for the project. The study took place at DePaul University, Chicago, Illinois, during 1974-75. The names of the students remain <u>confidential</u>.

Procedure of Study

The 254 students were divided into three groups, namely, a control group, which was administered a traditional final examination; an experimental group, administered an examination accompanied by music as a background (Rock and Roll music) and finally, a second experimental group taking an examination while accompanied by classical music. The examination took some 2½ hours to complete and all three groups took the same examination, approximately the same hours of the day, in the same room and with the same proctor administering and scoring the final examination.

Source: Blanchard, B.E., Journal of Sports Medicine 19:305, 1979.

The control and the two experimental groups were very carefully equated as to age, weight, and educational background. The only variables permitted to fluctuate, were the pulse-rate, blood-pressure, and the final grades earned in the examination.

The pulse-rate and blood-pressure were taken by a registered nurse and a medical technician, before, during, and after the final examination. All pulse-rates and blood-pressures were taken in the sitting position. In comparing the control and experimental groups, we accept the null hypothesis at the 1 percent [criterion] of significance.

Discussion

Table 1 provides a summary of the findings. It is interesting to note that prior to the examination, the pulse-rates of all three groups were relatively similar, with means of 69.1, 72.3, and 73.5, while the blood-pressure were 118/58, 122/65, and 131/68. During the examination, about 1½ hours of writing time, the blood-pressures of the control group and two experimental groups, rose to a mean of 152/113, 127/74, and 136/73, respectively. As one may note, the control group's mean systolic pressure increased by 34, while the diastolic pressure rose by 55.

Some three to four minutes following completion of the examination, the mean pulse-rate of the control group registered 80.4 (it was 69.1 at the start of the examination); the mean blood-pressure of the control group was 147/108. It was 118/58 when the exam began. The blood-pressure reading following the examination indicates an extremely poor condition of the recuperative power of the heart.

Both of the experimental groups, accompanied by music, displayed excellent recuperative activity of the heart. For example, the mean pulse-rates at the beginning of the examination registered 72.3 and 73.5; upon termination of the exam, some three to four minutes after completion of writing, the mean pulse-rates showed readings of 72.0 and 73.1. The mean blood pressure readings before and after the exam were 122/65 and 131/68 (before) and 122/68 and 131/69 (after).

In testing the differences between the means of the pulse-rates and blood-pressures of the control versus the two experimental groups at the conclusion of the examination, we must reject the null hypothesis at the 1 percent level, thus indicating a real statistical significant differences and not a chance variation.

It is interesting to note the findings of the control group mean examination score as compared to the two experimental group scores. The difference between the mean exam score of the control group, namely, 215.9 and the two experimental group mean scores of 250.9 and 253.2 are statistically significant at the 1 percent level. We must therefore reject the null hypothesis.

Conclusions

Academic competition for grades is conducted with such intensity in higher education that there is always the potential danger of over-exhaustion, nervous stress, anxiety, and uneasiness on the part of the examinee.

Higher education, as far as traditional examinations are concerned, may be considered a high risk factor, especially as it may relate to hypertension. University level testing may be exceeding the safety limit of student health. Colleges and universities may be the breeding ground for the socially-emotionally maladjusted and the neurotic. The traditional examination should be eliminated promptly.

Summary

The basic purpose of this study was to ascertain the effect that music might have on pulse-rate, blood-pressure, and final academic scores of a group of university students.

The vital importance of music is well-known to those professional people engaged in physical education as well as to the many dedicated individuals associated with clinics and hospitals who assist the mentally handicapped, the retarded, and those persons who may have emotional problems.

The sampling population in this study consisted of 254 university students between the ages of 20 and 31 who volunteered to participate in the research project. The study took place in an urban university during 1974-75.

The procedure involved in this study assembled the 254 students into three groups, namely, a control group (subject to no music), an experimental group (subject to Rock and Roll music) and a third experimental group (subject to classical music). The music was used as a background while the students engaged in taking a final examination in subject matter. All of the students were very carefully equated as to age, educational background, weight, and varied emotional tendencies. The pulse-rate and blood-pressure were taken of each student before, during, and following the final academic examination.

Results of the study appear to suggest several inferences, namely: (1) Music seems to act as a general factor in critical thinking by co-ordinating the thinking of students. For example, students earned higher grades who had music as an accompaniment; (2) Music tends to minimize the nervous states of students while taking an examination; (3) Colleges and universities may be the breeding grounds for the socially emotionally maladjusted and the neurotic and (4) Institutions of higher education may be a risk as far as health factors are concerned as traditional examinations (minus musical background) may be encouraging hypertension among our American youth.

Table 1. Comparative analysis: age, weight, pulse-rate, blood-pressure and final academic examination scores.

Groups	Type of measure	Age	Weight	Before exam		During exam BP[1]	After exam[2]		Scores: final academic exam[3]
				Pulse[1]	BP[1]		Pulse[2]	BP[2]	
Conventional exam, no music (#=82)	Range-Low -High Midpoint	21 31 25.3	109 165 130.5	58 78 69.1	110/55 126/63 118/58	146/108 159/119 152/113	70 91 80.4	138/106 156/111 147/108	181 265 215.9
Experimental exam, rock & roll (#=87)	Range-Low -High Midpoint	22 29 25.1	110 172 139.7	56 83 72.3	115/62 130/70 122/65	120/68 135/81 127/74	61 87 72.0	115/60 131/71 122/68	182 290 250.9
Experimental exam, classical (#=85)	Range-Low -High Midpoint	20 30 25.4	109 158 135.6	61 86 73.5	128/64 134/72 131/68	132/69 141/78 136/73	65 90 73.1	129/65 135/72 131/69	196 293 253.2

[1]The pulse-rate and blood-pressure were taken in the sitting position.
[2]The pulse-rate and blood-pressure were taken three to four minutes on completion of the exam.
[3]The maximum score attainable in the examination was 300.
R refers to the range; M refers to the mean; # refers to the number of individuals participating.

Question 2

Evaluate the article.

SUGGESTED RESPONSES
Exercise 13--Evaluation of Epidemiologic Studies

A. Second trimester abortion after vaginal termination of pregnancy.

The following discussion will focus on specific details of this study's design that could affect the quality of the clinical observations.

Purpose, background, and rationale

The purpose of the study was to determine if there was an increased risk of second-trimester abortion or premature labor in women with prior induced abortion. The intent is clearly to test an hypothesis but the authors do not state a null hypothesis. The rationale for the study is evident; there has been a marked increase in legal abortion in England after 1967, and there are two published papers calling attention to potential problems in subsequent pregnancy of women with a prior induced abortion.

Population and sample size needed for study

The correct denominators for this abortion study should be "all pregnant women with (cases) and without (controls) a history of induced abortion," or representative samples chosen at random from each of those populations. If one is to draw valid conclusions, the persons studied must satisfy these denominator requirements. It has not been demonstrated that the participants of this study were selected in any systematic or random manner, or that they are representative of either the "case" (exposed) or "control" (unexposed) populations. The only criterion stated for inclusion in the study is that they registered at the Queen Charlotte Maternity Hospital in 1971.

Furthermore, the presentation of data clearly marked "cases" and "controls" implies that those studied are similar with respect to all important variables affecting pregnancy outcome. Although cases and controls were matched for age, they have not been compared for other health, social, or demographic variables which might influence the rate of fetal loss, implying that the investigators believed no other variable except a history of induced abortion was important in the study of etiologic factors in fetal loss.

A series of highly selective factors including the quantity and quality of physicians, the patients, and their diseases, and the social and economic variables affect the operation of hospitals. Because these factors differ from place to place, data from different sources are not necessarily representative of the general population, or readily comparable. Selection of cases and/or controls from hospitals which reflect these complex factors may bias the clinical observations and lead to incorrect conclusions.

It is well known that the majority of induced abortions are performed on women who have living children, i.e., abortion is used to limit family size and/or achieve better spacing between pregnancies. To facilitate analysis, Wright et al. used criteria such that 91% of those categorized as cases were childless. Childless women with a previous "unwanted" pregnancy might be especially concerned about the outcome of a subsequent "wanted" pregnancy and therefore quite likely to seek early antenatal care and/or attend a sophisticated specialty hospital well known for excellent care. In order to overcome the difficulty of obtaining random or representative samples from single hospital sources, investigators should attempt to collect data from several sources and include a greater variety of patients among cases and controls. This would lend greater weight to the findings and make them more applicable to the general population.

Determination of sample size using established statistical sampling theory depends upon the level at which statistical significance is to be tested and power of the test used. The sample size may therefore vary with the hypothesis to be tested. Study of the sequelae of induced abortion would require a minimum of several hundreds of cases. A series of 91 cases is not a large enough sample of the prevalent population to draw valid conclusions about the sequelae of induced abortion.

Variables related to the selection of a cohort for prospective study

A cohort, or prospective study, is the most fruitful way to investigate the possible sequelae of induced abortion. Because age is known to be among the most important correlates in the etiology of spontaneous abortion, it should play a primary role in the selection of cases and controls. Furthermore, the implication that instrumental dilatation of the cervix during induced abortion produces irreversible changes raises the issue of the amount of dilatation used at the time of the induced abortion. It is not possible to document this variable except through examination of the operative records of that surgical procedure, which apparently were unavailable. However, due to the propensity for tissue to recover from injury, it is possible that the time interval between the induced abortion and subsequent pregnancy might affect the outcome of that pregnancy. This factor should have been addressed.

Several cohorts can be defined using the variables of age and interval prior to the subsequent pregnancy. Data reported for the eight cases who experienced second-trimester abortions reveals that they varied in age at the time of induced abortion (16-33) and in the interval between that abortion and the subsequent pregnancy whose outcome was studied (2-14 years). This indicates that women were not selected to represent a cohort of women with well-defined characteristics for these variables. The significance of the study's findings may be questioned because the data cannot be clearly related to variables that appear associated with pregnancy outcome.

Completeness of data

The estimates of the rate of spontaneous abortions among cases and controls are likely to be inaccurate because some data may have been lost to study. The following reasons are most likely to have occurred:

(a) Because some spontaneous abortion probably occurred prior to the date at which a woman might have registered, not all of the women who became pregnant were potentially available for registration.

(b) Not all women who registered were necessarily followed to the completion of pregnancy. Spontaneous abortions that may have occurred subsequent to the registration date could have been treated in places other than Queen Charlotte Maternity Hospital. Similarly, some women could have a completed pregnancy resulting in normal full-term delivery at a different hospital.

If these factors affected "cases" and "controls" to different degrees, the differences in rates between the groups could be either inflated or diminished.

The quality of the participants' responses at registration is also an important factor because it determines the classification of women regarding their induced-abortion status. Because of the difficulty of getting reliable pregnancy histories by interview, it is likely that some women would deny having an induced abortion when they actually had experienced such an operation. These women would be misclassified as "controls," and would increase the size of the control group. Since their pregnancies did not spontaneously abort, misclassification would lead to an underestimate of the spontaneous abortion rate among women without a history of an induced abortion. This would inflate any actual difference which might exist between spontaneous abortion rates in "true cases" and "true controls."

Estimates are not included about the completeness of their data or the effect of misclassification on the results.

Equal duration of observation among cases and controls

Reported data do not indicate the duration of observation for cases and controls. If cases and controls were not observed for equal periods of time antenatally, comparison of the groups is not theoretically or statistically valid. The group that was observed for a shorter period of time would be subject to lower rates of fetal loss compared to the group with longer observation. Patients who registered at earlier gestational age would have a longer exposure to the risk of pregnancy and greater likelihood of being selected in the study than those registering at later gestational age, because some of the latter may be lost to the study due to early spontaneous abortion.

Usefulness of "trimester of pregnancy" as an objective interval of risk

Both the length of gestation and the expected date of delivery (confinement-EDC) are determined from the date of the last menstrual period, which is used as an index of the date of conception. The fallacy of this assumption casts doubt on the clinicians' accuracy in determining the conception date. Furthermore, because pregnancy is a continuous process, the concept that it may be classified into separate trimesters with clearly identified cut-off points is both arbitrary and misleading, and would be difficult to support as a valid objective unit of measurement. Regardless of possible differences in the duration of observation for cases and controls, and in view of the continuous nature of pregnancy, it is reasonable to reexamine the data with respect to total spontaneous abortions (see revised Table 1 below). Such an analysis seriously weakens the validity of the study's conclusion.

It is also possible that patients who registered at earlier gestational age might have a more accurate determination of the length of gestation than patients who register at later gestational age. However, no useful information regarding the gestational age at entry into the study, for either cases or controls, is provided.

Revised Table 1. Spontaneous abortion by induced abortion status.

| | Number of Women | Spontaneous Abortion | | |
		First trimester	Second trimester	Total
Cases (Group A) with previous induced abortion	91	0	8	8
Controls (Broup B) no previous induced abortion	91	4	1	5

Circumstances of induced abortion

No information concerning the prior induced abortion is provided. This is disturbing since it is suggested that the surgical termination predisposes to fetal loss in subsequent pregnancy. Some of the women in the study who did suffer fetal loss, apparently had illegal induced abortions (performed prior to 1967 or done abroad) and some may have been performed by unqualified persons.

Etiology of spontaneous abortion

The authors do not indicate consideration of any of the multiple causes of spontaneous abortion that might, in fact, have caused the fetal loss among cases. These causes include maternal age, chromosome aberrations, Rh incompatibility between maternal and fetal blood, a variety of pelvic microorganisms, nutritional and metabolic factors, and smoking.

Discussion and conclusions

Data from the U.S. and other places do not show high complication rates for early legal terminations of pregnancy. This suggests that there may be differences in technical ability of abortionists. In addition, there are several techniques for terminating pregnancy, including dilatation and curettage (D&C) and suction or vacuum aspiration. Complication rates are somewhat higher in D&C than with suction. The reports of high complication rates that led to the research at Queen Charlotte's Hospital may reflect a high proportion of D&C rather than suction aspiration terminations. Lastly, there are some data to suggest that there may be an increased risk of second-trimester fetal loss in women who have had multiple prior induced abortions. It is difficult to interpret the present study's findings in comparison to other research because of several problems in study design.

The nonrandom selection of participants and/or factors apparently omitted from this study design could contribute to the differences in findings between the British and other studies, although it is not possible to specify which of the above account for the differences. Reexamination of the conclusions may be necessary, in view of the growing evidence that induced abortion is a relatively safe surgical procedure. One must wonder about the factors that contributed to higher morbidity among English women in this study.

The authors make a subtle transition in generalizing their findings from the past to the present. Their findings refer to some of the induced abortion that occurred in the past, and it should not be assumed that the risks are similar to those for induced abortions currently being performed. Factors such as improved surgical techniques (vacuum aspiration), better training and a greater amount of abortion experience on the part of physicians have combined to change the risks associated with induced abortion.

This study concluded that induced abortion might be causally related to second-trimester spontaneous abortion in the subsequent pregnancy. The implications are serious in view of the widespread use of induced abortion to terminate unwanted pregnancy. Because these findings disagree with other studies that show the relative safety of induced abortion, the effects of nonrandom selection of participants and/or other apparent omissions of epidemiological principles of study design must be considered. These omissions could have biased the data and erroneously led to the conclusion that fetal loss might be caused by a previous induced abortion.

Although this study may be criticized on many methodologic points, how much of the excess of second-trimester abortions to induced-abortion patients can be explained away because of the methodological problems? If some of the methodologic shortcomings act in opposite directions they might be expected to cancel out one another. However, a tenfold excess is not easily explained away. Although the study is not well designed, the association may be so strong that even a poorly designed study will uncover "the truth."

Reexamination of the data and also carefully conducted prospective studies would seem to be necessary.

B.   The effect of music on pulse-rate, blood pressure, and final exam scores of university students.

Purpose

The objective of this study is to determine whether music has an effect on blood pressure, pulse rates, and academic performance. The purpose of the study is not stated in the form of an hypothesis. However, it is obvious that the independent variable is music and that there are three dependent variables, namely, pulse rate, blood pressure, and examination scores of students.

Background, introduction, rationale for the study.

The introduction states an anecdotal observation and provides no review of the literature on this subject. While the observations are interesting, there is no scientific evidence presented to support or discredit the validity of the observations. Finally, the author makes no mention of a biologic mechanism through which music could exert its effects.

Research design

The population used for study is young adult university students. No mention is made of how the students were selected, although we might infer that this was either one large class or several smaller classes of students enrolled in the same course. There is no indication that the 254 students are a representative sample of the entire student enrollment of DePaul University or even that they are representative of all students taking a particular course. Furthermore, we are not told how the students were assigned to each of the three experimental groups. Was assignment voluntarily? Was it done randomly?

We are told that some procedure was used whereby the three groups were equated for age, weight, and educational background, although it is not clear whether the latter refers to the academic program, academic performance, or merely that the groups were composed of equal numbers of freshmen, sophomores, juniors, and senior year students. While these variables would have some relation to pulse rate, blood pressure, and final examination grades many other factors may also be related but have not been considered in the research design.

Observations to be made.

Blood pressures and pulse rates were measured by health professionals, but there is no indication that there was any standardized procedure followed, other than making observations of subjects in the sitting positon. Did the observers have any special training for taking blood pressure measurement? Were observers rated for digit preference? For visual and auditory acuity?

No mention is made about the type of equipment used and whether or not it was standardized? All of these points relate to the accuracy of the observations of blood pressure, i.e., the precision and validity of the measurements.

In order to achieve some uniformity, the examination was given in the same room, at the same hour of the day and with the same proctor. We do not know if the proctor was aware of the purpose of the study. If so, the proctor might score the exams subjectively if the exam included essay or open-ended questions. Of more importance is the fact that the exam had to be given on different days. It is possible that students of the first group communicated information about the exam to the second and/or third groups. No mention is made of precautions to prevent this possibility.

Finally, no mention is made about validation of test scores. Any one who has ever graded examinations is aware that the person grading may be subject to fatigue after reviewing a large number of tests. In addition, as one becomes familiar with the answers that students give, the grader's standard of excellence might change. Scores of exams graded earlier might be lower than those graded later. Unless the test is a short answer objective examination some grader bias might influence the test scores. No mention is made that test scores were validated or reproduced by a second grader.

With regard to the music selected, we do not know what compositions were played or at what sound level they were played. The terms "rock and roll" and "classical" music are vague. They imply loud, fast, rhythmic music contrasted with soft, melodic strains. Yet we can easily think of rock and roll tunes that are soft and not raucous, and classical music that is loud and unharmonious. Again, the procedure of study is notable for what we are not told. Finally, the statement regarding the null hypothesis implies that the error (type I error) is to be tested at the 0.01 criterion of significance. This implies that the sample size was explicitly calculated to be 254 in order to detect differences between control and experimental groups at this level of statistical significance. This is a somewhat different situation than that of testing the differences between scores of control and experimental groups and discovering that the p value is <0.01. The author is not clear whether or not the sample size has been calculated to detect differences with an α error of 1 percent or the test results fortuitously were statistically significant at p<0.01.

Presentation of findings

Number and age distributions of the three groups appears to be similar. The range in body weight is also similar but group 2 members are heavier than the control group.

Test results show that the controls did poorly compared to the music groups. Of interest is that the low scores of groups 1 and 2 were similar (181-182) and that the highest scores of groups 2 and 3 were similar (290-293). From the range we can say that the smarter students in groups 2 and 3 did better than the smart ones of group 1. The poorer students of groups 1 and 2 scored the same but the poorer students of group 3 did much better (196 vs. 181). We cannot exclude the possibility that students did communicate information about the exam to each other. Thus, if group 1 took the exam first, it might account for their poorer achievement.

In a different vein, if we propose that the soothing quality of music is related to academic performance we might expect to see a stepwise increase in score from the control (low score) to rock and roll (intermediate) to classical music groups (high score). The differences between mean scores of rock and roll and classical groups are negligible, however.

With regard to pulse and blood pressure scores all groups showed a rise during the exam and a decrease following the exam; however, the control groups rise was much greater. Pre- and postexam results were similar for groups 2 and 3. Of course, the presence of music may play a role in these results but if group 1 was the first to take the exam, then this might also be a factor. In addition to possible communication between students, groups 2 and 3 also had one or more days of additional study time to prepare for the final exams. This could also affect test results as well as contributing to the "anxiety" of control group students.

A subtle problem exists in presentation of blood pressure results. These are given as ranges for the group, rather than for individuals. It is unlikely that the systolic and diastolic scores are given for individuals. The data might better be presented as scatter diagrams, whereby we could see the change in blood pressure or pulse for individuals.

Conclusions and summary

The conclusions are not at all appropriate to this study. The students are not necessarily a representative sample of all university students. The sources of error and omissions in the study design raise doubts about the validity of the data. The biologic mechanism through which music might exert an effect has not been demonstrated. The conclusions (3 and 4) are unrelated to the original purpose of this study, and there is not a shred of evidence to support conclusions 3 and 4.

In summary, this article raises an interesting question but is unable to shed much light on the answer due to defects and omissions in the design. Improvement in the study design along the lines of the critical points indicated would be a useful endeavor.

EXERCISE 14. USES AND APPLICATIONS OF EPIDEMIOLOGY

You have completed the introduction to the basic principles of epidemiology and considered many of the issues of concern to epidemiologists. The purpose of this exercise is to demonstrate several applications and uses of epidemiology, which have not yet been discussed.

Goals

Upon completion of this exercise you should understand (1) the notion of surveillance, (2) the concept of risk factors in the prevention or control of disease, and (3) the relevance of epidemiology to health services activities and decision-making.

Methods

In order to achieve these goals you will need to understand

I.   WHO NEEDS EPIDEMIOLOGY?
II. SURVEILLANCE
III. RISK FACTORS AND PREVENTION OF DISEASE

    A.   A Study of Risk Factors In Fatal Coronary Heart Disease
    B.   The Coronary Risk Profile

IV. EPIDEMIOLOGY IN HEALTH SERVICES RESEARCH

Terms

Target population, high-risk group, risk factor, record linkage.

Suggested readings

Morris, J.N., Uses of Epidemiology, 3rd ed. E.S. Livingstone, London, 1975.
Langmuir, A.D., Evolution of the concept of surveillance in the U.S. Proc. Roy. Soc. Med. 64:681, 1971.
Langmuir, A.D., The surveillance of communicsble diseases of national importance, New Eng. J. Med. 268:182, 1963.
Langmuir, A.D., William Farr: Founder of modern concepts of surveillance, Int. J. Epidemiol. 5:13, 1976.
Acheson, E.D., and Fairbairn, A.S., Uses of Epidemiology in Planning Health Services, Int. Epidemiol. Association, 1973.

I.   WHO NEEDS EPIDEMIOLOGY?

An epidemiologist has stated his case for why the world and public health, and medicine in particular, need epidemiology and its methods (Morris, 1975).

> Epidemiology is the Cinderella of the medical sciences. The proposition might, however, be advanced that public health needs more epidemiology, and so does medicine as a whole, and, it may be said,

society at large. Public Health needs more epidemiology--this is the most obvious intellectual basis for its further advance. Epidemiology, moreover, as a tried instrument of research--with its modern developments in sampling and surveys, small-number statistics, the follow-up of cohorts, international comparisons, field experiment, and family study; and with its extensions to problems of genetics as well as environment, to physiological norms as well as disease, the psychological as well as the physical, morbidity as well as mortality-- epidemiology now offers the possibility of a new era of collaboration between public health workers and clinical medicine. Such a collaboration could be on equal terms, each making their particular contribution to the joint solving of problems.

One of the most urgent social needs of the day is to identify rules of healthy living that might do for us what Snow and others did for the Victorians, and help to reduce the burden of illness in middle and old age, which is so characteristic a feature of our society. There is no indication whatever that the experimental sciences alone will be able to produce the necessary guidance. Collaboration between clinician, laboratory scientist, and epidemiologist might be more successful. The possibilities are at present unlimited, if often neglected.

The applications of epidemiology involve looking at patterns of occurrence of disease in a population and the determinants of the occurrence, and provide information for these tasks:

1.   determining the etiology of disease
2.   determining causes of disease
3.   identifying high-risk persons
4.   controlling and preventing disease
5.   planning and evaluating health care delivery services with regard to the impact they have on the health of the population.

To accomplish these tasks epidemiologic methods are used in:

1.   investigation of outbreaks or epidemics
2.   studies with various designs and surveys to obtain incidence and prevalence measurements, risk, etc.
3.   experimental trials to determine the effectiveness of drugs, vaccines, or other types of therapy
4.   registries of people with known disease, i.e., cancer registries, birth defect registries
5.   early detection or screening for disease
6.   surveillance of a community for disease occurrence
7.   monitoring and evaluating the impact of health care systems.

Morris summarizes the applications and goals for epidemiology as follows:

1. To study the <u>history</u> of the health of populations, and of the rise and <u>fall of</u> diseases and changes in their character.
2. To <u>diagnose the health of the community</u>, and the condition of people, to measure the present dimensions and distribution of ill-health in terms of incidence, prevalence, and mortality.
3. To study the <u>working of health services</u> with a view to their improvement. Describe needs and demand, current supply of services, how they are utilized, success in reaching standards, success in improving health.
4. To estimate from the group experience what are the <u>individual risks</u> and chances (on average) of disease, accident, and defect.
5. To <u>complete the clinical picture</u> of chronic disease, and describe <u>its natural history</u>.
6. To <u>identify syndromes</u> by describing the distribution, association, and dissociation of clinical phenomena in the population.
7. To <u>search for causes</u> of health and disease by studying the incidence in different groups, defined in terms of their composition, their inheritance and experience, their behavior, and environment.

Although there are differences in how the "application pie" is cut, most epidemiologists agree that the major goal is to decrease the rate of morbidity and mortality in a population and to improve the health status of the community.

In the preceding exercises you have applied the principles and techniques of epidemiology to a variety of problems:

1. the study of disease patterns;
2. the investigation of epidemics;
3. the determination of etiology and criteria of causation of disease;
4. the assessment of risk;
5. the design of studies to describe, identify, and study factors associated with the occurrence of disease;
6. assessing the health of a population through the use of incidence and prevalence measures;
7. evaluating the quality of epidemiologic or other health and research reports.

II. SURVEILLANCE

Surveillance of disease refers to the continuing monitoring of all aspects of the occurrence and spread of a disease that are necessary to control that disease.

The fundamental difference between a health <u>survey</u> and <u>surveillance</u> is that a survey involves sampling at one point in time and provides a cross-sectional look at the situation, while surveillance calls for continuous, or longitudinal, observation of population groups.

Surveillance consists of data collection for a specified population and geographic area; tabulation, analysis, and interpretation of results; and periodic publication or distribution of findings to appropriate health personnel, agencies and the public.

The major sources or kinds of data relevant to disease surveillance include

1. mortality reports
2. morbidity reports
3. epidemic reports
4. reports of laboratory utilization
5. reports of individual case investigations
6. reports of epidemic investigations

7. special surveys (e.g., of hospital admissions, disease registers, serologic surveys)
8. information on animal reservoirs and vectors
9. demographic data
10. environmental data

The primary objective of disease surveillance is to determine the incidence or prevalence of diseases and the risk of disease transmission so control measures can be applied. Surveillance data must be current and complete in order to disclose the occurrence and distribution of disease. Disease surveillance is sometimes conducted even when control measures are not yet available. . . in anticipation of their development. The reasons for conducting surveillance under such circumstances are

1. to increase knowledge about the reservoir of disease and the modes of transmission so priorities can be established when control does become possible;

2. to assess the effect of control measures when they become available and are implemented.

Surveillance of family units has provided particularly useful information about etiologic factors, pathogenicity of infectious agents, and has helped describe the natural history of many infectious diseases. Surveillance of chronic diseases has contributed information about disease determinants or risk factors (such as smoking, blood pressure, serum levels of cholesterol and triglyceride in heart disease), and environmental hazards.

Government agencies and Health Departments prepare surveillance reports to provide current epidemiologic information about a variety of diseases. The numbers of case reports received during the current reporting period (week or month) are listed by disease, for the entire reporting area or political subdivisions within that area. The report disseminates information to the private and public health community and includes (1) information of current interest regarding the prevention, diagnosis, and treatment of selected diseases, and

(2) summaries of epidemologic investigations in progress or recently completed. A good example is the <u>Morbidity</u> <u>and</u> <u>Mortality</u> <u>Weekly</u> <u>Reports</u> (MMWR) published weekly by the Center for Disease Control. Excerpts from the MMWR are given below:

Surveillance Summary

Occupational Injury Surveillance—U.S.

The National Institute for Occupational Safety and Health (NIOSH), in conjunction with the Consumer Product Safety Commission (CPSC), recently developed a new surveillance system* to monitor all occupational injuries treated at a sample of 66 hospital emergency rooms, statistically selected to be representative of all U.S. hospital emergency rooms and placed in 5 categories according to hospital size and type. The number of sample hospitals selected from each category is proportional to the emergency-room usage for hospitals in that category.

Data in Table 1 show the types and estimated numbers of occupational injuries treated in U.S. hospital emergency rooms in the period September 24-30, 1981. In addition to these variables, detailed occupational injury information provided through this surveillance system includes treatment date, age, sex, type of accident, cause of accident, and disposition of case. As can be seen in Table 1, the most frequent type of injury is laceration (25.4%) Fingers are the most frequently injured body site (25.3%). Lacerations to the fingers (14.3%) are the most frequent type- and body site-specific occupational injury.

During a 3-month period beginning May 15, 1981, the estimated total number of occupational injuries (both lost-workday and nonlost-workday injuries) treated at all U.S. hospital emergency rooms was 839,061. This 3-month occupational injury experience extrapolates to a crude national estimate of 3.3 million occupational injuries treated in hospital emergency rooms for 1981. Seasonal differences are not addressed in this estimate.

*Based on the National Electronic Injury Surveillance System (NEISS) developed by CPSC in 1972.

Rubella—U.S., 1978-1981

A record low number of 3,904 cases of rubella was reported in the United States for 1980. This was 66.9% less than the 1979 total of 11,795 cases, the previous record low Between 1978 and 1980, the number of reported rubella cases declined 78.6% This trend continued throughout the first 35 weeks of 1981 (ending September 5), when 1,717 cases of rubella were reported, a 46.3% decline from the 3,196 cases reported for the same period in 1980 (Figure 1).

Age-specific data were available for 2,964 (76.0%) of the cases reported for 1980. The reported age-specific incidence rate of rubella has decreased for all age groups over the past 2 years, with the greatest decline being that for the 15- to 24-year-old group (Table 1). This has resulted in a marked change in the age-specific characteristics In 1978, the highest age-specific incidence rate was for 15- to 19-year olds. From 1978 through 1979, 73.8% of the reported cases of rubella were among persons ≥15 years old For 1980, only 46.6% of the cases were reported among persons ≥15 years old, and the highest incidence rate was for the <5-year olds.

Reported by Surveillance and Assessment Br, Immunization Div, Center for Prevention Services, CDC.

Editorial Note: Initially, rubella-control programs in the United States emphasized vaccination of preschool and elementary school children; vaccination of older individuals received only secondary emphasis. This strategy caused a dramatic decline in reported rubella and eliminated the characteristic 6- to 9-year cycle of epidemic rubella (1) There was also a marked change in the age characteristics for reported rubella cases. Whereas rubella was considered a disease of young children before vaccine licensure in 1969, from 1976 through 1979 approximately 70% of reported rubella cases were among individuals >15 years of age and the highest incidence rate was for the 15- to 19-year olds (2).

Current Trends

Ventricular Septal Defect

The number of reported cases of ventricular septal defect (VSD), a relatively common birth defect, has risen markedly in the United States over the last decade. The cause of this increase is unknown. This report updates results from 3 birth-defect monitoring systems in the United States: 1) the national Birth Defects Monitoring Program (BDMP), 2) the Metropolitan Atlanta Congenital Defects Program (MACDP), and 3) the Nebraska Birth Defects Prevention Program.

Data from these 3 programs show that the reported incidence of VSD has nearly tripled since the mid-1970s (Table 1). These reported rates can be used as a basis for estimating how many additional infants are born with VSD in the United States each year. A low estimate, derived from BDMP incidence data, would project 1,480 VSD infants (0.40/1,000 live births times the total of 3.7 million live births) born in the United States in 1970 and 4,248 (1.18/1,000 live births times the total of 3.6 million live births) in 1980, an excess of 2,768.

TABLE 1. Reported incidence of ventricular septal defect from three surveillance systems, United States, 1968-1980

Date	BDMP *		MACDP Atlanta **		Nebraska ***	
	Number of cases	Rate/1,000 total births	Number of cases	Rate/1,000 total births	Number of cases	Rate/1,000 total births
1968			31	1.17		
1969			33	1.20		
1970	342	0.40	29	0.98	3	0.12
1971	428	0.48	28	1.00	3	0.12
1972	496	0.54	37	1.45	5	0.21
1973	618	0.63	32	1.27	20	0.88
1974	717	0.66	52	2.10	25	1.06
1975	835	0.78	55	2.39	27	1.14
1976	895	0.85	66	2.91	25	1.05
1977	1,006	0.93	67	2.85	27	1.07
1978	937	0.96	68	2.79	30	1.20
1979	1,133	1.10	81	3.17	60	2.29
1980	909	1.18	70	2.60	38	1.37

* BIRTH DEFECTS MONITORING PROGRAM—Hospital discharge diagnosis survey of 25% of U.S. births since 1970

** METROPOLITAN ATLANTA CONGENITAL DEFECTS PROGRAM

*** THE NEBRASKA BIRTH DEFECTS PREVENTION PROGRAM

Nutrition Surveillance— U.S., 1980

The Coordinated Nutrition Surveillance Program of the Centers for Disease Control uses nutrition-related data collected by local health departments as part of routine delivery of child health services. During 1980, data were submitted for more than 250,000 children ages 6 months-10 years. These data concerned new patients at more than 1,300 clinics in 22 states.

The data consist primarily of identifying demographic information, height (length), weight, birth weight, and hemoglobin and/or hematocrit determinations. Data on height (length), weight, and age are converted to percentiles for height-for-age and weight-for-height, using the National Center for Health Statistics reference population (1). Levels <5th percentile height-for-age and weight-for-height and >95th percentile weight-for-height are reported as potentially abnormal values. Results based on these cutoff points are shown in Table 2. (Asians 6-10 years old are not represented because data for <100 children were reported.)

PNEUMONIA-INFLUENZA DEATHS IN 121 UNITED STATES CITIES

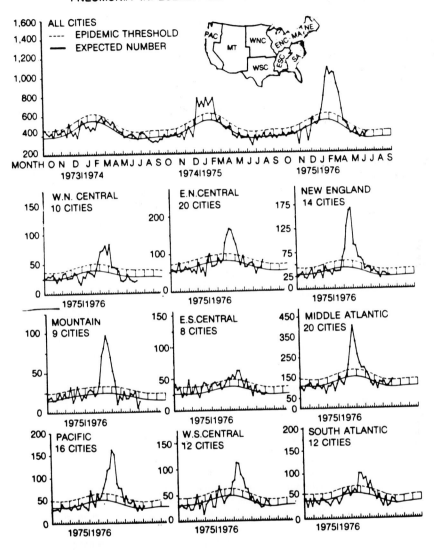

Methicillin-Resistant Staphylococcus aureus—U.S.

Over the past 5 years, there have been an increasing number of reports of infections with methicillin-resistant *Staphylococcus aureus* (MRSA) in U S hospitals (*1*) Review of the literature indicated that all reported MRSA problems in the United States have occurred in large, medical school-affiliated hospitals. This finding raised the question of whether MRSA infections are mainly confined to this group of hospitals, or whether the association is due to a reporting bias To study this question, rates were examined of MRSA occurrence among 63 hospitals that have been voluntarily reporting nosocomial infections and antimicrobial-susceptibility patterns to the National Nosocomial Infections Study (NNIS) regularly since 1974.

Defining an MRSA problem as methicillin resistance associated with more than 10% of the *S aureus* infections in one hospital in a given year, all MRSA problems in NNIS hospitals were found to occur in medical school-affiliated hospitals with more than 600 beds From 1974 to 1981, the percentage of all *S aureus* infections due to MRSA rose steadily in that group of large tertiary referral hospitals, whereas it remained below 4% for hospitals in all other categories (Figure 1).

Reported by Hospital Infections Program, Center for Infectious Diseases, CDC.

Childbearing and Abortion Patterns
Among Teenagers—U.S., 1978

Since 1976, CDC has been monitoring trends in childbearing and abortion patterns among teenagers, using data from its own abortion surveillance activities and vital statistics from the National Center for Health Statistics.

In 1978, females less than 20 years old continued to have relatively fewer births, more abortions, and more conceptions (live births and abortions combined) than they had in the previous 2 years. Births to teenagers represented a smaller proportion of total births in 1978 (16.6%) than in 1977 (17.2%). Similarly, abortions obtained by teenagers represented a smaller proportion of total abortions in 1978 (30.8%) than in 1977 (31.3%) These smaller proportions of births to and abortions among teenagers reflect decreasing numbers of 12- to 19-year olds in the population as a result of the low birth rates that began in the mid-1960s.

In 1978, the overall birth rate for teenagers declined to approximately the same level as in 1976 (34.6 births/1,000 women ages 12-19 years) It had risen in 1977 for the first time since 1970. The overall abortion rate for teenagers increased by 7.4%, (from 20.8 to 22.3 abortions/1,000 women ages 12-19 years.) a smaller percentage increase than in 1977. The overall conception rate (live births plus abortions/1,000 women ages 12-19 years) rose by 2% from 1977 to 1978, due entirely to an increase in the conception rate for women ages 18-19 years. The conception rate for 12- to 14-year olds did not change and for females ages 15-17 years, it declined

Teenagers in different age groups (≤14, 15-17, and 18-19) had different childbearing and abortion patterns.

Tuberculosis Among Indochinese Refugees—An Update

State tuberculosis control programs have reported that 3,895 Indochinese refugees were treated for tuberculosis during 1979 and 1980. The states reporting these cases received 96% of the 262,602 refugees who entered the United States during the 2-year period. Of the 3,895 patients, 3,330 (85.5%) entered the United States in 1979 or 1980, 103 (2.6%) entered in the period 1975-1978, and for 462 (11.9%) the year of entry was unknown. The states included 2,850 (73.2%) of these patients in their official tuberculosis morbidity count. The remaining 1,045 (26.8%) were added to tuberculosis case registers but were not counted as new or recurrent cases. Most areas also reported the number of refugees given preventive treatment. Geographic areas that received 90% of the refugees reported that 16.1% (42,217) had been given preventive therapy.

The estimated prevalence of tuberculosis among refugees at the time of entry was 1,138 cases/100,000 refugees. The annual incidence after arrival in the United States for refugees with no evidence of disease when screened overseas was 407/100,000 (Table 1). Prevalence rates were higher for males (1,371) than for females (852), as were the annual incidence rates (430 compared with 381) For refugees born in Laos, the prevalence and annual incidence rates of tuberculosis were about half the rates observed for refugees born in Vietnam and Kampuchea. For refugees who entered the United States in 1979, the annual incidence was greater in 1979 (719/100,000) than in 1980 (231/100,000).

Surveillance Summary

Surveillance of Childhood Lead Poisoning—U.S.

In the third quarter of fiscal year 1981, 62 childhood lead-poisoning prevention programs reported that 136,000 children were screened, and 4,900 were identified as having lead toxicity. Over 10,000 children were referred for follow up of other health problems, including iron deficiency and inadequate immunization.

Childhood lead-poisoning prevention programs are usually integrated components of local child health-care systems, and screening for lead toxicity is becoming a routine part of comprehensive health care for children ages 1-5. As a result, 70% of the children screened this quarter were tested by other local child-care providers such as Maternal and Child Health, Early Periodic Screening, Diagnosis, and Treatment Program, and Special Supplemental Food Program for Women, Infants, and Children.

Local childhood lead-poisoning prevention programs are designed to 1) screen high-risk children not served by clinic-based providers, 2) strengthen case-holding activities so that children with lead toxicity receive necessary long-term medical care, and 3) identify and eliminate sources of lead exposure for afflicted children.

In the third quarter of fiscal year 1981, programs 1) tested 15,000 high-risk children for lead toxicity in their homes, 2) kept 73% of children under pediatric management up-to-date in their scheduled medical follow up, and 3) completed environmental investigations at about 3,200 dwellings related to children with lead toxicity; identified lead hazards in 2,200 dwellings, and eliminated these hazards in 1,900 dwellings.

Reported by Environmental Health Svcs Div, Center for Environmental Health, CDC.

Human Plague—U.S., 1981

For 1981, 13 cases of human plague, 4 of them fatal, were reported from 5 states Arizona (4), California (1), Colorado (1), Oregon (1 fatal), New Mexico (6, 3 fatal) (Figure 2) Twelve cases were confirmed at CDC by fluorescent antibody testing and by bacteriologic identification and characterization; 1 case was confirmed serologically The patients ranged in age from 2 to 72 years with a mean age of 38.7 years. Seven patients (54%) were male, 6 were white, 6 were American Indian (5 Navajo, 1 Hopi), and 1 was Asian The clinical manifestations included bubonic plague (5 patients), septicemic plague (5), septicemic with confirmed secondary pneumonic plague (2), and presentation unspecified (1).

The various modes of infection were flea bite (5 cases), skinning an infected bobcat (1), rabbit hunting (1), bite of an infected domestic cat (1), and undetermined (5). The 5 cases acquired by flea bite occurred in relation to epizootic plague among prairie dogs (*Cynomys gunnisoni*) and rock squirrels (*Spermophilus variegatus*). Two patients with unknown source of infection resided in areas where an epizootic of plague was occurring in prairie dogs.

TABLE 3. Reported cases of human plague, by state, 1970-1981

State	Number of Cases
New Mexico	77
Arizona	21
California	16
Colorado	9
Oregon	7
Nevada	3
Utah	2
Wyoming	1
TOTAL	136

NOTIFIABLE DISEASES--SUMMARY OF REPORTED CASES, 1975-1980

DISEASES	1980	1979	1978	1977	1976	1975
U.S. total resident population (in thousands) 1980 census; July 1 est. 1971-1979	226,505	220,099	218,059	216,332	214,659	213,121
Amebiasis	5,271	4,107	3,937	3,044	2,906	2,775
Anthrax	1	—	6	—	2	2
Aseptic meningitis	8,028	8,754	6,573	4,789	3,510	4,475
Botulism, total	89	45	105	129	55	20
Foodborne	18	12	65	81	30	17
Infant	68	25	36	43	15	1
Brucellosis (undulant fever)	183	215	179	232	296	310
Chancroid	788	840	521	455	628	700
Chickenpox	190,894	199,081	154,089	188,396	183,990	154,248
Cholera	10	1	12	4	—	—
Diphtheria	3	59	76	84	128	307
Encephalitis, primary	264[1]	312[2]	290	341	530	2,362
Indeterminate	952[1]	1,192[2]	1,061	1,073	1,121	1,702
Post childhood infections	38[1]	84[2]	78	119	175	237
Gonorrhea	1,004,029	1,004,058[2]	1,013,436	1,002,219	1,001,994	999,937
Granuloma inguinale	51	76	72	75	71	60
Hepatitis A	29,087	30,407	29,500	31,153	33,288	35,855
Hepatitis B	19,015	15,452	15,016	16,831	14,973	13,121
Hepatitis, unspecified	11,894	10,534	8,776	8,639	7,488	7,158
Legionellosis	441[3]	578	761	359	235	
Leprosy	223	185	168	151	145	162
Leptospirosis	85	94	110	71	73	93
Lymphogranuloma venereum	199	250	284	348	365	353
Malaria	2,062	894	731	547	471	373
Measles (rubeola)	13,506	13,597	26,871	57,345	41,126	24,374
Meningococcal infections, total	2,840	2,724	2,505	1,828	1,605	1,478
Mumps	8,576	14,225	16,817	21,436	38,492	59,647
Pertussis (whooping cough)	1,730	1,623	2,063	2,177	1,010	1,738
Plague	18	13	12	18	16	20
Poliomyelitis, total	9	34	15	18	14	8
Paralytic	8	26	9	17	12	8
Psittacosis	124	137	140	94	78	49
Rabies, animal	6,421	5,119	3,254	3,130	3,073	2627
Rabies, human	—	4	4	1	2	2
Rheumatic fever, acute	432	629	851	1,738	1,865	2,854
Rubella (German measles)	3,904	11,795	18,269	20,395	12,491	16,652
Rubella congenital syndrome	50	62	30	23	30	30
Salmonellosis, excluding typhoid fever	33,715	33,138	29,410	27,850	22,937	22,612
Shigellosis	19,041	20,135	19,511	16,052	13,140	16,584
Smallpox						
Syphilis, primary and secondary	27,204	24,874	21,656	20,399	23,731	25,561
Total all stages	68,832	67,049	64,875	64,621	71,761	80,356
Tetanus	95	81	86	87	75	102
Trichinosis	131	157	67	143	115	252
Tuberculosis[4]	27,749	27,669	28,521	30,145	32,105	33,989
Tularemia	234	196	141	165	157	129
Typhoid fever (cases)	510	528	505	398	419	375
(Carriers)	62	71	62			
Typhus fever, flea-borne (endemic, murine)	81	69	46	75	69	41[2]
Typhus fever, tick-borne (Rocky Mountain spotted)	1,163	1,070	1,063	1,153	937	844
Yellow fever						

Smallpox — Last documented case occurred in 1949

Yellow fever — Last indigenous case reported 1911; last imported 1924

[1] Provisional data.
[2] Corrected data.
[3] Includes sporadic cases only
[4] Case data subsequent to 1974 are not comparable to prior years due to changes in reporting criteria which became effective in 1975.

*Not previously notifiable nationally

Data from surveillance of both infectious and noninfectious diseases are used for early detection of epidemics and for planning immunization campaigns and other activities. For example, after effective vaccines against poliomyelitis, measles, rubella, and other viral diseases became widely available, medical scientists, physicians, and laymen tended to assume that the vaccines were universally distributed to individuals, that the vaccines maintained protective titers of antibody, and hence that these diseases were no longer a serious health problem. These assumptions are far from correct, as demonstrated by several epidemics of these diseases since the introduction of the vaccines. For example, in 1968, after 5 years during which Houston, Texas, was free from the disease, 2 cases of paralytic poliomyelitis occurred. Results of serological study in 1968 indicated that a large proportion of children in low-income families were susceptible to polio virus. More than 50% of all low-income family children, ages 0 to 14 years, who were studied had incomplete protection, i.e., lacked antibody to at least one type of poliovirus.

Comparison with findings of a prior study (1963), conducted after Houston's 1962 mass oral polio virus vaccination campaign, indicated that a widespread absence or insufficient immunity was present among lower-income families. Polio vaccine was administered to virtually all children who were in the care of private physicians and was also freely available to low-income families, provided they attended public health clinics and asked for vaccine; however, no mass immunization programs and no surveys of immunity had been conducted between 1962 and 1968. Interviews conducted by the Houston City Health Department during February and March 1968 showed that the only polio vaccination of many children consisted of the single series of monovalent vaccines they received during the 1962 mass campaign.

Comparison of the 1968 findings with those in corresponding groups studied in 1963 is illustrated in Figure 1. Antibody data for the various age groups are shown as the percentage of children in each group who were missing one, two, or three antibody types.

Two factors contribute to the development of deficiencies in the immune status of populations: (1) failure to obtain proper vaccination can lead to the development of pockets of susceptibles even within a "well-vaccinated" community; and (2) decline of antibody levels in individuals with passage of time after vaccination. Both of these situations can and should be monitored by sur-veillance to detect groups at high risk before poliomyelitis epidemics reappear.

Question 1

a.   Compare the 1963 and 1968 graphs by age groups.

Exercise 14-12

Figure 1. Percentage of each age group in 1968 and 1963 who were susceptible to one or more types of polio virus, as measured by lack of antibody.

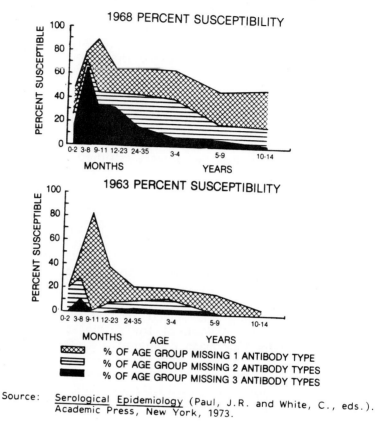

Source: Serological Epidemiology (Paul, J.R. and White, C., eds.). Academic Press, New York, 1973.

b. What accounts for the differences in susceptibility by age group between the two years?

c. Explain why the 3- to 8-month-old infants were at highest risk.

d. What would the results of the two graphs suggest to an epidemiologist?

Question 2

a.   If you were to set up a surveillance system to monitor polio immune status in Houston, what activities would have to be part of the surveillance process?

b.   What would be the major sources of data for your surveillance program?

c.   How complete do you believe your data collection would be?

d.   If polio epidemics reappear, they might be even more tragic than those of the 1940-1950 era.   Why?

Question 3

Assume that your surveillance system collects only 10-20% of the actual incidence cases (e.g., a venereal disease surveillance effort).   What alternatives are available to you to improve the level of surveillance?   Do you think you will raise the surveillance level using these procedures?

III. RISK FACTORS AND PREVENTION OF DISEASE

One objective of epidemiological studies is to provide information for identifying high-risk groups so that adverse outcomes can be prevented or their severity controlled.   Some examples are identification of women with early stages of cervical cancer to reduce the risk of death; protecting workers in asbestos factories to prevent development of asbestosis;   identification of persons at high risk of cardiovascular disease due to smoking, high blood pressure, or other factors.

The following exercise will examine risk factors in heart disease.

A.   A STUDY OF RISK FACTORS IN FATAL CORONARY HEART DISEASE*

Introduction

In an 18-year follow-up of 3263 longshoremen who had undergone multiphasic screening examinations in 1951, six characteristics were studied for their influence on risk of death from coronary heart disease (CHD) or stroke. Results of an earlier study were extended and amplified by attention to additional characteristics of high risk. Among the characteristics we found to be associated with increased death rates from CHD or stroke were reduced physical activity of work, indulgence in cigarette smoking, higher blood pressure level, increased weight-for-height, diagnosed heart disease, and abnormal glucose metabolism. Work activity attracted special attention because of the high energy expenditure demanded by some longshoring jobs.

The criterion for each characteristic was determined for men aged 35-64 years at the initial screening examination, in order to divide the total population of subjects into groups presumed to be at higher and lower risk. Cargo handlers, who comprised 68% of the study population, represent the more physically active longshoremen, the remaining one-third were regarded as less active. Cigarette smoking of one or more packs per day was identified in 39% of the longshoremen; systolic blood pressure above the mean, in 44%; weight-for-height above the mean, in 50%; diagnosed heart disease (causes 410-443, International Classification of Diseases, seventh revision), in 7%; and abnormal glucose metabolism (diagnosed diabetes mellitus or a blood-sugar of 205 mg% or more one hour after a 50 gm sucrose load), in 5%.

Longshoremen expend more energy in the conduct of their jobs than workers in most other industries. Estimated energy and oxygen costs of cargo-handling and of less active longshoring tasks were done in 1951, using energy requirements on holdmen handling a variety of cargo, and similar data from other work forces. Weighting the results for the proportional contribution of specific job classifications, it was found that cargo handlers used 6.7 calories per minute (1.34 liters of oxygen), and less active longshoremen used 2.8 calories per minute (0.56 liters of oxygen) during comparable work periods. Considering both work and rest periods, a difference in energy expenditure of about 925 calories during an eight-hour work day was found between cargo handlers and those less active.

Decedents were identified from records of the International Longshoremen's and Warehousemen's Union-Pacific Maritime Association Welfare Fund. The starting population was traced by death clearance procedures, with less than one percent loss to 18-year follow-up observations. Official death certificates identified CHD and stroke deaths occurring between the initial screening examination of 1951 and termination of the study in 1969.

---

*Paffenbarger, R.S., et al., Am. J. Public Health 61:1362, 1971. Adapted for use as a teaching exercise and used with permission of Dr. D.I. Clemmer, Tulane University School of Public Health.

Subjects were stratified into presumed high- and low-risk groups, and person-years of experience were compiled by single years of age and the results combined into 10-year age classes to steady the numbers. The cause-specific death rates per 10,000 person-years experience were compared by group. Age-specific or age-adjusted rates (direct method) by 10-year age classes were computed. Differences in rates between high- and low-risk groups are given as: (a) risk-ratios, which compare death rates in the presence vs. the absence of a characteristic (multiplied by 100), and (b) relative death ratios, which show the effect of two or more characteristics present in combination as compared with death rates in their absence.

Results

Of the 3263 longshoremen aged 35-64 years at time of examination in 1951, a total of 1098 were known to be dead by the 1969 follow-up. Among them were 350 who died from an underlying cause of coronary heart disease (cause 420, I.C.D.) and 93 who died from stroke (46 of underlying cause I.C.D. 330 or 331, and 47 of I.C.D. cause 332 or 334). These totals represent CHD and stroke death rates of 69.7 and 18.5, respectively, per 10,000 person-years experience in the 18-year period. The mean (± standard deviation) age at death was 62 (± 9) for coronary heart disease and 64 (± 8) for stroke, while survivors ranged in age from 53 to 82 years.

Work activity

Figure 2 shows age-adjusted and age-specific death rates per 10,000 person-years among San Francisco longshoremen during the 18-year follow-up period by physical activity and age at death. The figure also presents death risk-ratios, which are obtained by dividing rates for less active longshoremen by rates for cargo handlers. In effect, these risk-ratios are the relative risk.

Question 4

a. Why were person-years rather than persons used as a denominator for CHD death rates shown in Figure 2?

b. Why was it necessary to age-adjust the rates for the "all ages" category?

c. Summarize the relationship between age, physical activity, and CHD.

Figure 2. Death rates from CHD among San Francisco longshoremen, by physical activity of work at initial examination (1951), and age at death.

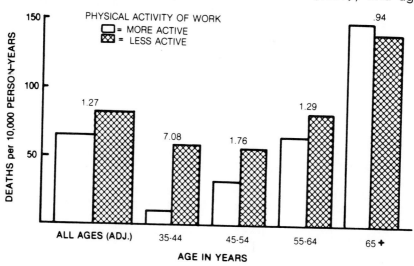

[Risk ratios above pairs of bars represent rates for less active longshoremen divided by rates for the more active cargo handlers.]

d.   Can you suggest some explanations of the reversal of the rate relationship for "more" and "less" active groups in the oldest age category?

Characteristics of high risk

Figure 3 gives age-adjusted death rates from CHD for each of six characteristics (risk factors) of high risk assessed at the initial examination. Age-specific rates are not given since, with the exception of work activity (already discussed), no trend with age was observed for the remaining five chacteristics. The figure also gives risk-ratios computed by dividing rates of groups with these high-risk characteristics by rates of groups with low risk.

Question 5

From the data in Figure 3, rank the six risk factors from highest to lowest according to the observed excess mortality. [Remember to observe the significance criterion of each factor ($p < 0.05$ means the difference is statistically significant at the 95% and $p < 0.01$ at the 99% criterion of significance).]

Figure 3. Age-adjusted death rates from CHD among San Francisco longshore-men, by six characteristics assessed in 1951.

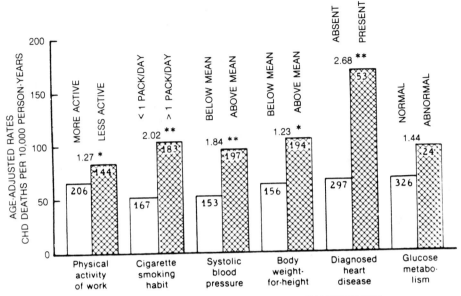

CHARACTERISTICS AT INITIAL EXAMINATION

[Risk ratios above pairs of bars represent rates for longshoremen with higher risk divided by rates for those with lower risk. *indicates p < 0.05, **indicates p < 0.01. Numbers within bars are numbers of decedents.]

Work activity and other characteristics

Figure 4 gives age-adjusted death rates from CHD in the 18-year follow-up for combinations of work activity and each of the five other characteristics studied. The figure also gives risk-ratios obtained by dividing rates for less active longshoremen by rates for cargo handlers for each of the characteristics.

Question 6

a. Describe the relationship between CHD mortality rates, work activity, and the other 5 risk factors shown in Figure 4?

b. Less physical activity combined with the presence of which other factor(s) appears to increase the risk of fatal CHD most?

Exercise 14-18

Figure 4. Age-adjusted death rates and risk-ratios from CHD among San Francisco longshoremen by combinations of physical activity of work and five other characteristics assessed in 1951.

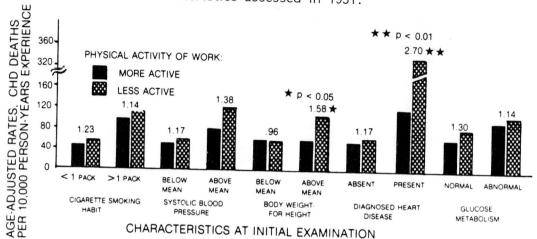

[Risk ratios above pairs of bars represent rates for less active longshoremen divided by rates for the more active cargo handlers.]

In general, a combination of diagnosed heart disease, smoking one or more packs of cigarettes per day, and higher systolic blood pressure produced the strongest effects when they occurred together or in combination with any of the remaining three characteristics.

The effect on CHD mortality rates of unspecified combinations of any two to five of the six characteristics is shown in Figure 5. Relative death ratios represent rates for longshoremen with various combinations of characteristics divided by rates for those without these characteristics.

Question 7

a.   What effect does the addition of risk factors have on the relative death ratio?

b.   What implications does this study have for the prevention of CHD deaths?

c.   At what point might intervention be most effective?

Figure 5. Relative death ratios of age-adjusted death rates from CHD among San Francisco longshoremen, by unspecified combinations of six characteristics assessed in 1951.

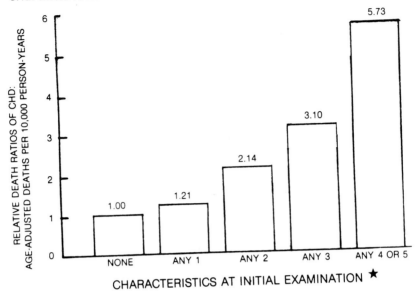

★Less physical activity; cigarettes >1 pk/day; systolic BP above mean; weight above mean; diagnosed heart disease; and abnormal glucose metabolism.

B.   THE CORONARY RISK PROFILE

The American Heart Association, using data on Caucasians participating in a long-term prospective study of residents of Framingham, Massachusetts, has produced The Coronary Risk Handbook, which has the purpose of "providing" the physician with a method for easily estimating the risk of CHD and for guiding his choice of preventive management in patients who have no clinical evidence of that disease.

The following section of the exercise is based on the handbook.

Need for reducing coronary mortality

Premature death from CHD among men and women in their productive years continues to be a major public health problem. The most common mode of death in persons with either symptomatic or presymptomatic coronary artery disease is sudden death. Sudden death accounts for more than half of all coronary fatalities under age 65. Of these fatalities, over 65% are unheralded by prior symptoms and occur unexpectedly. More than half of all coronary deaths occur outside the hospital before cardiac resuscitation teams can reach victims.

Associated risk factors in coronary heart disease

A number of risk factors are associated with an increased risk of CHD (sudden coronary death, myocardial infarction, and angina pectoris). The Framingham and other epidemiological studies have shown that a prediction of the likelihood of developing CHD can be made for groups of persons well in advance of the appearance of symptoms. Among the risk factors identified are sex, age, cigarette smoking, elevated blood pressure, high levels of serum cholesterol, glucose intolerance, and ECG abnormalities. These factors are not the only risk factors that might be considered in assessing risk of coronary heart disease, but they are a set with proven merit that can be readily measured without hazard or trauma to the patient.

Developing the coronary risk profile

In general, the more risk factors present, or the greater the degree of abnormality of any factor, the greater the risk. Tables in the Handbook combine the five risk factors for each age-sex group and facilitate assessment of risk for persons whose blood pressure or cholesterol values do not always reach some arbitrary value set as "abnormal." When the tables are used, fewer persons will be misclassified at low risk because they have borderline values for blood pressure and cholesterol.

The tables have been computed for combinations of the set of variables for each sex and age group, and provide a synthesis of this information expressed as the probability of a coronary event in a specified period of time. The tables allow presymptomatic assessment of coronary vulnerability, and the development of a coronary risk profile. They do not necessarily apply to persons who already have coronary heart disease. Figures 6 and 7 illustrate the use of risk factor data.

For each sex and age group, the figures give the probability, in chances per 100, of developing CHD in six years. For those whose blood pressure or serum cholesterol value lies between those given, choose the nearest figure from the tables. If more precise values are desired, a linear interpolation or specific formulas to compute these probabilities are provided in the original Framingham report. Remember that these probabilities have been computed from age- and sex-specific rates similar to those you calculated in earlier exercises of this guide. Thus, the risk profile is an application of rates.

To obtain the probability of developing CHD from the table section being used:

1. Round the patient's cholesterol (CHOL) and systolic blood pressure (SBP) values to levels closest to those in the margins of the tables.

2. Find the risk probability at the intersection of the patient's cholesterol and systolic blood pressure in the body of the appropriate table section.

Using the risk profile

While the tables are easy to use, an example of their use may help. A 45-year-old man who does not smoke cigarettes, does not have glucose intolerance or evidence of left ventricular hypertrophy on an electrocardiograph test (LVH-ECG), and who has a systolic blood pressure of 165 and cholesterol of 285, will have a probability of developing coronary heart disease in six years of 7.8 in 100 (7.8%) as estimated from Figure 6 (upper left section). A man the same age who has a similar blood pressure and cholesterol but who smokes cigarettes and has impaired glucose tolerance and LVH-ECG will have a risk of 14.7 in 100 (14.7%) (probability given in the lower right section of the table). This average risk is not the actual risk for any particular person, but it does provide a standard of comparison for a group of persons of the same age and sex.

Question 8

A man presents himself with the following characteristics:

a. age 45 years
b. smoker
c. systolic blood pressure = 171 mg Hg

d. negative ECG findings
e. no glucose intolerance
f. CHOL = 310 mg %

a. What is his risk of developing CHD within 6 years? (Use Figure 6.)

b. What does this mean?

c. What happens to his risk if he stops smoking?

d. What else could be done to reduce this man's risk of developing CHD? Which factor, if eliminated, would most reduce his risk?

Figure 6. Probability (per 100) of developing coronary heart disease in six years according to specified characteristics: 45 year old man.

Does not smoke cigarettes and LVH-ECG Negative

Glucose tolerance absent

CHOL ↓ \ Systolic Blood Pressure →	150	165	180	195
185	2.5	3.1	3.7	4.4
210	3.2	3.9	4.6	5.5
235	4.1	4.9	5.9	7.0
260	5.2	6.2	7.4	8.7
285	6.5	7.8	9.2	10.9
310	8.2	9.8	11.5	13.6
335	10.3	12.2	14.3	16.7

Smokes cigarettes and LVH-ECG Negative

CHOL ↓ \ Systolic Blood Pressure →	150	165	180	19
185	3.9	4.7	5.6	6.
210	5.0	5.9	7.1	8.
235	6.3	7.5	8.9	10.
260	7.9	9.4	11.1	13.
285	9.9	11.7	13.7	16.
310	12.3	14.5	16.9	19.
335	15.2	17.8	20.7	23.

Glucose tolerance present

CHOL ↓ \ Systolic Blood Pressure →	150	165	180	195
185	3.3	3.9	4.7	5.6
210	4.2	5.0	6.0	7.1
235	5.3	6.3	7.5	8.9
260	6.7	7.9	9.4	11.1
285	8.4	9.9	11.7	13.8
310	10.5	12.3	14.5	17.0
335	13.0	15.3	17.9	20.8

CHOL ↓ \ Systolic Blood Pressure →	150	165	180	19
135	5.1	6.0	7.2	8.
210	8.4	7.6	9.0	10.
235	8.0	9.5	11.2	13.
260	10.0	11.9	14.0	16.
285	12.5	14.7	17.2	20.0
310	15.5	18.1	21.0	24.3
335	19.0	22.0	25.4	29.1

Source: American Heart Association, Coronary Risk Handbook, 1973.

Question 9

a.   What is the risk for a woman with the same characteristics as the man? (Use Figure 7.)

b.   If she stops smoking, what happens to her risk?

c.   Although the woman's rate is low to begin with, suggest hypotheses (besides sex) to explain why a woman's risk does not decrease as much as a man's after cessation of smoking.

Figure 7. Probability (per 100) of developing coronary heart disease in six years according to specified characteristics: 45 year old woman.

not smoke cigarettes and LVH-ECG Negative

Systolic Blood Pressure	→150	165	180	195
CHOL ↓				
185	0.9	1.1	1.4	1.7
210	1.1	1.4	1.7	2.1
235	1.3	1.7	2.1	2.6
260	1.6	2.0	2.6	3.2
285	2.0	2.5	3.1	3.9
310	2.4	3.1	3.8	4.7
335	3.0	3.7	4.6	5.8

(left margin: ...se ...erance ...nt)

Smokes cigarettes and LVH-ECG Negative

Systolic Blood Pressure	→150	165	180
CHOL ↓			
185	0.9	1.2	1.5
210	1.1	1.4	1.8
235	1.4	1.8	2.2
260	1.7	2.1	2.7
285	2.1	2.0	3.3
310	2.6	3.2	4.0
335	3.1	3.9	4.9

Systolic Blood Pressure	→150	165	180	195
CHOL ↓				
185	1.3	1.7	2.1	2.6
210	1.6	2.0	2.6	3.2
235	2.0	2.5	3.1	3.9
260	2.5	3.1	3.8	4.8
285	3.0	3.7	4.7	5.8
310	3.7	4.6	5.7	7.0
335	4.5	5.5	6.9	8.5

(left margin: ...ose ...erance ...ent)

Systolic Blood Pressure	→150	165	180
CHOL ↓			
135	1.4	1.8	2.2
210	1.7	2.2	2.7
235	2.1	2.6	3.3
260	2.6	3.2	4.0
285	3.1	3.9	4.9
310	3.8	4.8	5.9
335	4.7	5.8	7.2

rce: American Heart Association, Coronary Risk Handbook, 1973.

Question 10

a. What risk will the man have if several factors change, e.g., he reduces his systolic blood pressure to 150 mg Hg, cuts out smoking, and reduces his cholesterol to 210 mg %?

b. What risk will the woman have if she does the same?

c.   What are the problems involved in interpreting the meaning of the risk assigned to a person by this screening method?

d.   Do you think this risk profile is of much value in preventing coronary heart disease? Why?

IV.   EPIDEMIOLOGY IN HEALTH SERVICES RESEARCH

Epidemiology in health services research is directed at conducting studies of community needs and resources, utilization of services, the effectiveness of services to improve community health, and for setting priorities for services and research.

The entire spectrum of health services activities can be included: hospital admission, discharge and length of stay, treatment, diagnostic methods, mortality, outcome of treatment, availability, accessibility and use of health services, etc.   Many questions can be studied:

Does the distribution of surgery for cardiac patients reflect a pattern of selection for certain geographic areas or income groups?
Are children in urban areas at higher risk of losing their tonsils than their country cousins?
Does a radical mastectomy increase a woman's survival more than a simple mastectomy?
How many people need services and are not receiving them?
Are the rates of morbidity and mortality lower under a socialized medical system than in a fee-for-service system?
Is the treatment worse than the disease?

A.   COMPARISON OF HOSPITALS

To compare teaching and nonteaching hospitals for case-fatality from various diseases, examine Figures 8 and 9.

Question 11

a.   Give reasons for the differences based on your suppositions or knowledge about the make-up of teaching hospitals as opposed to nonteaching hospitals.

Figure 8. Case-fatality in teaching and nonteaching hospitals in England and Wales, 1956-59.

Admission diagnosis	Teaching hospital percent fatality	Nonteaching hospital percent fatality†
Emergency admissions		
Ischemic heart disease	23.0	29.0**
Perforated ulcer	8.1	10.0
Hernia with obstruction	6.1	9.7**
Hyperplasia of prostate	9.4	13.0*
Head injury	2.7	3.4*
Other admissions		
Ischemic heart disease	9.5	25.0***
Peptic ulcer with surgery	1.1	1.9*
Hernia	0.3	0.3
Hyperplasia of prostate	3.5	6.0**
Head injury	14.0	4.4***

*p <0.05   **p <0.01   ***p <0.001

†Standardized for age and sex of teaching hospital admissions.

Source: Lipworth, L., et al., Medical Care 1:71, 1963.

Figure 9. Case-fatality by selected cause, teaching and nonteaching hospitals in England and Wales, 1953-1959.

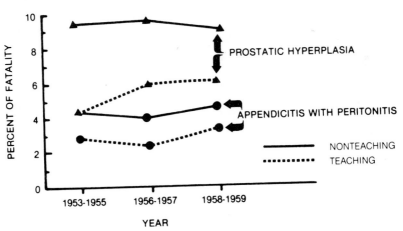

Source: Lipworth, L., et al., Medical Care, 1:71, 1963.

b.   Why are the data standardized by age and sex?

c.   How might these data be used by hospital administrators?

d.   What other data might you wish to have, to better understand the reasons for the differences?

B.   THE FREQUENCY AND IMPORTANCE OF SURGICAL PROCEDURES IN A
POPULATION

When organs are surgically removed the risk of certain diseases may be decreased to zero since disease cannot develop in a removed organ. However,
the risk may increase for other diseases as a result of organ removal. For
example, anemia may develop in persons with gastrectomy, while persons with
thyroidectomy may develop myxedema and hypoparathyroidism. Need for
follow-up of persons with certain types of surgery has implications for the
health service system, in terms of surveillance and treatment of the sequelae
of prior surgery.

How frequent are certain types of surgical procedures? In England, the
Oxford Record Linkage Study* (O.R.L.S.) used a population of 320,000 in
central rural England to study the question. Information on the population at
risk was obtained from the census; deaths and discharges from hospitals were
reported to O.R.L.S. with pertinent information about diagnosis, treatment,
and surgical procedures. The risk of organ removal was calculated by age
and sex from data collected over a 4-year period.

The frequency of different organ removal operations is shown in Figure 10.

Question 12

a.   Which operations are most frequent for women and men?

b.   What are the two most common operations for the entire population?

---

*Adapted from Acheson, E.D., and Fairbairn, A.S., in Uses of Epidemiology
in Planning Health Services, Vol. I. Int. Epidemiol. Assoc., January 1973.

Figure 10. Operations for organ removal, Oxford Record Linkage Area, 1962-1965, excluding malignant conditions, crude rates for all ages per 1000 person-years.

Operation	Organ removal Operation code	Males		Females	
		No. of operations	Rate per 1000 person-years	No. of operations	Rate per 1000 person-years
Tonsillectomy	261-262	2460	3.57	2471	3.61
Hysterectomy	722-724		---	1755	2.56
Appendectomy	441	1299	1.89	1195	1.74
Prostatectomy	672-677	379	0.55		---
Cholecystectomy	521	176	0.26	544	0.79
Partial gastrectomy	423	179	0.26	63	0.09
Subtotal thyroidectomy	071	42	0.06	226	0.33
Oophorectomy	702		---	160	0.23
Nephrectomy	606	30	0.04	48	0.07
Lower limb amputation	890-892	65	0.09	33	0.05
PERSON-YEARS AT RISK, 1962-1965		689,024		685,046	

c. Persons having organ removal due to malignant disease were excluded from data presented in Figure 10. Why?

Figures 11a to 11c compare the rate and cumulative risk of the most frequent operations in this population.

Question 13

Which age group and sex (if applicable) has the highest frequency of each of the operations shown in Figures 11a, b, and c? Explain each pattern.

a. tonsillectomy:

b. hysterectomy:

c. appendectomy:

Figure 11a. Tonsillectomy rate and cumulative risk percent by age and sex, Oxford Record Linkage Area, 1962-1965.

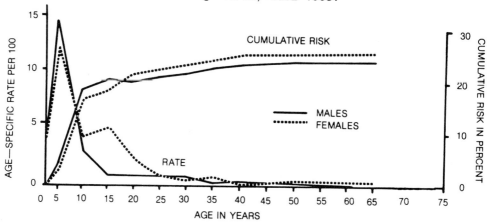

Figure 11b. Hysterectomy rate and cumulative risk percent by age and sex, Oxford Record Linkage Area, 1962-1965.

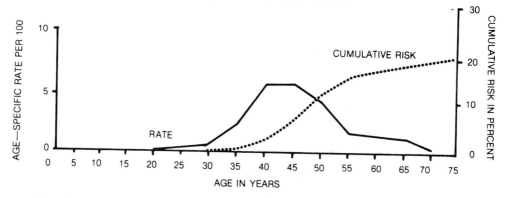

Figure 11c. Appendectomy rate and cumulative risk percent by age and sex, Oxford Record Linkage Area, 1962-1965.

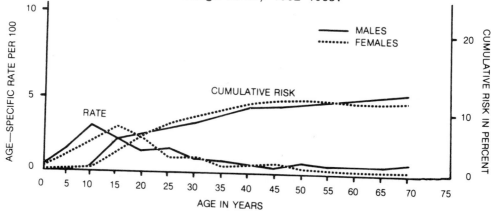

Question 14

By age 55, 15% of English women have a hysterectomy for nonmalignant reasons.

a.   What effect might that have on cervical cancer screening rates, i.e., the rate of positive PAP smears in women?

b.   Suppose that the mortality rate from cervical cancer declined after the start of the cervical cancer screening program. Would you agree that the screening program was responsible? Explain.

A study was conducted to examine the effect of an increasing frequency of hysterectomy and a decreasing population at risk on uterine cancer rates in the U.S. Hysterectomy is a common operative procedure in the U.S. with an estimated 690,000 operations performed in 1973. (Tonsillectomy was the most frequent surgical procedure performed in 1973--834,000 operations.)

Figure 12a. Annual hysterectomy operative rates per 100,000 women in the United States, as estimated by the Hospital Discharge Survey of the National Center for Health Statistics.

Age (years)	1965	1968	1973
15-24	42	79	93
25-34	651	754	1176
35-44	1358	1547	2011
45-64	761	825	1084
65+	303	324	261
All ages	439	490	651

Source: Lyon, J.L. and Gardner, J.W., The rising frequency of hysterectomy: its effect on uterine cancer rates. Am. J. Epidemiol. 105:439, 1977.

Figure 12b shows the result of that increase. The corrected rate excludes women with hysterectomy from the denominator.

Figure 12b. White U.S. uterine cancer mortality, 1960-1973. Age-adjusted
mortality rates (1970 U.S. standard population) uncorrected and
corrected for removal of women, by hysterectomy, from the population at risk.

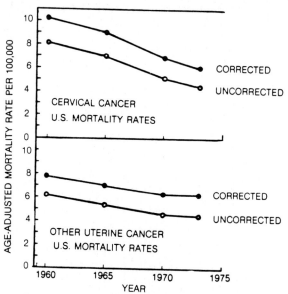

Source: Lyon, J.L. and Gardner, J.W., The rising frequency
of hysterectomy: its effect on uterine cancer rates.
Am. J. Epidemiol. 105:439, 1977.

These examples have demonstrated some health statistics that may be useful for
planning and for evaluating the effects of health services. Such information
provides an opportunity to understand what is going on inside the health
facility as well as in the community outside it.

This concludes the guide. We know you have worked hard to learn the principles of epidemiology. We hope you have enjoyed your initiation into the
world of epidemiology and that this guide will continue to be of value to you in
the future.

The appendices that follow contain an extensive bibliography of epidemiologic
references and a suggested format for test questions.

SUGGESTED RESPONSES
Exercise 14--Uses and Applications of Epidemiology

1a. In 1963 susceptibility was mainly concentrated in children under 3 years, particularly in those <12 months of age. Most of those susceptible had partial immunity, meaning that they were missing only one antibody type. Few children were totally lacking immunity.

In 1968, the proportion susceptible had increased in all age groups. While the largest proportion susceptible continued to be among the under 2 age group, there was a large increase among the 2-14 year olds. There was a large increase in the proportions missing one, two, and three antibody types.

1b. With no immunization compaign in the interim, there would be decreasing immunity over time (deterioration) among those who had prior immunization. In the years after 1963 new infants were born who may not have been immunized at all.

1c. There was a decrease in passively acquired maternal antibodies without further immunization of the child.

1d. High-risk groups have been identified. A vaccination campaign is necessary; start in children <1 year of age and revaccinate older children.

2a. Collection of data, tabulation, analysis, dissemination of results, maintaining close contact with hospitals, medical society, practicing physicians, laboratories, public schools, etc. Adequate publicity, quality control of laboratories, training and supervision of field staff would also be major activities.

2b. Serologic surveys, Health Department reports of illness, hospital admission reports, school reports on immunization status of those entering school and school absence records would be appropriate sources.

2c. It depends upon how aggressive your surveillance system is, and whether or not you have continuing cooperation from community resources. Although many diseases are legally "reportable," collection of information depends upon voluntary efforts of practitioners.

2d. Because vaccines are available to prevent the disease, there is less natural and acquired immunity, particularly in the urban areas. Thus, many more people might develop the disease.

3. Publicity, education of local physicians about the purpose of surveillance and the need for their cooperation might improve reporting. You could prepare seminars or other educational programs in conjunction with the county medical society to gain cooperation. Special surveys of high-risk

groups would help to identify prevalent cases. Interviews of cases would help to determine contacts who might also be at risk or who may have the disease (or be infected). Success would depend upon the initiative and creativity of the program director and cooperation of community health resources. A major problem with any surveillance system is underreporting of cases or incomplete data. A successful system will keep these problems to a minimum.

4a. Due to deaths and mobility, individuals in the study were <u>observed for different lengths of time</u> rather than all for 18 years. Also, because the age of the men ranged from <u>35 to 64 years</u> at the time they entered the study, they contributed different numbers of years of observation to various age categories depending on age at entry. For these reasons the age distribution of the cohort also shifts over time.

4b. The outcome being measured (CHD) varies with age; the age composition of the "more" and "less" active groups must have been different. There are probably more young people categorized in the "more" active group.

4c. CHD rate increases with age in both activity groups.

The more active group had lower CHD rates than the less-active group, except for the 65+ age group. After 65+ years, the rate for the more-active group was slightly higher than less active.

4d. The CHD-prone persons in the less active group may have died earlier because of lower physical activity level or other factors such as having diagnosed heart disease. Those who survive would be a relatively CHD-"resistant" population in the 65+ age group. Their CHD death rate would be lower than anticipated.

Men could have switched groups. Perhaps men initially in the more active group took less active jobs later on, and showed the effects of inactivity. After retirement, those in the "more active" group may have resumed a "less-active" life style.

More physical activity might exert a delaying action rather than a preventive action on CHD. The CHD-prone persons in the more active group may eventually succumb, although, overall mortality rates are lower for this group, and so, in this study, CHD in the more-active group never reaches the rate of the less-active group.

5.   1. Diagnosed heart disease
     2. Cigarettes >1 pack per day
     3. High blood pressure
     4. Less physical activity
     5. Overweight
     6. Abnormal glucose (although the ratio is greater than some other factors it is not statistically significant and is ranked lower).

6a.   Except for mean body weight-for-height, rates are higher for less active men regardless of whether the other factor is present or absent.

6b.   Less physical activity + diagnosed heart disease
Less physical activity + overweight

7a.   Adding risk factors results in increase in CHD mortality rates.

7b.   No one factor seems to be the culprit; rather a number of factors can act in a potentiating manner, some having a stronger effect than others. This suggests the necessity of multiple points of intervention, i.e., a change of lifestyle.

7c.   Early intervention, before heart disease becomes symptomatic.   A program based on reduced smoking, increased physical activity, and control of weight and blood pressure is required.   Screening programs to detect abnormal glucose metabolism also might be included.

8a.   The probability is 14.5%.

8b.   It means he has about 15 chances in 100 of developing CHD by the time he is 51 years old.

8c.   The probability drops to 9.8%.

8d.   Control of other risk factors such as blood pressure would reduce the risk.   Cholesterol reduction would appear to help greatly.

9a.   The probability is 3.2%.

9b.   There would not be much change; her risk is 3.1%.

9c.   Men may have smoked for a longer time.
Men may have smoked more cigarettes or inhaled more than women.
Women's risk is low to start with, so that eliminating just one factor won't
     have much effect.

10a. The probability is reduced to 3.2%.

10b. The probability is reduced to 1.1%.

10c. These data are not predictions for individuals.   The risks are based on grouped data.   This does not necessarily represent any specific individual's risk, but rather the average risk of the group to which an individual belongs.

The profile leaves out other factors, e.g., weight, activity, genetic inheritance, personality type, and stress.

There may be problems of sensitivity and specificity of measurements. There may be many false positives and negatives; none of this is addressed in the handbook.

The decrease may not be appropriate if the effects of smoking are irreversible. Persons who quit would continue to remain at higher risk. The person who has never smoked may always be at lower risk due to total absence of the factor.

10d. It depends upon whether or not people are willing to modify their lifestyles and habits to reduce exposure to these risk factors. Changing habits is difficult to sustain and requires dedication on the part of the individual as well as societal commitment to creating an environment that emphasizes reduced risk. There has been a decrease in CHD mortality in the U.S. for the past several years. Perhaps the facts about CHD risk factors are being accepted by the general population.

11a. Professional staff-to-patient ratios are higher in teaching hospitals, which means that patient care is likely to be better for complicated cases.

Teaching hospitals may admit a greater proportion of low-risk patients for any given category of disease. Teaching hospitals may have access to better or newer diagnostic or treatment equipment, and also newer techniques for diagnosis or treatment.

A higher proportion of patients from upper classes may be admitted to teaching hospitals. This could mean that the basic health status of patients is better than for nonteaching hospital patients. Because England and Wales have a socialized system of medical care, ability to pay for care might not influence admission policy.

11b. Age and sex distributions are probably different for each type of hospital.

11c. Unless they had asked for this study, the nonteaching hospital administrators might not like it. They might reject the data as "biased" or use these data to justify increased spending on new equipment or to raise salaries in order to attract better trained professional and nonprofessional staff.

11d. Useful information would include staffing patterns, demographic characteristics of patients, severity of admissions, type of staff training, age, type, and utilization of equipment.

12a. Women: tonsillectomy, hysterectomy, appendectomy. Men: tonsillectomy, appendectomy, prostatectomy.

12b. The tonsillectomy rate is 3.59 and appendectomy is 1.82 per 1000 person-years, respectively, when the data for males and females are combined.

12c. Persons with organ removal for malignant disease have a reduced life expectancy compared to persons with nonmalignant disorders. Thus, a person with lung cancer at age 40 will usually not be alive to be operated upon for diseases expected to occur after age 50. The exclusion was made to avoid bias.

13a. Ages 5-9 in both sexes have high frequency, but males are higher; a second peak occurs for females at age 15. Cumulative risk is higher for females.

Young males may have more severe illness from tonsillitis than young females. The second peak for females may be related to puberty or adolescent lifestyle, or it may indicate a cohort phenomenon.

13b. Ages 40-45 years are highest, it may have to do with menopause. The increase after age 30 may result from sequelae of pregnancy or birth control practices, or may represent inappropriate surgery.

13c. Highest rates are in males at age 10 and females at age 15. Males may be less tolerant of or suffer more severe abdominal pain, and have surgical intervention more readily than females. Dietary differences, physical activity, or injury may also be factors. Females with onset of menses around puberty may receive inappropriate surgery for pain that is actually of gynecological origin. Cumulative risk is higher for males than females. Appendectomy may be performed routinely with other abdominal surgery particularly in adult life.

14a. It skews the rates, because not all women in the denominator are truly at risk of cervical cancer, i.e., those who have had hysterectomy that included cervix removal are no longer at risk. The observed rates would be lower than the true rate because the denominator, with hysterectomized women included, would be larger than it should be.

14b. No; if the frequency of hysterectomy were rising, it might be enough to cause the observed decrease in the mortality rates by inflating the denominator.

In order for the screening test to be effective, it must be used by women who are at high risk of the disease, i.e., those who married young, those with multiple partners and those infected with Herpes virus. Cervical cancer mortality might not be markedly affected if the screening was used primarily by women with low risk of acquiring the disease.

APPENDIX I
Bibliography of Readings in Epidemiology and Public Health

Abramson, J. H.   The Cornell Medical Index as an Epidemiological Tool. Am. J. Publ. Health 56:287, 1966.

Abramson, J. H., and C. Hopp. The Control of Cardiovascular Risk Factors in the Elderly. Prev. Med. 5:32,1976.

Acheson, E. D. Medical Record Linkage. London: Oxford Univ. Press, 1967.

Ackerknecht, E. H. Anticontagionism between 1821 and 1867. The Fielding H. Garrison Lecture. Bull. Hist. Med., 22:562, 1948.

Ackerknecht, E. H. History and Geography of the Most Important Diseases. New York: Hafner, 1965.

Adams, F., The Genuine Works of Hippocrates. London: Sydenham Society, 1849. Reprinted, Baltimore: Williams & Wilkins, 1939.

American Heart Association. The Coronary Drug Project: Design, Methods and Baseline Results. New York: Am. Heart Assoc., Monogr. No. 38, 1973.

American Heart Association. Coronary Risk Handbook. New York: Am. Heart Assoc., 1973.

American Public Health Association. Guide for the Followup of Tuberculosis: Cases, Contacts, Suspects. New York: Am. Publ. Health Assoc., 1963.

American Public Health Association. Diagnostic Procedures for Virus and Rickettsial Diseases, 4th Ed. New York: Am. Publ. Health Assoc., 1969.

American Public Health Association. Diagnostic Procedures and Reagents, 5th ed. New York: Am. Publ. Health Assoc., 1970.

American Public Health Association. Diagnostic Procedures for Bacterial, Mycotic and Parasitic Infections. New York: Am. Publ. Health Assoc., 1970.

American Public Health Association. International Conference on Nosocomial Infections. Atlanta: CDC, 1970.

American Public Health Association. Recommended Procedures for the Examination of Seawater and Shellfish, 4th Ed. New York: Am. Publ. Health Assoc., 1970.

American Public Health Association. Syphilis and Other Venereal Diseases. Cambridge: Harvard Univ. Press, 1970.

American Public Health Association. Intersociety Committee for a Manual of Methods of Air Sampling and Analysis. Washington, D. C.: U.S. Government Printing Office, 1972.

American Public Health Association. Minority Health Chart Book. Washington, D. C.: U.S. Government Printing Office, 1974.

American Public Health Association. Standard Methods for Examination of Water and Waste Water, 14th ed. New York: Am. Publ. Health Assoc., 1976.

American Public Health Association. Intersociety Agency Committee on Micro-biological Methods for Foods. Washington, D. C.: U.S. Government Printing Office, 1976.

American Public Health Association. Standard Methods for Examination of Dairy Products, 14th ed. New York: Am. Publ. Health Assoc., 1978.

American Public Health Association. Control of Communicable Diseases in Man, 13th ed. New York: Am. Publ. Health Assoc., 1981.

Anderson, L. J., G. M. Baer, J. S. Smith, W. G. Winkler, and R. C. Holman. Rapid Antibody Response to Human Diploid Rabies Vaccine. Am. J. Epidemiol. 114:270,1981.

Andrews, J. M., and A. D. Langmuir. Philosophy of Disease Eradication. Am. J. Pub. Health 53:1, 1963.

Austin, D. F., and S. B. Werner. Epidemiology for the Health Sciences. Springfield: Thomas Publ. Co., 1974.

Austin, M. A., S. Berreyesa, J. L. Elliott, R. B. Wallace, E. Barrett-Conner, and M. H. Criqui. Methods for Determining Long Term Survival in a Population Based Study. Am. J. Epidemiol. 110:747,1979.

Austin, M. A., M. H. Criqui, E. Barrett-Conner, and M. J. Holdbrook. The Effect of Response Bias on the Odds Ratio. Am. J. Epidemiol. 114:137, 1981.

Aycock, W. L., G. E. Lutman, and G. I. Folet. Seasonal Prevalence as a Principle in Epidemiology. Am. J. Med. Sciences 209:395, 1945.

Aykroyd, W. R. Conquest of Deficiency Diseases: Achievements and Prospects. World Health Organization, FFHC Basic Study No. 24. Geneva: WHO, 1970.

Bailey, N. T. J. The Mathematical Theory of Epidemics. New York: Hafner Publ. Co., 1957.

Bailey, N. T. J. Statistical Methods in Biology. New York: Wiley, 1959.

Baker, G. Endemial Colic of Devonshire. 1767 Facsimile, Delta Omega ed. New York: Am. Pub. Health Assoc., 1958.

Baker, S. P. On Lobbies, Liberty and the Public Good. Am. J. Pub. Health 70:533,1980.

Ball, K. P., and R. Turner. Realism in the Prevention of Coronary Heart Disease. Prev. Med. 4:390,1975.

Barclay, G. W. Techniques of Population Analysis. New York: Wiley, 1958.

Barker, D. J. P., and G. Rose. Epidemiology in Medical Practice, 2nd ed. New York: Churchill Livingstone, 1979.

Barr, M. Environmental Contamination of Human Breast Milk. Am. J. Pub. Health 71:124,1981.

Barrett-Conner, E. Epidemiology for the Infection Control Nurse. St. Louis: Mosby, 1978.

Barrett-Conner, E. Infectious and Chronic Disease Epidemiology: Separate and Unequal? Am. J. Epidemiol. 109:245,1979.

Bates, M. The Natural History of Yellow Fever in Colombia. Sci. Monthly 63:42, 1946.

Bates, M. The Nature of Natural History. New York: Scribner, 1950.

Bates. M. The Forest and the Sea. New York: Random House, 1960.

Bearman, J. E., and B. W. Brown. The Relevance of Modern Clinical Trial Methodology to the Practice of Medicine. Perspect. Biol. Med. 10:259, 1967.

Beebe, G. W. Record Linkage Systems--Canada vs. the United States. Am. J. Pub. Health 70:1246,1980.

Belloc, N. B. Validation of Morbidity Survey Data by Comparison with Hospital Records. J. Am. Statist. Assoc. 49:832, 1954.

Berkson, J. Limitations of the Application of Fourfold Table Analysis to Hospital Data. Biometrics Bull. 2:47, 1946.

Beveridge, W. I. B. Influenza: The Last Great Plague: An Unfinished Story of Discovery. New York: Prodist, 1977.

Blum, R. H. The Patient's Definition of Illness. In The Management of the Doctor-Patient Relationship, pp. 1-28. New York: McGraw-Hill, 1960.

Boyd, M. F., ed. Malariology: A Comprehensive Survey of All Aspects of This Group of Diseases from a Global Standpoint. Philadelphia: Saunders, 1949.

Brachman, P. S., S. A. Plotkin, E. H. Blumford, and M. M. Atchison. An Epidemic of Inhalation Anthrax: The First in the Twentieth Century. II. Epidemiology. Am. J. Hygiene 72:6, 1960.

Breslow, L. Epidemiology as a Tool in Cancer Research. In Proc. 3rd Cancer Conf., Am. Cancer Soc., pp. 15-26. Philadelphia: Lippincott, 1957.

Breslow, L. A History of Cancer Control in the United States, 1946-1971. USDHEW, National Cancer Institute, 1977.

Breslow, L., and D. W. Roberts, eds. Symposium on Screening for Asymptomatic Disease. J. Chronic Dis. 2(4), 1955.

Breslow, N.E. The Analysis of Case-Control Studies: Statistical Methods in Cancer Research. Lyon: International Agency for Research in Cancer, 1980.

Brinton, L. A., M. P. Vessey, R. Flavel, and D. Yeates. Risk Factors for Benign Breast Disease. Am. J. Epidemiol. 113:203, 1981.

Brockington, C. A Short History of Public Health. London: Churchill, 1956.

Brodman, K., and L. S. Goldstein. The Medical Data Screen: An Adjunct for the Diagnosis of 100 Common Diseases. Arch. Environ. Health 14:821, 1967.

Brothwell, D., and A. T. Sandison, eds. Diseases in Antiquity. Springfield: Thomas, 1967.

Budd, W. Typhoid Fever: Its Nature, Mode of Spreading, and Prevention. Originally published in London in 1874. New York: Am. Pub. Health Assoc., 1931. Reprinted, Metuchen: Arno Press, 1977.

Buechley, R. W. A Formulation of Some Logical Problems in Epidemiology. Am. J. Epidemiol. 107:265, 1978.

Burnet, F. M. Viruses and Man. Baltimore: Penguin, 1953.

Burnet, F. M., and D. O. White. Natural History of Infectious Disease, 4th ed. London: Cambridge Univ. Press, 1972.

Camus, A. The Plague. Translated from the French by Stuart Gilbert. New York: Modern Library, 1948.

Canadian Cooperative Stroke Study Group. A Randomized Trial of Aspirin and Sulfinpyrazone in Threatened Stroke. New Engl. J. Med. 299:53, 1978.

Carpenter, B. H., J. R. Chromy, W. D. Bach, D. A. LeSourd, and D. G. Gillette. Health Costs of Air Pollution: A Study of Hospitalization Costs. Am. J. Pub. Health 69:1232, 1979.

Cassel, J. Occupation and Physical Activity and Coronary Heart Disease. Arch. Int. Med. 128:920, 1971.

Cassel, J. The Contribution of the Social Environment to Host Resistance. Am. J. Epidemiol. 104:107, 1976.

Cassel, J., R. Patrick, and D. Jenkins. Epidemiologic Analysis of the Health Implications of Culture Change: A Conceptual Model. Ann. N.Y. Acad. Sci. 84:938, 1960.

Central Committee for Medical and Community Program of the American Heart Association. Risk Factors and Coronary Disease. New York: Am. Heart Assoc., 1968.

Chadwick, E. Report on the Sanitary Condition of the Laboring Population of Great Britain, 1842, reprinted with an introduction by M.W. Flinn. Edinburgh: Univ. Press, 1965.

Chapin, C. V. Papers of Charles V. Chapin, M.D. In Principles of Epidemiology, pp. 172-205. New York: Commonwealth Fund, 1934.

Chase, G., and M. R. Klauber. A Graph of Sample Sizes for Retrospective Studies. Am. J. Pub. Health 55:1993, 1965.

Chase, H. C. The Study of Infant Mortality from Linked Records: Methods of Study and Registration Aspects, United States. National Center for Health Statistics, Public Health Service Publication, No. 1000-ser. 20, No. 7. Washington, D.C.: USGPO, 1970.

Chiang, C. L. An Index of Health: Mathematical Models. Public Health Service Publication No. 1000-ser. 2, no. 5. Washington D.C.: USGPO, 1965.

Christianson, R. E. The Relationship between Maternal Smoking and the Incidence of Congenital Anomalies. Am. J. Epidemiol. 112:684, 1980.

Cobb, S. The Frequency of Rheumatic Diseases. American Public Health Assn. Vital and Health Statistics Monographs. Cambridge: Harvard Univ. Press, 1972.

Cobb, S., P. M. Densen, J. Elinson, D. M. Spain, and M. T. Bellows. Potentialities and Limitations in Field Study Methods and Needs for Improvement, Conference on Epidemiology of Atherosclerosis and Hypertension. Harriman, New York: American Heart Association and National Heart Institute, 1956.

Cochran, W. G. Matching in Analytical Studies. Am. J. Pub. Health 43:684, 1953.

Cockburn, A. The Evolution and Eradication of Infectious Diseases. Baltimore: Johns Hopkins Press, 1963.

Cockrill, W. R. Patterns of Disease. (Zoonoses.) Vet. Rec. 78:1, 1966.

Cole, P. The Evolving Case-Control Study. J. Chronic Dis. 12:15-27, 1979.

Cole, P., and B. MacMahon. Attributable Risk Percent in Case-Control Studies. Br. J. Prev. Soc. Med. 25:242-244, 1971.

Collaborative Group for the Study of Stroke in Young Women. Oral Contraception and Increased Risk of Cerebral Ischemia or Thrombosis. N. Engl. J. Med. 288:871, 1973.

Colombo, F., S. Shapiro, D. Slone, and G. Tognoni, eds. Epidemiological Evaluation of Drugs. Littleton, Massachusetts: PSF Publ., 1977.

Colvez, A., and M. Blanchet. Disability Trends in the United States Population 1966-1976: Analysis of Reported Causes. Am. J. Pub. Health 71:464, 1981.

Comparability in International Epidemiology. Milbank Mem. Fund Quart. 43: No. 2, Part 2, April 1965.

Comstock, G. W. Frost Revisited: The Modern Epidemiology of Tuberculosis. Am. J. Epidemiol. 101:363, 1975.

Comstock, G. W. Uncontrolled Ruminations on Modern Controlled Trials. Am. J. Epidemiol. 108:81, 1978.

Cooper, B., and H. G. Morgan. Epidemiological Psychiatry. Springfield: Thomas Publ. Co., 1973.

Cornfield, J., and K. Detre. Selection on Atherosclerosis as an Explanation of the Attenuated Cholesterol-Mortality Relation in Coronary Heart Disease. Am. J. Epidemiol. 110:716, 1979.

Cornfield, J., and W. Haenszel Some Aspects of Retrospective Studies. J. Chronic Dis. 11:523, 1960.

Cornfield, J., and S. Mitchell. Selected Risk Factors in Coronary Disease: Possible Intervention Effects. Arch. Environ. Health 19:382, 1969.

Cox, D. R. Planning of Experiments. New York: Wiley, 1958.

Creech, J. L. Angiosarcoma of the Liver among Polyvinyl Chloride Workers-- Kentucky. Morbidity Mortality Weekly Rep. 23:49, 1974.

Creighton, C. A History of Epidemics in Britain, Vol. 1, From 66 A.D. to Extinction of Plague; Vol. 2, From the Extinction of Plague to the Present Time. Cambridge: Univ. Press, 1894.

Crosby, A. W. Epidemic and Peace, 1918. Westport: Greenwood Press, 1976.

Cruikshank, R., K. L. Standard, and H. B. L. Russell, eds. Epidemiology and Community Health in Warm Climate Countries. New York: Churchill Livingstone, 1976.

Cumston, C. G. An Introduction to the History of Medicine: From the Time of the Pharoahs to the End of the XVIII Century. London: Dawsons of Pall Mall, 1968.

Cutler, S. J. The Role of Morbidity Reporting and Case Registers in Cancer Control. Pub. Health Rep. 65:1084, 1950.

Cutler, S. J., S. W. Greenhouse, J. Cornfield, and M. A. Schneiderman. The Role of Hypothesis Testing in Clinical Trials. J. Chronic Dis. 19: 857, 1966.

Dalenius, T. (ed.). Bibliography on Non-sampling Errors in Surveys, I (A-G); II (H-Q). Intern. Statist. Rev. 45:71-89, 1977, I (A-G); 45:181- 197, 1977, II (H-Q); 45:303-317, 1977, III (R-Z).

Dauer, C. C., R. F. Korns, F., and L. M. Schuman. Infectious Diseases. Vital and Health Statistics Monographs. New York: American Public Health Assoc., 1968.

Davis, C. E. The Effect of Regression to the Mean in Epidemiologic and Clinical Studies. Am. J. Epidemiol. 104:493, 1976.

Dawber, T. R., G. F. Meadors, and E. J. Moore, Jr. Epidemiological Approaches to Heart Disease: The Framingham Study. Am. J. Pub. Health 41:279, 1951.

Dean, H. T., F. S. McKay, and E. Elvove. Mottled Enamel Survey of Bauxite, Arkansas, 10 Years After a Change in the Common Water Supply. Pub. Health. Rep. 53:1736, 1938.

Dean, H. T., F. A. Arnold, and E. Elvove. Domestic Water and Dental Caries V. Pub. Health Rep. 57: 1155, 1942.

DeCoufle, P., T. L. Thomas, and L. W. Pickle. Comparison of the Proportionate Mortality Rates and Standardized Mortality Ratio Risk Measures. Am. J. Epidemiol. 111:263, 1980.

DeKruif, P. Microbe Hunters. New York, Harcourt Brace, 1935.

Dixon, C. W. Smallpox. London: Churchill, 1962.

Dobson, A. J., R. W. Gibberd, D. J. Wheeler, and S. R. Leeder. Age-Specific Trends in Mortality from Ischemic Heart Disease and Cerebrovascular Disease in Australia. Am. J. Epidemiol. 113:404, 1981.

Dolan, E. F., and H. T. Silver. William Crawford Gorgas: Warrior in White. New York: Dodd, Mead, 1968.

Doll, R., ed. Methods of Geographic Pathology: Report of the Study Group Convened by the Council for International Organizations of Medical Sciences. Springfield, Ill.: Thomas, 1959.

Dorn, H. Some Applications of Biometry in the Collection and Evaluation of Medical Data. J. Chronic Dis. 1:638:, 1955.

Dorn, H. F. A Classification System for Morbidity Concepts, Pub. Health Rep. 72:1043, 1957.

Dorn, H. F. Mortality, pp. 437-471. In Study of Population: An Inventory and Appraisal, P. Hauser, and O. D. Duncan, eds. Chicago: Univ. of Chicago Press, 1959.

Dorn, H. F. Some Problems Arising in Prosective and Retrospective Studies of the Etiology of Disease. N. Engl. J. Med. 261:571, 1959.

Douglas, M. Purity and Danger: An Analysis of Concepts of Pollution and Taboo. London: Routledge & Kegan Paul, 1966.

Downes, J., and S. D. Collins. A Study of Illness Among Families in the Eastern Health District of Baltimore. Milbank Mem. Fund Quart. 18:5, 1940.

Doyle, D. M. Accuracy of Selected Items of Blue Cross Information. Inquiry 3:16, 1966.

Dubois, G. Comparison of Relative Risks Computed from Prevalence and Incidence Studies. Am. J. Epidemiol. 104:222, 1976.

Dubos, R. Mirage of Health. New York: Harper, 1959.

Dubos, R. Man Adapting. New Haven: Yale Univ. Press, 1965.

Dubos, R. Man, Medicine and Environment. New York: Praeger, 1968.

Dubos, R., and J. Dubos. The White Plague: Tuberculosis, Man and Society. Boston: Little Brown, 1952.

Dubos, R. J., and J. G. Hirsch, eds. Bacterial and Mycotic Infections of Man, ed. 4. Philadelphia: Lippincott, 1965.

Duffy, J. Sword of Pestilence, Baton Rouge: Louisiana State Univ. Press, 1966.

Dunn, H. L. Points of Attack for Raising the Levels of Wellness. J. Nat. Med. Assoc. 49:225, 1957.

Dunn, H. L., and W. Shackley. Comparison of Cause-of-Death Assignments by the 1929 and 1938 Revisions of the International List: Deaths in the United States, 1940. Vital Statist. Spec. Rep., 19:14, 153, 1944.

Dunn, J. E. The Use of Incidence and Prevalence in the Study of Disease Development in a Population. Am. J. Pub. Health 52:1107, 1962.

Dupree, E. A., and M. B. Meyer. Role of Risk Factors in Complications of Diabetes Mellitus. Am. J. Epidemiol. 112:100, 1980.

Ederer, F. Practical Problems in Collaborative Clinical Trials. Am. J. Epidemiol. 102:111, 1975.

Edsall, G. The Swine Flu Affair: Decision-Making on a Slippery Disease. Am. J. Epidemiol. 110:522, 1979.

Elandt-Johnson, R. C. Definition of Rates: Some Remarks on Their Use and Misuse. Am. J. Epidemiol. 102:267, 1975.

Elder, R. and R. M. Acheson. New Haven Survey of Joint Diseases, XIV. Social Class and Behavior in Response to Symptoms of Osteoarthritis. Milbank Mem. Fund Quart. 48:449, 1970, pt. 1.

Emerson, H. Reliability of Statements of Cause of Death from Clinical and Pathological Viewpoints. Am. J. Pub. Health 6:680, 1916.

Engel, L. W., J. A. Strauchen, L. Chiazze, and M. Heid. Accuracy of Death Certification in an Autopsied Population with Specific Attention to Malignant Neoplasms and Vascular Diseases. Am. J. Epidemiol. 111:99, 1980.

Epidemic of Poliomyelitis in New York, New York City Dept. of Health Monograph Reprinted, Metuchen: Arno Press, 1977.

Epidemiologic Evaluation of Drugs, Proc. Intern. Symp. Milan, Italy, May 1977. Biomedical Press, 1977.

Epidemiologic Impact of Psychotropic Drugs, Proc. Intern. Symp. Milan, Italy. New York: Elsevier, North Holland Biomedical Press, 1981.

Epidemiologic Reviews, Am. J. Epidemiol (Annual), 1979, 1980, 1981.

Epidemiology of Abortion and Fertility Regulation in Latin America. PAHO, 1975.

Epidemiology of Aging. National Institutes of Health Conference, 1977.

Epidemiology of Anencephalus and Spina Bifida, Elwood, J. M. New York: Oxford Univ. Press, 1980.

Epidemiology of Arterial Blood Pressure, Kesteloo, H., and J. V. Joossens, eds. Boston: Nijhoff, 1980.

Epidemiology of Cerebrovascular Diseases, Kurtzke, J. F. Springer Press, 1969.

Epidemiology of Chronic Digestive Disease, Langman, M. J. S. Chicago: Year Book Medical Publishers, 1979.

Epidemiology of Chronic Lung Diseases in Children, Gordis, L. Baltimore: Johns Hopkins Press, 1973.

Epidemiology of Chronic Respiratory Disease, Higgins, I. T. T. Ann Arbor: Univ. Michigan Press, 1974.

Epidemiology of Dementia, Mortimer, J. A. and L. M. Schuman, eds. New York: Oxford Univ. Press, 1981.

Epidemiology of Diabetes and Its Vascular Lesions, West, K. M. New York: Elsevier, North Holland Biomedical Press, 1978.

Epidemiology of Drug Abuse, Greene, M. H. and R. L. DuPont, 1974.

Epidemiology of Drug Abuse, Conference on the Current Issues, Richards, L. G. and L. B. Blevens, eds. Miami Beach: NIH, NIDA, 1977.

Epidemiology of Epilepsy, Alter, M. and W. A. Hauser, eds. Bethesda: NIH, NINDS, 1971.

Epidemiology of Hospital Associated Infections, Fuchs, P. C. Chicago: Am. Soc. Clin. Pathologists, 1979.

Epidemiology of Human Mycotic Diseases, Al-Doory, Y., ed. Springfield: Thomas, 1975.

Epidemiology of Multiple Sclerosis, Alter, M. and J. F. Kurtzke. Springfield: Thomas, 1968.

Epidemiology of Neurologic and Sense Organ Disorders, Kurland, L. T., J. K. Kurtzke, and I. D. Goldberg. Cambridge: Harvard Univ. Press, 1973.

Epidemiology of Prematurity, Proc. NIH Conf., Reed, D. M. and F. J. Stanley, eds. Baltimore: Urban and Schwartzenberg, NICHD, 1977.

Epidemiology of Road Traffic Accidents: Report on a Conference. Copenhagen: WHO, 1976.

Epidemiology of Stomach Cancer: Meeting on the Future Inquiries into Its Epidemiology. Hirayama, T., ed. Tokyo: WHO, 1976.

Epidemiologic Studies in Viral Hepatitis. Am. J Epidemiol. 105:91-162, 1977. (Entire issue)

Epstein, F. H. Predicting Coronary Heart Disease. J. Am. Med. Assoc. 201:795, 1967.

Epstein, F. H. Epidemiologic Aspects of Atherosclerosis. Atherosclerosis 14:1, 1971.

Ernster, V. On the Teaching of Epidemiology to Medical Students. Am. J. Epidemiol. 109:617, 1979.

Evans, A. S. The Need for Serologic Evaluation of Immunization Programs. Am. J. Epidemiol. 112:725, 1980.

Evans, D., and D. S. Lane. Long Term Outcome of Smoking Cessation Workshops. Am. J. Pub. Health 70:725, 1980.

Fanshel, S. and J. W. Bush. A Health-Status Index and Its Application to Health Services Outcomes. Oper. Res. 18:1021, 1970.

Farr, W. Vital Statistics: Memorial Volume of Selections from the Reports and Writings of Wm. Farr (1885), Humphreys, N. A., ed. Metuchen: Arno Press, 1975.

Feinleib, M., R. J. Garrison, R. Fabsitz, J. C. Christian, Z. Hrubec, N. O. Borhani, W. B. Kannel, R. Rosenman, J. T. Schwartz, and J. O. Wagner. The NHLBI Twin Study of Cardiovascular Disease Risk Factors: Methodology and Summary of Results. Am. J. Epidemiol. 106:284, 1977.

Feinstein, A. R. Clinical Judgment. Baltimore: Williams & Wilkins, 1967.

Feinstein, A. R. Methodologic Problems and Standards in Case-Control Research. J. Chronic Dis. 32:35-41, 1979.

Feldman, J. J. Barriers to the Use of Health Survey Data in Demographic Analysis. Milbank Mem. Fund Quart. 36:203, 1958.

Feldman, J. J. The Household Interview Survey as a Technique for the Collection of Morbidity Data. J. Chronic Dis. 11:535, 1960.

Fields, W. S., N. A. Lemak, R. F. Frankowski, and R. J. Hardy. Controlled Trial of Aspirin in Cerebral Ischemia. Stroke 8:301, 1977.

Fine, P. E. M. A Commentary on the Mechanical Analogue to the Reed-Frost Epidemic Model. Am. J. Epidemiol. 106:87, 1977.

Fisher, R. A. The Design of Experiments, 7th ed. New York: Hafner Publ., 1971.

Fleiss, J. L. Statistical Methods for Rates and Proportions. New York: Wiley, 1981.

Foley, D. L. Census Tracts in Urban Research. J. Am. Statist. Assoc. 48:733, 1953.

Fox, J.P., C. E. Hall, and L. R. Elveback. Epidemiology: Man and Disease. New York: MacMillan, 1970.

Framingham Study (Multiple Volumes). Washington: USGPO.

Francis, T., Jr. An Evaluation of the 1954 Poliomyelitis Vaccine Trials-- Summary Report. Am. J. Pub. Health 45:1, 1955.

Francis, T., Jr. Evaluation of the 1954 Field Trial of Poliomyelitis Vaccine: Final Report. Michigan: Edwards, 1957.

Frankel, L. K., and L. I. Dublin. A Sickness Survey of North Carolina. Pub. Health Rep. 31:2820, 1916.

Fraumeni, J.F., ed. Persons at High Risk of Cancer. New York: Academic Press, 1975.

Freeman, J. Prevalence, Incidence and Duration. Am. J. Epidemiol. 112:696, 1980.

Friedman, G. D. Medical Usage and Abusage: "Prevalence" and "Incidence." Ann. Int. Med. 84:502, 1976.

Friedman, G.D. Primer of Epidemiology, 2nd ed. New York: McGraw-Hill, 1980.

Froelicher, V. Analysis of Epidemiologic Studies of Physical Inactivity as a Risk Factor for Coronary Heart Disease. Prog. Cardiovasc. Dis. 15:41, 1972.

Frost, W. H. Papers of Wade Hampton Frost. New York: Commonwealth Fund, 1941. Republished, Metuchen: Arno Press, 1977.

Gafafer, W. M., ed. Occupational Diseases: A Guide to Their Recognition. PHS Pub. No. 1097. Washington: USGPO, 1964.

Gale, A. H. Epidemic Diseases. Baltimore: Penguin, 1959.

Galen's Hygiene. Translated by R. M. Green, Springfield: Thomas, 1951.

Gangarosa, E. J., and G. A. Faich. Cholera: The Risk to American Travelers. Ann. Intern. Med. 74:412,1971.

Gent, M., and I. Shigematsu. Epidemiological Issues in Reported Drug-Induced Illnesses--SMON and Other Examples; Hamilton: McMaster Univ. Library Press, 1978.

Gilliam, A. Opportunities for Application of Epidemiologic Method to Study of Cancer. Am. J. Pub. Health 43:1247, 1953.

Gilliam, A. Epidemiology in Non-Communicable Disease. Pub. Health Rep. 69:907, 1954.

Gladen, B., and W. J. Rogan. Misclassification and the Design of Environmental Studies. Am. J. Epidemiol. 109:607, 1979.

Glasser, J. The Quality and Utility of Death Certificate Data. Am. J. Pub. Health 71:231, 1981.

Gold, R., and B. Yankaskas, eds. Epidemiology and Public Health: Pretest Self-Assessment and Review, 2nd ed. New York: McGraw-Hill, 1980.

Goldberger, J. Goldberger on Pellagra. Terris, M., ed. Baton Rouge: Louisiana State Univ. Press, 1964.

Goldston, I., ed. Beyond the Germ Theory: The Roles of Deprivation and Stress in Health and Disease. New York: Health Education Council, 1954.

Gordis, L. Assuring the Quality of Questionnaire Data in Epidemiologic Research. Am. J. Epidemiol. 109:21, 1979.

Gordis, L. Challenges to Epidemiology in the Coming Decade. Am. J. Epidemiol. 112:315, 1980.

Gordon, J. Epidemiology, the Diagnostic Discipline of Public Health. J. Roy. San. Inst. 74:445, 1954.

Gordon, J. Epidemiology in Modern Perspective. Proc. Roy. Soc. Med. 47:22, 1954.

Gordon, T. Symptoms as a Diagnostic Tool, in Three Views of Hypertension and Heart Disease, pp. 9-10. PHS Publ. No. 1000-ser. 2, No. 22 Washington: USGPO, 1967.

Gorgas, M. D., and B. J. Henrick. William Crawford Gorgas: His Life and Work. Garden City: Doubleday Page, 1924.

Graham, S., and C. Mettlin. Diet and Colon Cancer. Am. J. Epidemiol. 109:1, 1979.

Graunt, J. Natural and Political Observations Made upon the Bills of Mortality. London, 1662. Reprinted as Foundations of Vital Statistics, Vol. 3, Part 8, Chap. 1, pp. 1421-1436. In Newman, J.R. The World of Mathematics. New York: Simon & Schuster, 1956.

Greenhouse, S. Some Epidemiologic Issues for the 1980s. Am. J. Epidemiol. 112:269, 1980.

Greenland, S. Response and Follow-up Bias in Cohort Studies. Am. J. Epidemiol. 106:184, 1977.

Greenland, S. The Effect of Misclassification in the Presence of Covariates. Am. J. Epidemiol. 112:564, 1980.

Greenwood, M. Epidemiology: Historical and Experimental. Baltimore: John Hopkins Press, 1932.

Greenwood, M. Epidemic and Crowd Diseases. London: Williams & Norgate, Ltd., 1935.

Greenwood, M. Medical Statistics from Graunt to Farr. London: Cambridge Univ. Press, 1948.

Greenwood, M., A. B. Hill, W. W. C. Topley, and J. Wilson. Experimental Epidemiology, p. 7-63 and 193-203. Medical Research Council, Special Report Series, No. 209, London: His Majesty's Stationery Office, 1936.

Hackett, L. W. Malaria in Europe: An Ecological Study. London: Oxford Univ. Press, 1937.

Haenszel, W., ed. Epidemiological Approaches to the Study of Cancer and Other Chronic Diseases. National Cancer Institute Monogr. No. 19. Washington: USGPO, 1966.

Hammond, E. C. Some Preliminary Findings on Physical Complaints from a Prospective Study of 1,064,004 Men and Women. Am. J. Pub. Health 54:11, 1964.

Hardy, R. J., and C. White. Matching in Retrospective Studies. Am. J. Epidemiol. 93:75, 1971.

Harris, M. Mutagenicity of Chemicals and Drugs. Science 171:51, 1971.

Hartunian, N. S., C. N. Smart, and M. Thompson. The Incidence and Economic Costs of Cancer, Motor Vehicle Injuries, Coronary Heart Disease and Stroke: A Comparative Analysis. Am. J. Pub. Health 70:1249, 1980.

Haynes, S. G., and M. Feinleib. Women, Work and Coronary Heart Disease: Prospective Findings from the Framingham Heart Study. Am. J. Pub. Health 70:133, 1980.

Hecker, J. F. The Epidemics of the Middle Ages. London: Sydenham Society, 1844.

Henderson, B. E., R. J. Gordon, H. Menck, J. SooHoo, S. P. Martin, and M. C. Pike. Lung Cancer and Air Pollution in Southcentral Los Angeles County. Am. J. Epidemiol. 101:477, 1975.

Henderson, D. A. Epidemiology in the Global Eradication of Smallpox. Int. J. Epidemiol. 1:25, 1972.

Henle, J. On Miasmata and Contagia, 1840 (George Rosen, transl.). Baltimore: The Johns Hopkins Press, 1938.

Henry, S. A. Landmarks in the History of Cancer of the Scrotum. Cancer of the Scrotum in Relation to Occupation. New York: Oxford Univ. Press, 1946.

Herbst, A. L., R. J. Kurman, R. E. Scully and D. C. Poskanzer. Clear Cell Adenocarcinoma of the Genital Tract in Young Females. N. Engl J. Med. 287:1259, 1972.

Hirsch, A. Handbook of Geographical and Historical Pathology, Vol. 1 (C. Creighton, transl.). London: New Sydenham Society, 1883.

Hirst, L. F. The Conquest of Plague: A Study of the Evolution of Epidemiology. Oxford: Clarendon Press, 1953.

Hobsen, W. World Health and History. Bristol: John Wright, 1963.

Holland, W. W., ed. Data Handling in Epidemiology. London: Oxford Univ. Press, 1970.

Holland, W. W. and S. Gilderdale. Epidemiology and Health. Chicago: Year Book Med. Publ., 1977.

Holland, W. W., and L. Karhausen, eds. Health Care and Epidemiology. Boston: G. K. Hall, 1979.

Holland W. W., A. E. Bennett, I.R. Cameron, C. du V. Florey, S. R. Leader, R. S. F. Schilling, A. V. Swan, and R .E. Waller. Health Effects of Particulate Pollution: Reappraising the Evidence. Am. J. Epidemiol. 110:525, 1979 (special issue).

Holmes, O. W. The Contagiousness of Puerperal Fever. In Medical Essays (1842-1882). Boston: Houghton, Mifflin, 1883.

Hoppenbrouwers, T., M. Calub, K. Arakawa, and J. E. Hodgman. Seasonal Relationship of Sudden Infant Death Syndrome and Environmental Pollutants. Am. J. Epidemiol. 113:623, 1981.

Horsfall, F. L., Jr., and I. Tamm, ed. Viral and Rickettsial Infections of Man, 4th ed. Philadelphia: Lippincott, 1965.

Horvitz, D. G. Methodological Considerations in Evaluating the Effectiveness of Programs and Benefits. Inquiry 2:96, 1965.

Horwitz, O., and C. E. Palmer. Epidemiological Basis of Tuberculosis Morbidity and Mortality. Bull. World Health Organization 30:609, 1964.

Huebner, R. J. The Virologist's Dilemma: Part V. Criteria for Etiologic Association of Prevalent Viruses With Prevalent Diseases. In Viruses In Search of Disease. Ann N.Y. Acad. Sci. 67:430, 1956-1957.

Huff, D. How to Lie With Statistics. New York: Norton, 1954.

Hypertension Detection and Follow-up Program Cooperative Group. Reduction in Mortality of Persons with High Blood Pressure, Including Mild Hypertension. J. Am. Med. Assoc. 242:2562, 1979.

Ibrahim, M. A., ed. The Case-Control Study: Consensus and Controversy. London: Pergamon Press, 1979.

International Classification of Diseases Adapted, 10 Editions (9th Revision) Univ. Michigan Press, 1978.

International Symposium on Coronary Heart Disease: Proceedings. Stockholm: Association against Heart and Lung Disease, 1972.

Iskrant, A. P., and P. V. Joliet. Accidents and Homicide. Vital and Health Statistics Monographs. New York: Am. Pub. Health Assoc., 1968.

Israel, R. A., and A. J. Kelbba. A Preliminary Report on the Effect of Eighth Revision ICDA On Cause of Death Statistics. Am. J. Pub. Health 59:1651, 1969.

Jacobs, D. R., J. T. Anderson, and H. Blackburn. Diet and Serum Cholesterol: Do Zero Correlations Negate the Relationship? Am. J. Epidemiol. 110:77, 1979.

Jacobsen, R. R. The Epidemiology of Leprosy. USPHS Hospital, Carville, Louisiana, 1967.

Jacques, P. F., S. C. Hartz, R. W. Tuthill, and C. Hollingsworth. Elimination of "Lead Time" Bias in Assessing the Effect of Early Breast Cancer Diagnosis. Am. J. Epidemiol. 113:93, 1981.

James, G., R. E. Patton, and A. S. Heslin. Accuracy of Cause of Death Statements on Death Certificates. Pub. Health Rep. 70:39, 1955.

James, M. T., and R. F. Harwood. Herm's Medical Entomology, 6th ed. New York: Macmillan, 1969.

Jenkins, C. D. Psychologic and Social Prescursors of Coronary Disease. Part I. N. Engl. J. Med. 284:244, 1971. Part II. N. Engl. J. Med. 284:307, 1971.

Jick, H. The Commission on Professional and Hospital Activities--Professional Activity Study. A National Resource for the Study of Rare Illnesses. Am. J. Epidemiol. 109:625, 1979.

Jick, H., and M. P. Vessey. Case-Control Studies in the Evaluation of Drug-Induced Illness. Am. J. Epidemiol. 107:1, 1979.

Jick, H., A. M. Walker, R. N. Watkins, D. C. D'Ewart, J. R. Hunter, A. Danford, S. Madsen, B. J. Dinan, and K. J. Rothman. Oral Contraceptives and Breast Cancer. Am. J. Epidemiol. 112:577, 1980.

Jick, H., A. M. Walker, and K. J. Rothman. The Epidemic of Endometrial Cancer: A Commentary. Am. J. Pub. Health 70:164, 1980.

Kahn, C. History of Smallpox and Its Prevention. Am. J. Dis. Child. 106:597, 1963.

Kahn, H. The Relationship of Reported Coronary Heart Disease Mortality to Physical Activity of Work. Am. J. Pub. Health 53:1058, 1663.

Kaminsky, R., J. Brockert, J. Sestito, and T. Frazier. Occupational Information on Death Certificates: a Survey of State Practices. Am. J. Pub. Health 71:525, 1981.

Kannel, W. Profile of the Coronary Prone Individual, the Framingham Study. Proc. Med. Soc. 55:74, 1967.

Kantor, A. F. Upton Sinclair and the Pure Food and Drug Act of 1906. Am. J. Pub. Health 66:1202, 1976.

Kark, S. L. Epidemiology and Community Medicine. New York: Appleton-Century-Crofts, 1974.

Kass, E.H., ed. Preventive Approaches to Chronic Disease: Proceedings of a Conference on Chronic Diseases, 1969. Milbank Mem. Fund Quart. 47(3): 1969, Part 2.

Katz, S., A. B. Ford, R. W. Moskowitz, B. A. Jackson, and M. W. Jaffe. Studies of Illness in the Aged: The Index of ADL, A Standardized Measure of Biological and Psychosocial Function. J. Am. Med. Assoc. 185: 914, 1963.

Katz, S., A. B. Ford, T. D. Downs, and M. Adams. Chronic Disease Classification in Evaluation of Medical Care Programs. Med. Care 7:139, 1969.

Kemper, J. T. Error Sources in the Evaluation of Secondary Attack Rates. Am. J. Epidemiol. 112:457, 1980.

Kessler, I. I., and M. L. Levin. The Community as an Epidemiologic Laboratory: A Casebook of Community Studies. Baltimore: Johns Hopkins
Press, 1970.

Keys, A., C. Aravanis, H. Blackburn, F. S. P. Van Buchem, R. Buzina,
B. S. Djordjevic, A. S. Dontas, F. Fidanza, M. J. Karvonen, N. Kimura,
D. Lekos, M. Monti, V. Puddu, and H. L. Taylor. Epidemiologic Studies
Related to Coronary Heart Disease: Characteristics of Men Aged 40-59 in
Seven Countries. Acta Medica Scand., Suppl. 460, 1966.

Keys, A., C. Aravanis, H. Blackburn, F. S. P. Van Buchem, R. Buzina,
B. S. Djordjevic, F. Fidanza, M. J. Karvonen, A. Menotti, V. Puddu,
and H.L. Taylor. Coronary Heart Disease: Overweight and Obesity as
Risk Factors. Ann. Int. Med. 77: 15, 1972.

Kirchheimer, W. F. Leprosy (Hansen's Disease). In: CRC Handbook Series in
Zoonoses, Steele, J. H., ed. Boca Raton: CRC Press, 1979.

Kleinbaum, D. G., H. Morgenstern, and L. L. Kupper. Selection Bias in
Epidemiologic Studies. Am. J. Epidemiol. 113:452, 1981.

Kleinman, J. C., J. J. Feldman, and M. A. Monk. The Effects of Changes in
Smoking Habits on Coronary Heart Disease Mortality. Am. J. Pub. Health
69:795, 1979.

Klingberg, M. A., and J. A. C. Weatherall. Epidemiologic Methods for Detect-
ing Teratogens. Basel: Karger, 1979.

Knox, E. G., and R. M. Acheson. Epidemiology in Health Care Planning: A
Guide to the Uses of a Scientific Method. New York: Oxford Univ.
Press, 1979.

Kotin, P., and L. A. Gaul. Smoking in the Workplace: A Hazard Ignored.
Am. J. Pub. Health 70:575, 1980.

Kramer, M. A. Discussion of the Concepts of Incidence and Prevalence as
Related to Epidemiologic Studies of Mental Disorders. Am. J. Pub. Health
47:826, 1957.

Kuller, L., and D. M. Reisler. An Explanation for Variations in Distribution
of Stroke and Arteriosclerotic Heart Disease Among Populations and Racial
Groups. Am. J. Epidemiol. 93:1, 1971.

Kuller, L., J. Neaton, A. Caggiula, and L. Falvo-Gerard. Primary Prevention
of Heart Attacks: the Multiple Risk Factor Intervention Trial. Am. J.
Epidemiol. 112:185, 1980.

Kurlander, A. B., E. H. Hill, and P. E. Enterline. An Evaluation of Some
Commonly Used Screening Tests for Heart Disease and Hypertension. J.
Chronic Dis. 2:427, 1955.

Kurtzke, J. F. Epidemiology of Cerebrovascular Disease. New York:
Springer-Verlag, 1969.

Kurtzke, J. F. International Classification of Diseases 9: A Regression. Am.
J. Epidemiol. 109:383, 1979.

Laird, N. M., M. C. Weinstein, and W. B. Stason. Sample-Size Estimation: A
Sensitivity Analysis in the Context of a Clinical Trial for Treatment of
Mild Hypertension. Am. J. Epidemiol. 109:408, 1979.

Lambert, R. Sir John Simon. 1816-1904. London: MacGibbon & Kee, 1963.

Lane, J. M., F. L. Ruben, J. M. Neff, and J. D. Milar. Complications of
Smallpox Vaccination, 1968: National Surveillance in the U.S. N. Engl.
J. Med. 281:1201, 1969.

Langmuir, A. D. The Surveillance of Communicable Diseases of National Importance. N. Engl. J. Med. 268:182, 1963.

Langmuir, A. D. William Farr: Founder of Modern Concepts of Surveillance. Int. J. Epidemiol. 5:13, 1976.

Langmuir, A. D., N. Nathanson, and W. J. Hall. The Surveillance of Poliomyelitis in the United States in 1955. Am. J. Pub. Health 46:75, 1956.

Lapage, G. Animals Parastic to Man. Baltimore: Penguin, 1963.

Last, J. M. Primary Medical Care: Record Keeping. Milbank Mem. Fund Quart. 43(2): 1965.

Last, J. M., ed. Maxcy-Rosenau Public Health and Preventive Medicine, 11th ed. New York: Appleton-Century-Crofts, 1980.

Lee, D. H. K., and D. Minard, ed. Physiology, Environment and Man: The Bretton Woods Symposium on Physiological Characterization of Health Hazards in Man's Environment. New York: Academic Press, 1970.

Leske, M. C., F. Ederer, and M. Podgor. Estimating Incidence from Age-Specific Prevalence in Glaucoma. Am. J. Epidemiol. 113:606, 1981.

Levin, M. L. Screening for Asymptomatic Disease: Principles and Background. J. Chronic Dis. 2:367, 1955. (Entire issue)

Levin, M. L., H. Goldstein, and P. R. Gerhardt. Cancer and Tobacco. A Preliminary Report. J. Am. Med. Assoc. 143:336, 1950.

Lew, E. A. Heart Disease Mortality: Changing Terminology, Diagnostic Fashions and Capabilities. Am. J. Pub. Health 70:411, 1980.

Lilienfeld, A. M. Epidemiological Methods and Inferences in Studies of Non-Infectious Diseases. Pub. Health Rep. 72:51, 1957.

Lilienfeld, A. M. The Epidemiology of Mongolism. Baltimore: Johns Hopkins Press, 1969.

Lilienfeld, A. M., ed. Reviews in Cancer Epidemiology, Vol. 1. New York: Elsevier-North Holland, 1980.

Lilienfeld, A. M., ed. Times, Place and Persons. Baltimore: Johns Hopkins Press, 1980.

Lilienfeld, A. M. The Humean Fog: Cancer and Cholesterol. Am. J. Epidemiol. 114:1, 1981.

Lilienfeld, A. M. and A. J. Gifford, eds. Chronic Diseases and Public Health. Baltimore: Johns Hopkins Press, 1966.

Lilienfeld, A. M. and D. E. Lilienfeld. Foundations of Epidemiology, 2nd Ed. New York: Oxford Univ. Press, 1980.

Lilienfeld, A. M., E. Pedersen, and J. E. Dowd. Cancer Epidemiology: Methods of Study. Baltimore: Johns Hopkins Press, 1967.

Lilienfeld, A. M., M. L. Levin, and I. I. Kessler. Cancer in the United States. Cambridge: Harvard Univ. Press, 1972.

Lilienfeld, D. E. and A. M. Lilienfeld. Epidemiology: A Retrospective Study. Am. J. Epidemiol. 106:445, 1977.

Lin, F. Y., and C. C. Standely. The Scope of Epidemiology in Psychiatry. Geneva: World Health Organization, Public Health Papers No. 16, 1962.

Lind, J. An Essay on the Effectual Means of Preserving the Health of Seamen in the Royal Navy (1757). London: A. Millar, 1957.

Lind, J. A. Treatise on the Scurvy (1753) C. P. Stewart and D. Guthrie, eds., Edinburgh: Univ. Press, 1953.

Linos, A., J. W. Worthington, W. M. O'Fallon, and L. T. Kurland. The Epidemiology of Rheumatoid Arthritis in Rochester, Minnesota: A Study of Incidence, Prevalence, and Mortality. Am. J. Epidemiol. 111:87, 1980.

Liu, K., R. Cooper, J. McKeever, P. McKeever, R. Byington, I. Soltero, R. Stamler, F. Gosch, E. Stevens, and J. Stamler. Assessment of the Association between Habitual Salt Intake and High Blood Pressure: Methodological Problems. Am. J. Epidemiol. 110:219, 1979.

Longmate, N. King Cholera: The Biography of a Disease. London: Hamish Hamilton, 1966.

Lovel, R. The Aetiology of Infectious Diseases. East Lansing: Michigan State Univ. Press, 1959.

Lowe, C. R., and J. Kostrezewski, eds. Epidemiology: A Guide to Teaching Methods. London: Churchill-Livingstone, 1973.

Lowell, A. M. Tuberculosis in the World. USDHEW, PHS, Washington: USGPO, 1976.

Lubs, H. A., and F. H. Ruddle. Chromosomal Abnormalities in the Human Population: Estimation of Rates Based on the New Haven Newborn Study. Science 169:495, 1970.

MacDonald, G. The Epidemiology and Control of Malaria. London: Oxford Univ. Press, 1957.

MacMahon, B., T. M. Lin, C. R. Lowe, A. Mirra, B. Ravnihar, E. J. Salber, D. Trichopoules, V. G. Valaoras, and S. Yuasa. Lactation and Cancer of the Breast: A Summary of an International Study. Bull. World Health Organization 42:185, 1970.

MacMahon, B., and T. Pugh. Epidemiologic Methods. Boston: Little, Brown, 1970.

Mainland, D. Notes on the Planning and Evaluation of Research, with Examples from Cardiovascular Investigation. Part I. Am. Heart J. 55:644, 1958; part II. 55:824, 1958.

Mainland, D. Elementary Medical Statistics, 2nd ed. Philadelphia: Saunders, 1963.

Mainland, D. Lecture Notes in Medical Statistics (Miller, M. C., ed.). Ann Arbor: Biometry Imprint Series Press, 1979.

Major, R. Classic Descriptions of Disease. Baltimore: Thomas, 1939.

Major, R. Fatal Partners: War and Disease. Garden City: Doubleday, Doran, 1941.

Major, R. Disease and Destiny. Logan Clendening Lectures on the History and Philosophy of Medicine--Series 8. Lawrence: Univ. of Kansas Press, 1958.

Manchee, R. J., M. G. Broster, J. Melling, R. M. Henstridge, and A. J. Stagg. Bacillus Anthracis on Gruinard Island. Nature 294:254, 1981.

Mantel, N., and W. Haenszel. Statistical Aspects of the Analysis of Data from Retrospective Studies of Disease. J. Nat. Cancer Inst. 22:719, 1959.

Mantel, N., C. Brown, and D. P. Byar. Tests for Homogeneity of Effect in an Epidemic Investigation. Am. J. Epidemiol. 106:125, 1977.

Marks, G. and W. K. Beatty. Epidemics. New York: Scribner, 1976.

Marmot, M. Facts, Opinions and Affaires du Coeur. Am. J. Epidemiol. 103:519, 1976.

Mausner, J., and A. K. Bahn. Epidemiology: An Introductory Text. Philadelphia: Saunders, 1974.

Maxcy, K. F. An Epidemiological Study of Endemic Typhus (Brill's Disease) in the Southeastern United States with Special Reference to Its Mode of Transmission. Am. J. Epidemiol. 85:333, 1967.

May, J. M. The Ecology of Human Disease. New York: M.D. Publications Inc., 1958.

May, J. M. Studies in Disease Ecology, Vol. 2. New York: Hafner, 1961.

McKay, F. S., and G. V. Black. An Investigation of Mottled Teeth: An Endemic Developmental Imperfection of the Enamel of the Teeth Heretofore Unknown in the Literature of Dentistry. Dent. Cosmos. 58:477-484, 1916 (Part I); 58:627-644, 1916 (Part II); 58:781-792, 1916 (Part III); 58:894-904, 1916 (Part IV).

McMullen, D. B., and H. W. Harry. Comments of the Epidemiology and Control of Bilharziasis. WHO Bull. 18:1037, 1958.

Mechanic, D. Medical Sociology: A Selective View. New York: Free Press, 1968.

Meier, P. Safety Testing of Poliomyelitis Vaccine. Science 125:1067, 1957.

Meyer, K. F. The Zoonoses in Their Relation to Rural Health. Publications in Public Health, Vol. 3. Berkeley: Univ. of California Press, 1955.

Miettenen, O. S. Matching and Design Efficiency in Retrospective Studies. Am. J. Epidemiol. 91:111, 1970.

Miller, D. C. Handbook of Research Design and Social Measurement, 2nd ed. New York: David McKay, 1970.

Miller, J. R. The Use of Registers and Vital Statistics in the Study of Congenital Malformations. In Second Scientific Conference on Congenital Malformations, pp. 334-340. New York: International Medical Corps, 1963.

Milunsky, A. Alpha-fetoprotein and the Prenatal Detection of Neural Tube Defects. Am. J. Pub. Health 69:552, 1979.

Mishler, E. G., and N. A. Scotch. Sociocultural Factors in the Epidemiology of Schizophrenia. Inter. J. Psychiatry 1:258, 1965.

Modell, W. Mass Drug Catastrophes and the Roles of Science and Technology. Science 156:346, 1967.

Modell, W. Malaria and Victory in Vietnam. Science 162:1346, 1968.

Monath, T. P., ed. St. Louis Encephalitis. Washington: Am. Pub. Health Assoc., 1980.

Monson, R. R. Occupational Epidemiology. Boca Raton: CRC Press, 1980.

Moore, W. S. Classifying Morbidity. Inquiry 7:41, 1970.

Moriyama, I. M. Development of the Present Concept of Cause of Death. Am. J. Pub. Health 46:426, 1956.

Moriyama, I. M. Problems in the Measurement of Health Status. In Indicators of Social Change (Eleanor Sheldon and Wilbert Moore, eds.). New York: Russell Sage Foundation, 1968.

Moriyama, I. M. Classification of Disease: A Fundamental Problem. J. Chronic Dis. 11:462, 1970.

Moriyama, I. M., D. E. Kreuger, and J. Stamler. Cardiovascular Diseases in the United States. Cambridge: Harvard Univ. Press, 1971.

Morris, J. Incidence and Prediction of Ischemic Heart Disease in London Busmen. Lancet 2:553, 1966.

Morris, J. N. Uses of Epidemiology, 3rd ed. London: Livingstone, 1975.

Morton, N. E. <u>Outline of Genetic Epidemiology</u>. New York: Karger, 1981.

Morton, R. F., and J. R. Hebel. <u>A Study Guide to Epidemiology and Biosta-</u><u>tistics including 100 Multiple Choice Questions</u>. Baltimore: Univ. Park Press, 1979.

Moses, L. E., and F. Mosteller. Institutional Differences in Postoperative Death Rates. Commentary on Some of the Findings of the National Halothane Study. <u>J. Am. Med. Assoc</u>. 203:492, 1968.

Naeye, R. Causes of Fetal and Neonatal Mortality by Race in a Selected U.S. Population. <u>Am. J. Pub. Health</u> 69:857, 1979.

Nathanson, N., and J. R. Martin. The Epidemiology of Poliomyelitis: Enigmas Surrounding Its Appearance, Endemicity and Disappearance. <u>Am. J. Epi-</u><u>demiol</u>. 110:672, 1979.

<u>National Center for Health Statistics Publications</u>
    <u>Fertility Tables for Birth Cohorts by Color</u> (annual)
    Health Examination Data (Series)
    Health Interview Survey (Series)
    Health in the United States, a Chartbook (Series)
    Hospital Discharge Survey (Series)
    Hospital Utilization (Series)
    Marriage and Divorce (Annual)
    Maternal and Child Health Studies Project (Series)
    Mortality and Natality (Annual)
    State Estimates of Disability and Utilization of Medical Services: U.S. (Series)
    Vital and Health Statistics (Series)

National Center for Health Statistics. <u>Use of Hospital Data for Epidemiologic</u> <u>and Medical Care Research</u>. A Report of the United States National Committee on Vital and Health Statistics. PHS Publ. No. 1000-ser. 4, no. 11 Washington: USGPO, 1969.

National Center for Health Statistics. <u>The 1970 Census and Vital and Health</u> <u>Statistics: A Study Group Report the Public Health Conference on Rec-</u><u>ords and Statistics</u>. PHS Publ. No. 1000-ser. 4, no. 10, Washington: USGPO, 1969.

National Institute of Mental Health Office of Program Planning and Evaluation. <u>Biological Rhythms in Psychiatry and Medicine</u>. PHS Publ. No. 2088. Washington: USGPO, 1970.

National Library of Medicine. <u>Bibliography of the History of Medicine</u>. Washington: USGPO, 1964 (issued annually with 5-year cumulations).

National Research Council. <u>Drug Efficacy Study: Final Report of the Com-</u><u>missioner of Food and Drugs, Food and Drug Administration</u>. Washington: UGSPO, 1969.

Neel, J. V., M. W. Shaw, and W. J. Schull. <u>Genetics and the Epidemiology of</u> <u>Chronic Disease</u>. PHS Publ. No. 1163, Washington: USGPO, 1965.

NIOSH. <u>Criteria for a Recommended Standard</u>.... [for] occupational exposure (series). U.S. Dept. of Health Education and Welfare (Dept. of Health and Human Services), National Institute for Occupational Safety and Health.

Nohl, J. <u>The Black Death</u>. London: Unwin Books, 1961.

Office on Smoking and Health. <u>The Health Consequences of Smoking: Cancer</u>. A Report of the Surgeon General. Rockville: PHS, USDHHS, 1982.

Oglesby, P., ed. International Symposium on the Epidemiology of Hypertension. New York: Stratton Intercontinental Medical Books, 1974.

Panum, P. L. Observations Made During the Epidemic of Measles on the Faroe Island in the Year 1846. Translated from Danish, Delta Omega Society, 1940. Another translation in Med. Classics 3:803, 1939.

Park, C. B. Attributable Risk for Recurrent Events: An Extension of Levin's Measure. Am. J. Epidemiol. 113:491, 1981.

Patterson, J. E. Assessing the Quality of Vital Statistics. Am. J. Pub. Health 70:944, 1980.

Paul, J. R. Clinical Epidemiology. Chicago: Univ. of Chicago Press, 1966.

Paul, J. R., and C. White. Serologic Epidemiology. New York: Academic Press, 1973.

Pavloskii, E. N. Human Diseases and Natural Foci (B. Rottenberg, transl.). Moscow: Foreign Languages Publishing House, 1964.

Pelton, W. J., J. B. Dunbar, R. S. McMillan, P. Moller, and A. E. Wolff. The Epidemiology of Oral Health. American Public Health Association Vital and Health Statistics Monographs. Cambridge: Harvard Univ. Press, 1969.

Percy, C., E. Stanek, and L. Gloeckler. Accuracy of Cancer Death Certificates and Its Effect on Cancer Mortality Statistics. Am. J. Pub. Health 71:242, 1981.

Peterson D.R., ed. Epidemiology and Clinical Problems. New York: MSS Information Corp., 1973.

Pettenkofer, M. The Value of Health to a City. 1873. (H. E. Sigerist, transl.). Baltimore: Johns Hopkins Press, 1941.

Pickles, W. N. Epidemiology in Country Practice. Baltimore: Williams & Wilkins, 1949.

Poland, J. D., and A. M. Barnes. Plague. In: CRC Handbook of Zoonoses (Steele, J. H., ed.). Boca Raton: CRC Press, 1979.

Polissar, L. The Effect of Migration on Comparison of Disease Rates in Geographic Studies in the United States. Am. J. Epidemiol. 111:175, 1980.

Pott, P. Cancer Scroti. In Chiururgical Works of Percival Pott: A New Edition With His Last Corrections. London: Johnson, 1970.

Primary Prevention of the Atherosclerotic Diseases. Report by ICHD, Circulation, Vol. XLII, December 1970. Revised, April 1972.

Principles for the Clinical Evaluation of Drugs. WHO, Technical Report Series, No. 403, 1968.

Prinzing, F. Epidemics Resulting from Wars. Oxford: Clarendon Press, 1916. Facsimile copy, Univ. Microfilms, 1971.

Ramazzini, B. Diseases of Workers. (The Latin Text of 1713, De Morbis Artificum Revised With Translation and Notes by Wilmer Cave Wright). Chicago: Univ. of Chicago Press, 1940.

Rawls, W.E., W. A. F. Tompkins, and J. L. Melnick. The Association of Herpesvirus Type 2 and Carcinoma of the Uterine Cervix. Am. J. Epidemiol. 89:547, 1969.

Reed-Frost Symposium on Biostatistics and Epidemiology. Am. J. Epidemiol. 104:363-492, 1976. (entire issue)

Reid, D. D. Epidemiological Methods in the Study of Mental Disorders. World Health Organization, Public Health Papers No. 2, 1960.

Reid, D. D. International Studies in Epidemiology. <u>Am</u>. <u>J</u>. <u>Epidemiol</u>. 102: 469, 1975.

Reinberg, A., and M. H. Smolensky. <u>Biological</u> <u>Rhythms</u>, <u>Metabolism</u>, <u>and</u> <u>Medicine</u>. New York: Springer-Verlag, 1983.

Remington, R. D. Editorial: Statistics: How Many Experimental Subjects? Or One Good Question Deserves Another. <u>Circulation</u> 39:431, 1969.

Remington, R. D., and M. A. Schork. <u>Statistics</u> <u>With</u> <u>Applications</u> <u>to</u> <u>the</u> <u>Bio-</u> <u>logical</u> <u>and</u> <u>Health</u> <u>Sciences</u>. Englewood Cliffs: Prentice-Hall, 1970.

Report of Inter-Society Commission for Heart Disease Resources: Primary Prevention of Atherosclerotic Diseases. <u>Circulation</u>, Vol. 42, December 1970.

Reves, R., D. Blakey, D. E. Snider, and L. S. Farer. Transmission of Multiple Drug-Resistant Tuberculosis: Report of a School and Community Outbreak. <u>Am</u>. <u>J</u>. <u>Epidemiol</u>. 113:423, 1981.

Robertson, L. S. Automobile Safety Regulations and Death Reductions in the United States. <u>Am</u>. <u>J</u>. <u>Pub</u>. <u>Health</u> 71:818, 1981.

Roemer, M. I., A. T. Moustafa, and C. E. Hokins. A Proposed Hospital Quality Index: Hospital Death Rates Adjusted for Case Severity. <u>Health</u> <u>Services</u> <u>Res</u>. 3:95, 1968.

Rolleston, J. D. <u>The</u> <u>History</u> <u>of</u> <u>the</u> <u>Acute</u> <u>Exanthemata</u>. London: William Heinemann (Medical Books), 1937.

Rose, G. A., and H. Blackburn. <u>Cardiovascular</u> <u>Survey</u> <u>Methods</u>. WHO Monogr. Ser. No. 56. Geneva: World Health Organization, 1968.

Rosen, G. <u>A</u> <u>History</u> <u>of</u> <u>Public</u> <u>Health</u>. New York: M.D. Publications, 1958.

Rosenburg, C. E. <u>The</u> <u>Cholera</u> <u>Years</u>: <u>The</u> <u>United</u> <u>States</u> <u>in</u> <u>1832</u>, <u>1849</u>, <u>and</u> <u>1866</u>. Chicago: Univ. of Chicago Press, 1962.

Rothman, K. J. A Pictorial Representation of Confounding in Epidemiologic Studies. <u>J</u>. <u>Chronic</u> <u>Dis</u>. 28:101, 1975.

Rothman, K., and J. D. Boice. <u>Epidemiologic</u> <u>Analysis</u> <u>with</u> <u>a</u> <u>Programmable</u> <u>Calculator</u>. Washington: USGPO, 1979.

Rothman, K. J., S. Greenland, and A. M. Walker. Concepts of Interaction. <u>Am</u>. <u>J</u>. <u>Epidemiol</u>. 112:467, 1981.

Roueche, B. <u>Eleven</u> <u>Blue</u> <u>Men</u> <u>and</u> <u>Other</u> <u>Narratives</u> <u>of</u> <u>Medical</u> <u>Detection</u>. Boston: Little, Brown, 1953.

Roueche, B. <u>The</u> <u>Incurable</u> <u>Wound</u> <u>and</u> <u>Further</u> <u>Narratives</u> <u>of</u> <u>Medical</u> <u>Detec-</u> <u>tion</u>. New York: Little, Brown, 1957.

Roueche, B. <u>Curiosities</u> <u>of</u> <u>Medicine</u>: <u>An</u> <u>Assembly</u> <u>of</u> <u>Medical</u> <u>Diverson</u> (1552-1962). Boston: Little, Brown, 1963.

Roueche, B. <u>Annals</u> <u>of</u> <u>Epidemiology</u>. Boston: Little, Brown, 1967.

Sanders, B. S. Completeness and Reliability of Diagnosis in Therapeutic Prac-tice. <u>J</u>. <u>Health</u> <u>Human</u> <u>Behav</u>. 5:84, 1964.

Saracci, R. Interaction and Synergism. <u>Am</u>. <u>J</u>. <u>Epidemiol</u>. 112:465, 1980.

Sartwell, P. E. Some Approaches to the Epidemiologic Study of Chronic Dis-ease. <u>Am</u>. <u>J</u>. <u>Pub</u>. <u>Health</u> 45:609, 1955.

Sartwell, P. E. On the Methodology of Investigations of Etiologic Factors in Chronic Disease: Further Comments. <u>J</u>. <u>Chronic</u> <u>Dis</u>. 11:61, 1960.

Sartwell, P. E. Oral Contraceptives and Thromboembolism: A Further Report. <u>Am</u>. <u>J</u>. <u>Epidemiol</u>. 94:192, 1971.

Sartwell, P. E., and M. Merrell. Influence of the Dynamic Character of Chronic Disease on the Interpretation of Morbidity Rates. Am. J. Pub. Health 42: 579, 1952.

Sauer, H. I., and P. E. Enterline. Are Geographic Variations in Death Rates for the Cardiovascular Diseases Real? J. Chronic Dis. 10:513, 1959.

Schnurrenberger, P. R., and W. T. Hubbert. Reporting of Zoonotic diseases. Am. J. Epidemiol. 112:23, 1980.

School of Salernum, Regimen Sanitatis Salerni, English Version by Sir John Harrington, numerous editions.

Schuman, L. M., ed. Research Methodology and Potential in Community Health and Preventive Medicine. Ann. N.Y. Acad. Sci. 107:471, 1963.

Schwabe, C. W., H. P. Rieman, and C. E. Franti. Epidemiology in Veterinary Practice. Philadelphia: Lea & Febiger, 1977.

Schwartz, D., R. Flamant, and J. Lellouch, eds. Clinical Trials (M. J. R. Healy, transl.). New York: Academic Press, 1980.

Scott, H. H. A History of Tropical Medicine. London: Arnold, 1939.

Serfling, R. E. Historical Review of Epidemic Theory. Human Biol. 24:145, 1952.

Sever, J. L. Rubella as a Teratogen. Adv. Teratol. 2:127, 1967.

Shapiro, S., E. R. Schlesinger, and R. E. L. Nesbitt, Jr. Infant, Perinatal, Maternal, and Childhood Mortality in the United States. Vital and Health Statistics Monogr. American Public Health Assoc., 1968.

Shattuck, G. C. Diseases of the Tropics. New York: Appleton-Century-Crofts, 1951.

Shattuck, L. The Sanitary Condition of Boston. The Report of a Medical Commission, 1850. Reprinted, Metuchen: Arno Press, 1977.

Sheps, M. C. On the Person-Years Concept in Epidemiology and Demography. Milbank Mem. Fund Quart. 44:1:69, 1966.

Shryock, R. H. Medicine in America: Historical Essays. Baltimore: Johns Hopkins Press, 1966.

Sigerist, H. E. Medicine and Human Welfare. New Haven: Yale Univ. Press, 1941.

Sigerist, H. E. Civilization and Disease. Ithaca: Cornell Univ. Press, 1943.

Sigerist, H. E. Landmarks in the History of Hygiene. Univ. of London Heath Clark Lectures 1952, delivered at The London School of Hygiene and Tropical Medicine. New York: Oxford Univ. Press, 1956.

Silverman, C. The Epidemiology of Depression. Baltimore: Johns Hopkins Press, 1968.

Simmons, J. S., T. F. Whayne, G. W. Anderson, and H. M. Harock. Global Epidemiology: A Geography of Disease and Sanitation. Philadelphia: Lippincott, 1954.

Simon, J. English Sanitary Institutions. London: Cassell, 1890.

Simon, J. Filth Diseases and their Prevention, 1876. Reprinted, Metuchen: Arno Press, 1977.

Sinclair, U. The Jungle. New York: Doubleday Page, 1906.

Slaughter, F. G. Epidemic! Garden City: Doubleday, 1961.

Smillie, W. G. Public Health, Its Promise for the Future. A Chronicle of the Development of Public Health in the United States, 1607-1914. New York: Macmillan, 1955.

Smith, A. H., R. J. Waxweiler, and H. A. Tyroler. Epidemiologic Investigation of Occupational Carcinogenesis Using a Serially Additive Expected Dose Model. Am. J. Epidemiol. 112:787, 1980.

Smith, B. Community Health: An Epidemiological Approach. New York: Macmillan, 1979.

Smith, G. Plague on Us. New York: The Commonwealth Fund, 1941.

Smith, T. Parasitism and Disease. Princeton Univ. Press, 1934. Reprinted, New York: Hafner, 1963.

Smith, W. E. Minamata. New York: Holt, Rinehart & Winston, 1975.

Smoking and Health: A Report of the Advisory Committee to the Surgeon General of the Public Health Service. Public Health Service Publ. No. 1103, US DHEW; Washington: USGPO, 1964.

Smoking and Health: A Report of the Surgeon General. US DHEW, Washington: USGPO, 1979.

Snow, J. Snow on Cholera. New York: Hafner, 1965.

Stallones, R. A. Theory and Methods of Epidemiologic Study of Home Accidents. Ann. N.Y. Acad. Sci. 107:647, 1963.

Stallones, R. A. Epidemi(olog)^{2}y. Am. J. Pub. Health 53:82, 1963.

Stallones, R. A. The Rise and Fall of Ischemic Heart Disease. Sci. Am. 243:53, 1980.

Stallones, R. A. To Advance Epidemiology. Annu. Rev. Pub. Health 1:69, 1980.

Stamler, J. Epidemiology of Coronary Heart Disease. Med. Clin. North America 57:5, 1973.

Stamler, J., R. Stamler, and T. N. Pullman, eds. The Epidemiology of Hypertension: Proceedings of an International Symposium. New York: Grune & Stratton, 1967. 2nd International Symposium, Chicago: Grune & Stratton, 1974.

Stamler, J., C. Fields, and S. L. Andelman. Epidemiology of Cancer of the Cervix. Am. J. Pub. Health 57:791, 1967.

Steele, J.H., ed. CRC Handbook Series in Zoonoses. Section A: Bacterial, Rickettsial and Mycotic Diseases (1979); Section B: Viral Disease (1981); Section C: Parasitic Diseases (1982); Section D: Antibiotic and Sulfa Drugs (1983). Boca Raton: CRC Press.

Stellman, S. D., H. Austin, and E. L. Wynder. Cervix Cancer and Cigarette Smoking: A Case-Control Study. Am. J. Epidemiol. 111:383, 1980.

Stewart, G. T., ed. Trends in Epidemiology: Application to Health Service Research and Training. Springfield, Ill.: Thomas, 1972.

Straus, L. G. Disease in Milk: The Life Work of Nathan Straus. Metuchen: Arno Press, 1977.

Strode, G. K., ed. Yellow Fever. New York: McGraw-Hill, 1951.

Suchman, E. A., B. S. Phillips, and G. F. Streib. An Analysis of the Validity of Health Questionnaires. Soc. Forces 36:223, 1958.

Sullivan, D. F. Conceptual Problems in Developing an Index of Health. National Center for Health Statistics-P.H.S. Publication No. 100-ser. 2. no. 17, Washington: USGPO, 1966.

Sullivan, D. F. Disability Components for an Index of Health. National Center for Health Statistics, PHS Publication No. 1000-ser. 2, no. 42, Washington: USGPO, 1971.

Susser, M. <u>Causal Thinking in the Health Sciences</u>. New York: Oxford Univ. Press, 1973.

Susser, M. An Introduction to the Work of William Farr. <u>Am</u>. <u>J</u>. <u>Epidemiol</u>. 101:469, 1975.

Susser, M. Judgment and Causal Inference: Criteria in Epidemiologic Studies. <u>Am</u>. <u>J</u>. <u>Epidemiol</u>. 105:1, 1977.

Sussman, M. B. The Indiscriminate State of Social Class Measurement. <u>Soc</u>. <u>Forces</u> 49:549, 1971.

Sutton, H. E. and M. I. Harris. <u>Mutagenic Effects of Environmental Contaminants</u>. New York: Academic Press, 1972.

Sydenstricker, E. A Study of Illness in a General Population Group. Hagerstown Morbidity Studies No. 1: The Method of Study and General Results. <u>Pub</u>. <u>Health Rep</u>. 41:2069, 1926.

Sydenstricker, E. <u>Health and Environment</u>. New York: McGraw-Hill, 1933.

Sydenstricker, E. <u>The Challenge of Facts</u> (R.V. Kasius, ed.). New York: Prodist (Milbank Mem. Fund), 1974.

Syme, S. L. Contributions of Social Epidemiology to the Study of Medical Care Systems: The Need for Cross-Cultural Research. <u>Med</u>. <u>Care</u> 9:203, 1971.

Syme, S. L., and L. F. Berkman. Social Class, Susceptibility and Sickness. <u>Am</u>. <u>J</u>. <u>Epidemiol</u>. 104:1, 1976.

Symposium on Coronary Heart Disease Prevention Trials: Design Issues in Testing Lifestyle Intervention. <u>Am</u>. <u>J</u>. <u>Epidemiol</u>. 108:85-111, 1978.

<u>Symposium on Epidemiologic Studies and Clinical Trials in Chronic Diseases</u>, PAHO Advisory Committee on Medical Research. Washington, 1972.

Symposium on Normality. Article 2 in Biology of Human Variation. <u>Ann</u>. <u>N.Y</u>. <u>Acad</u>. <u>Sci</u>. 134:505-591, 1966.

Taylor, H. L. Death Rates Among Physically Active and Sedentary Employees of the Railroad Industry. <u>Am</u>. <u>J</u>. <u>Pub</u>. <u>Health</u> 52:1697, 1962.

Taylor, I., and J. Knowelden. <u>Principles of Epidemiology</u>. Boston: Little, Brown, 1964.

Thompson, D. J. On Getting the Most Out of Multivariate Data Analyses. <u>Am</u>. <u>J</u>. <u>Pub</u>. <u>Health</u> 69:851, 1979.

Thorner, R. M., and Q. R. Remein <u>Principles and Procedures in the Evaluation of Screening for Disease</u>. PHS Publ. No. 846, P.H. Monogr. No. 67, Washington: USGPO, 1961.

Topley, W. W. C. The Biology of Epidemics. <u>Proc</u>. <u>Roy</u>. <u>Soc</u>. <u>London</u> 130: 337, 1942.

Trussell, R. E., J. Elinson, and M. L. Levin. Comparison of Various Methods of Estimating the Prevalence of Chronic Disease in a Community-The Hunterdon County Study. <u>Am</u>. <u>J</u>. <u>Pub</u>. <u>Health</u> 46:173, 1956.

Vaughn, W. T. Influenza: An Epidemiologic Study. <u>Am</u>. <u>J</u>. <u>Hygiene</u> 7:260, 1921, <u>Am</u>. <u>J</u>. <u>Hygiene</u> Monogr. Ser. No. 1.

Vogt, T. M., and R. E. Johnson. Recent Changes in the Incidence of Duodenal and Gastric Ulcer. <u>Am</u>. <u>J</u>. <u>Epidemiol</u>. 111:713, 1980.

Wallenstein, S. A Test for Detection of Clustering Over Time. <u>Am</u>. <u>J</u>. <u>Epidemiol</u>. 111:367, 1980.

Walter, S. D. Prevention for Multifactorial Diseases. <u>Am</u>. <u>J</u>. <u>Epidemiol</u>. 112:409, 1980.

Webster, L. T. Experimental Epidemiology. <u>Medicine</u> 11:321, 1952.

Weinblatt, E., S. Shapiro, and C. W. Frank. Prognosis of Women with Newly Diagnosed Coronary Heart Disease--A Comparison with Course of Disease Among Men. Am. J. Pub. Health 63:577, 1973.

Weiss, N. S. Inferring Causal Relationships: Elaboration of the Criterion of "Dose-Response." Am. J. Epidemiol. 113:487, 1981.

Weissman, M. M., and G. L. Klerman. Epidemiology of Mental Disorders: Emerging Trends in the United States. Arch. Gen. Psychiatry 35:705, 1978.

Whipple, G. C. Typhoid Fever: Its Causation, Transmission, and Prevention. New York: Wiley, 1908.

White, C., and J. Bailar. Retrospective and Prospective Methods of Studying Association in Medicine. Am. J. Pub. Health 46:35, 1956.

White, K. L., and M. M. Henderson, ed. Epidemiology as a Fundamental Science. New York: Oxford Univ. Press, 1976.

Wilson, J. M. G., and G. Jungner. Principles and Practice of Screening for Disease. Public Health Papers, No. 34. Geneva: World Health Organization, 1968.

Wilson, R. W. Do Health Indicators Indicate Health? Am. J. Pub. Health 71:461, 1981.

Winslow, C. E. A., W. G. Smillie, J. A. Doull, and J. E. Gordon. In The History of American Epidemiology (F. H. Top, ed.). St. Louis: Mosby, 1952.

Winslow, C. E. A. The Conquest of Epidemic Disease. Madison: Univ. of Wisconsin Press, 1980.

Winslow, D. J., and D. H. Connor. Human Malaria. Med. Times 95:593, 1967.

Witts, L. J. (ed.). Bibliography on Observer Error and Variation. In Medical Surveys and Clinical Trials, pp. 43-49. London: Oxford Univ. Press, 1964.

World Health Organization. Symposium on Biological Effects of Low-Level Radiation Pertinent to Protection of Man and His Environment. Vienna: International Atomic Energy Agency, 1976.

World Health Organization. Cancer Registration and Its Techniques (MacLennon, R., tech. ed.). Lyon: Int. Agency Res. on Cancer, 1978.

Wylie, C. M. The Definition and Measurement of Health and Disease. Pub. Health Rep. 85:100, 1970.

Yellow Fever: A Compilation of Various Publications. Senate Documents, Vol. 61, No. 822, Washington: USGPO, 1911.

Yerushalmy, J., and C. E. Palmer. On the Methodology of Investigations of Etiologic Factors in Chronic Diseases. J. Chronic Dis. 10:27, 1959.

Yorke, J. A., N. Nathanson, G. Pianigiani, and J. Martin. Seasonality and the Requirements for Perpetuation and Eradication of Viruses in Populations. Am. J. Epidemiol. 109:103, 1979.

Zarafonetis, C. J. D. Drug Abuse: Proceedings of the International Conference. Philadelphia: Lea & Febiger, 1972.

Zborowski, M. Cultural Components in Response to Pain. J. Soc. Issues 8:16, 1952.

Zdeb, M. S. The Probability of Developing Cancer. Am. J. Epidemiol. 106:6, 1977.

Zinsser, H. Rats, Lice and History. Boston: Little, Brown, 1935.

The following publications contain articles or reports of interest to epidemiologists:

AMA Archives of Environmental Health
American Cancer Society. Cancer Facts and Figures. (Annual)
American Journal of Epidemiology (formerly, Am. J. Hygiene)
American Journal of the Medical Sciences
American Journal of Public Health
American Journal of Tropical Medicine and Hygiene
British Journal of Preventive and Social Medicine
British Medical Journal
Bulletin of the World Health Organization
Ca--A Cancer Journal for Clinicians, American Cancer Society
Clio Medica
Excerpta Medica, Section XVIII (Public Health, Social Medicine and Hygiene)
International Journal of Epidemiology
Journal of Chronic Diseases
Journal of Hygiene, Cambridge
Journal of Occupational Medicine
Morbidity and Mortality Weekly Report (MMWR), Published Weekly [and Annual
    Summary] by Center for Disease Control
New England Journal of Medicine
Preventive Medicine
Proceedings of the Royal Society of Medicine
Proceedings of the Royal Statistical Society
Public Health, London
Public Health Reports
Surveillance Reports for (selected) Infectious and Noninfectious Diseases,
    Induced Abortions and Family Planning, Published Annually or as Necessary by Center for Disease Control
The Lancet
Transactions Epidemiological Society of London
WHO Expert Committee Reports
WHO World Health Statistics Annual
WHO Task Group on Environmental Health Criteria
WHO Technical Reports Series

APPENDIX II
Suggested Examination Questions for Coursework Evaluation

A. ANALYSIS OF A DISEASE OUTBREAK

The Problem

You have been contacted by a local health officer to assist in an investigation of 34 cases of jaundice.
1. What information would you try to determine prior to undertaking a field investigation?
2. List some preliminary hypotheses that you would investigate.

Analysis of data:
Students are presented clinical and demographic information and activities of ill individuals.

3. Calculate attack rates by age and other appropriate host characteristics.
4. Graph the epidemic curve or spot map to locate the outbreak in time and place.
5. How would you define a case in this outbreak?
6. Describe the pattern(s) that are evident.
7. Identify an appropriate population or group of nonill or unexposed persons.

Students are presented with appropriate information for a comparison group of persons.

8. Calculate appropriate illness or exposure rates for the comparison group. Calculate the relative risk.
9. What is the likely source of the outbreak? What is the mode of transmission? Can you identify the etiologic agent?
10. What measures would you recommend to control this outbreak or to prevent future outbreaks?

B. EVALUATION OF AN EPIDEMIOLOGIC REPORT
Students are provided an epidemiologic report selected from a clinical or public health journal. They should prepare a detailed evaluation of the report that addresses these questions:

1. What is the purpose of the study?
2. What type of study design was used?
3. Is there a suitable comparison group? Are case (exposed) and comparison (unexposed) groups similar for important variables?
4. What are the major findings of the study?
5. Are there sources of bias or error that could have produced a spurious association? What steps were taken to avoid bias or error?
6. To what population do the conclusions refer? Are the conclusions justified? Has the study question been answered?
7. Are the findings consistent with other known evidence or biologic theory?
8. How could the study have been improved?

Academic Press, Inc.

(Harcourt Brace Jovanovich, Publishers)

ORLANDO   SAN DIEGO   NEW YORK   LONDON
TORONTO   MONTREAL   SYDNEY   TOKYO

Academic Press, Inc., Orlando, Florida 32887

Academic Press, Inc. (London) Ltd.
24/28 Oval Road, London NW1 7DX, England

Academic Press Canada
55 Barber Greene Road, Don Mills, Ontario M3C 2A1, Canada

Academic Press Australia
P.O. Box 300, North Ryde, N.S.W. 2113, Australia

Academic Press Japan, Inc.
Iidabashi Hokoku Bldg., 3-11-13, Iidabashi, Chiyoda-ku, Tokyo 102, Japan

ISBN 0–12–593180–8